T0226796

Sarcoma

Editors

CHANDRAJIT P. RAUT
ALESSANDRO GRONCHI

SURGICAL ONCOLOGY CLINICS OF NORTH AMERICA

www.surgonc.theclinics.com

Consulting Editor
TIMOTHY M. PAWLIK

July 2022 • Volume 31 • Number 3

ELSEVIER

1600 John F. Kennedy Boulevard • Suite 1800 • Philadelphia, Pennsylvania, 19103-2899

http://www.theclinics.com

SURGICAL ONCOLOGY CLINICS OF NORTH AMERICA Volume 31, Number 3
July 2022 ISSN 1055-3207, ISBN-13: 978-0-323-84930-2

Editor: John Vassallo (j.vassallo@elsevier.com)
Developmental Editor: Diana Ang

Surgical Oncology Clinics of North America (ISSN 1055-3207) is published quarterly by Elsevier Inc., 360 Park Avenue South, New York, NY 10010-1710. Months of publication are January, April, July, and October. Business and Editorial Offices: 1600 John F. Kennedy Blvd., Ste. 1800, Philadelphia, PA 19103-2899. Customer Service Office: 3251 Riverport Lane, Maryland Heights, MO 63043. Periodicals postage paid at New York, NY and additional mailing offices. Subscription prices are $325.00 per year (US individuals), $776.00 (US institutions) $100.00 (US student/resident), $363.00 (Canadian individuals), $803.00 (Canadian institutions), $100.00 (Canadian student/resident), $470.00 (foreign individuals), $803.00 (foreign institutions), and $205.00 (foreign student/resident). Foreign air speed delivery is included in all *Clinics* subscription prices. All prices are subject to change without notice. **POSTMASTER**: Send address changes to *Surgical Oncology Clinics of North America*, Elsevier Health Science Division, Subscription Customer Service, 3251 Riverport Lane, Maryland Heights, MO 63043. **Customer Service: 1-800-654-2452 (US and Canada). 314-447-8871 (outside US and Canada). Fax: 314-447-8029. E-mail: journalscustomerservice-usa@elsevier.com (for print support); journalsonline support-usa@elsevier.com (for online support).**

Reprints. For copies of 100 or more, of articles in this publication, please contact the Commercial Reprints Department, Elsevier Inc., 360 Park Avenue South, New York, New York 10010-1710. Tel. 212-633-3874; Fax: 212-633-3820; E-mail: reprints@elsevier.com.

Surgical Oncology Clinics of North America is covered in *MEDLINE/PubMed (Index Medicus)* and *EMBASE/Excerpta Medica, Current Contents/Clinical Medicine,* and *ISI/BIOMED.*

Contributors

CONSULTING EDITOR

TIMOTHY M. PAWLIK, MD, PhD, MPH, MTS, MBA, FACS, FRACS (Hon)
Professor and Chair, Department of Surgery, The Urban Meyer III and Shelley Meyer Chair for Cancer Research, Professor of Surgery, Oncology, Health Services Management and Policy, Surgeon in Chief, The Ohio State University, Wexner Medical Center, Columbus, Ohio, USA

EDITORS

CHANDRAJIT P. RAUT, MD, MSc, FACS, FSSO
Chief, Division of Surgical Oncology, Department of Surgery, BWH Distinguished Chair in Surgical Oncology, Brigham and Women's Hospital, Surgery Director, Center for Sarcoma and Bone Oncology, Dana-Farber Cancer Institute, Professor of Surgery, Harvard Medical School, Boston, Massachusetts, USA

ALESSANDRO GRONCHI, MD, FSSO
Surgical Oncologist, Professor of General Surgery, Chair Sarcoma Service–Department of Surgery, Fondazione IRCCS Istituto Nazionale dei Tumori, Milano, Italy

AUTHORS

ALBIRUNI R. ABDUL RAZAK, MB, BCh
Princess Margaret Cancer Centre, University Health Network, Toronto, Ontario, Canada

SAMEER S. APTE, MDCM, FRCSC
Department of Surgical Oncology, Peter MacCallum Cancer Centre, Melbourne, Victoria, Australia

MARCO BAIA, MD
The Sarcoma Unit, Queen Elizabeth Hospital Birmingham NHS Foundation Trust, Edgbaston, Birmingham, United Kingdom

SEBASTIAN BAUER, MD
Department of Medical Oncology, Sarcoma Center, West German Cancer Center, University Duisburg-Essen, Medical School, Essen, Germany; DKTK Partner Site Essen, German Cancer Consortium (DKTK), Heidelberg, Germany

MARCUS Q. BERNARDINI, MD, MSc
Princess Margaret Cancer Centre, University Health Network, Department of Obstetrics and Gynaecology, University of Toronto, Toronto, Ontario, Canada

JEAN-YVES BLAY, MD, PhD
Professor of Medicine, General Director, Centre Leon Berard, Lyon, France

MEHDI BRAHMI, MD, PhD
Centre Leon Berard, Lyon, France

JEFFREY M. BROWN, MD
Departments of Orthopaedics and Oncological Sciences, Huntsman Cancer Institute, University of Utah School of Medicine, Salt Lake City, Utah, USA

JESSICA BURNS, MD
Division of Molecular Pathology, Institute of Cancer Research, London, United Kingdom

DARIO CALLEGARO, MD
Department of Surgery, Fondazione IRCCS Istituto Nazionale dei Tumori, Milan, Italy

GIULIA CAPELLI, MD
Department of Surgical, Oncological and Gastroenterological Sciences (DiSCOG), First Surgical Clinic, University of Padua, Padua, Italy

KENNETH CARDONA, MD, FACS, FSSO
Patricia R. Reynolds Professor in Sarcoma, Professor of Surgery, Division of Surgical Oncology, Department of Surgery, Lead, Sarcoma Disease Team, Winship Cancer Institute, Associate Chief of Surgery, Emory University Hospital Midtown, Emory University School of Medicine, Atlanta, Georgia, USA

BRANDON COPE, MD
Department of Surgical Oncology, The University of Texas MD Anderson Cancer Center, Houston, Texas, USA

AIMEE M. CRAGO, MD, PhD, FACS, FSSO
Associate Attending Surgeon, Department of Surgery, Gastric and Mixed Tumor Service, Memorial Sloan Kettering Cancer Center, New York, New York, USA

SANDRA P. D'ANGELO, MD
Memorial Sloan Kettering Cancer Center and Weill Cornell Medical College, New York, New York, USA

MARC DE PERROT, MD, MSc
Department of Surgery, University of Toronto, Division of Thoracic Surgery, Princess Margaret Cancer Centre/University Health Network, Toronto, Ontario, Canada

ELIZABETH G. DEMICCO, MD, PhD
Department of Pathology and Laboratory Medicine, Mount Sinai Hospital, Department of Laboratory Medicine and Pathobiology, Sinai Health System, University of Toronto, Toronto, Ontario, Canada

NICOLAS DEVAUD, MD
Instituto Oncologico Fundacion Arturo Lopez Perez (FALP), Santiago, Chile

ARMELLE DUFRESNE, MD, PhD
Department of Medical Oncology, Centre Leon Berard, Lyon, France

MARCO FIORE, MD, FACS, FEBSh
Sarcoma Service - Department of Surgery, Fondazione IRCCS Istituto Nazionale dei Tumori, Milan, Italy

SAMUEL FORD, MD, PhD, FRCS
The Sarcoma Unit, Queen Elizabeth Hospital Birmingham NHS Foundation Trust, Birmingham, United Kingdom

ANNA MARIA FREZZA, MD
Medical Oncology, Fondazione IRCCS Istituto Nazionale Tumori, Milan, Italy

CLAUDIA GIANI, MD
Medical Oncology, Fondazione IRCCS Istituto Nazionale Tumori, Milan, Italy

REBECCA A. GLADDY, MD, PhD
Princess Margaret Cancer Centre, University Health Network, Division of General Surgery, Sinai Health System, University of Toronto, Toronto, Ontario, Canada

MRINAL GOUNDER, MD
Sarcoma Medical Oncology, Memorial Sloan Kettering Cancer Center and Weill Cornell Medical College, New York, New York, USA

ALESSANDRO GRONCHI, MD, FSSO
Surgical Oncologist, Professor of General Surgery, Chair Sarcoma Service–Department of Surgery, Fondazione IRCCS Istituto Nazionale dei Tumori, Milano, Italy

DAVID E. GYORKI, MBBS, MD, FRACS
Department of Surgical Oncology, Peter MacCallum Cancer Centre, Melbourne, Victoria, Australia

RICK L. HAAS, MD, PhD
Department of Radiotherapy at the Netherlands Cancer Institute, Amsterdam, the Netherlands; Department of Radiotherapy at the Leiden University Medical Center, Leiden, the Netherlands

NADIA HINDI, MD
Department of Oncology, Fundación Jimenez Diaz University Hospital and Hospital General de Villalba, Health Research Institute Fundación Jimenez Díaz, Universidad Autonoma de Madrid (IIS-FJD, UAM), Madrid, Spain

PAUL H. HUANG, PhD
Division of Molecular Pathology, Institute of Cancer Research, London, United Kingdom

KEVIN B. JONES, MD
Departments of Orthopaedics and Oncological Sciences, Huntsman Cancer Institute, University of Utah School of Medicine, Salt Lake City, Utah, USA

ROBIN L. JONES, MBBS, MRCP, MD
Medical Oncology, Fondazione IRCCS Istituto Nazionale Tumori, Milan, Italy; Sarcoma Unit, The Royal Marsden NHS Foundation Trust, London, United Kingdom

BERND KASPER, MD, PhD
Sarcoma Unit, Mannheim University Medical Center, University of Heidelberg, Mannheim, Germany

KARINEH KAZAZIAN, MD, PhD
Department of Surgery, University of Toronto, Toronto, Ontario, Canada

EMILY Z. KEUNG, MD, AM, FACS
Department of Surgical Oncology, The University of Texas MD Anderson Cancer Center, Houston, Texas, USA

KOROSH KHALILI, MD
Joint Department of Medical Imaging, University of Toronto, Toronto, Ontario, Canada

TERESA S. KIM, MD
Department of Surgery, University of Washington, Seattle, Washington, USA

HANNA KOSEŁA-PATERCZYK, MD, PhD
Maria Sklodowska-Curie National Research Institute of Oncology, Deputy for Clinical Oncology Unit in Department of Soft Tissue/Bone, Sarcoma and Melanoma, Warsaw, Poland

YAN LEYFMAN, MD
Department of Hematology Oncology, Icahn School of Medicine at Mount Sinai, New York, New York, USA

VALENTINA MESSINA, MD
Sarcoma Service - Department of Surgery, Fondazione IRCCS Istituto Nazionale dei Tumori, Milan, Italy

CRISTINA MITRIC, MD
Princess Margaret Cancer Centre, University Health Network, Department of Obstetrics and Gynaecology, University of Toronto, Toronto, Ontario, Canada

CRISTIAM MORENO TELLEZ, MD
Department of Medicine, University of Colorado School of Medicine, Aurora, Colorado, USA

ANDREA NAPOLITANO, MD, PhD
Sarcoma Unit, The Royal Marsden NHS Foundation Trust, London, United Kingdom

CHANDRAJIT P. RAUT, MD, MSc, FACS, FSSO
Chief, Division of Surgical Oncology, Department of Surgery, BWH Distinguished Chair in Surgical Oncology, Brigham and Women's Hospital, Surgery Director, Center for Sarcoma and Bone Oncology, Dana-Farber Cancer Institute, Professor of Surgery, Harvard Medical School, Boston, Massachusetts, USA

VINOD RAVI, MD
Department of Sarcoma Medical Oncology, The University of Texas MD Anderson Cancer Center, Houston, Texas, USA

CHRISTINA L. ROLAND, MD, MS, FACS
Associate Professor of Surgery, Vice Chair for Research, Department of Surgical Oncology, Chief, Sarcoma Section, The University of Texas MD Anderson Cancer Center, Houston, Texas, USA

PIOTR RUTKOWSKI, MD, PhD
Maria Sklodowska-Curie National Research Institute of Oncology, Head of Department of Soft Tissue/Bone, Sarcoma and Melanoma, Warsaw, Poland; Deputy Director for National Oncological Strategy and Clinical Trials

INGA-MARIE SCHAEFER, MD
Assistant Professor, Department of Pathology, Brigham and Women's Hospital, Harvard Medical School, Boston, Massachusetts, USA

ASHWYN K. SHARMA, MD
Department of Surgery, Division of Surgical Oncology, University of California, San Diego, San Diego, California, USA; Moores Cancer Center, University of California, San Diego, La Jolla, California, USA

JASON K. SICKLICK, MD, FACS
Department of Surgery, Division of Surgical Oncology, University of California, San Diego, San Diego, California, USA; Professor of Surgery and Pharmacology, Moores Cancer Center, University of California, San Diego, La Jolla, California, USA

CAROLINE C.H. SIEW, MBBS, MMed (Surgery), FRCS
Department of Surgical Oncology, The Netherlands Cancer Institute – Antoni van Leeuwenhoek, Amsterdam, the Netherlands; Department of General Surgery, Tan Tock Seng Hospital, Singapore

NEETA SOMAIAH MD
Associate Professor and Deputy Chair, Sarcoma Medical Oncology, The University of Texas MD Anderson Cancer Center, Houston, Texas, USA

GAYA SPOLVERATO, MD
Department of Surgical, Oncological and Gastroenterological Sciences (DiSCOG), First Surgical Clinic, University of Padua, Padua, Italy

DIRK STRAUSS, MD
Sarcoma Unit, Department of Academic Surgery, Royal Marsden Hospital, Royal Marsden NHS Foundation Trust, London, United Kingdom

APARNA SUBRAMANIAM, MBBS, MPH
Department of Sarcoma Medical Oncology, The University of Texas MD Anderson Cancer Center, Houston, Texas, USA

CAROL J. SWALLOW, MD, PhD
Department of Surgery, University of Toronto, Department of Surgical Oncology, Princess Margaret Cancer Centre/Mount Sinai Hospital, Toronto, Ontario, Canada

PRAPASSORN THIRASASTR, MD
The University of Texas MD Anderson Cancer Center, Houston, Texas, USA

WINAN J. VAN HOUDT, MD, PhD, MS
Department of Surgical Oncology, The Netherlands Cancer Institute – Antoni van Leeuwenhoek, Amsterdam, the Netherlands

OLGA VORNICOVA, MD
Princess Margaret Cancer Centre, University Health Network, Toronto, Ontario, Canada

BREELYN A. WILKY, MD
Department of Medicine, University of Colorado School of Medicine, Aurora, Colorado, USA

Contents

The 2020 WHO Classification of Soft Tissue and Bone Tumors features revisions based on recent advances in the histopathologic and molecular diagnostic workup of soft tissue tumors. We herein highlight select new entities in the categories of adipocytic tumors, fibroblastic and myofibroblastic tumors, smooth muscle tumors, vascular tumors, and tumors of uncertain differentiation, a novel category for undifferentiated round cell sarcomas of bone and soft tissue, and revisions to nomenclature, grading, and risk stratification. This article provides an overview on revised diagnostic criteria, state-of-the-art genetic and immunohistochemical markers, and prognostication with an impact on clinical management. In addition, we discuss challenging aspects in the diagnosis and/or prognostication of select well-established entities that will be discussed in more detail in other articles of this book.

In the past few years, the sarcoma community has successfully completed several trials in patients with soft tissue sarcoma (STS) or gastrointestinal stromal tumor (GIST). The current review summarizes recently reported relevant trials or trial updates investigating radiotherapy, chemotherapy, and targeted therapy in patients with localized extremity or superficial trunk STS, retroperitoneal sarcoma, and GIST.

Sarcoma and locally aggressive connective tissue tumors are a complex group of diseases with a growing number of histotypes in the most recent WHO classification. Most of these tumors are rare (incidence $<6/10^5$/y) or ultrarare ($<1/10^6$/y). Despite their rarity, sarcomas are often good models for the development of personalized medicine, and a large number of new clinical trials in select histotypes and molecular subsets were reported during the past 5 years, leading to a faster rate of new drug approvals. We analyzed the published literature and the abstracts reported in major congresses dedicated to sarcoma and connective tissue tumor management in the last 5 years. Several targeted therapies, cytotoxic treatments, and immunotherapies have demonstrated activity in dedicated histologic and molecular subtypes of sarcomas. The majority of the studies for ultrarare entities are uncontrolled studies, as a consequence of the rarity of histotypes, but randomized controlled trials were available in the less rare histotypes. Most successful trials were based on biomarker selection, which were often driver molecular alterations, while a large number of ongoing research programs aim to identify biomarkers in parallel to new drug development. Availability of the new agents varies across countries. This article describes the new drugs that made it through to the finish line and new agents with promising activity that are in later stages of investigation in the large family of malignant connective tissue tumors.

Early experiences with modern immunotherapy have been disappointing in trials of unselected sarcoma subtypes. However, remarkable efficacy has been observed with immune checkpoint inhibitors (ICIs) in a subset of patients, with the most promising outcomes to date in alveolar soft part sarcoma, cutaneous angiosarcoma, undifferentiated pleomorphic sarcoma (UPS), and dedifferentiated liposarcoma (dLPS). Adoptive cellular therapies targeting cancer testis antigens have shown promising activity, but only synovial sarcoma (SS) and myxoid/round cell liposarcomas reliably express these targets. The majority of sarcomas are immunologically "cold" with sparse immune infiltration, which may explain the poor response to immunotherapy. Current immunotherapy trials for sarcomas explore combination therapies with checkpoint inhibitors to overcome immune evasion and novel targets in adoptive cellular therapies. The role of tertiary lymphoid structures, PD-L1 expression, tumor mutational burden, microsatellite instability, and tumor lymphocytes as biomarkers for response are areas of active investigation. In this review, we highlight prior and ongoing clinical efforts to improve outcomes with immunotherapy and discuss the current state of understanding for biomarkers to select patients most likely to benefit from this approach.

Retroperitoneal liposarcomas are a rare entity and are comprised mostly of the well-differentiated and dedifferentiated subtypes. Eight-year survival ranges from 30% to 80% depending on histologic subtype and grade. Surgery is the cornerstone of treatment and compartment resection is the current standard. Mesenteric liposarcomas are extremely rare and comprise more high-grade lesions, with poorer prognosis of 50% 5-year overall survival. They are managed with a similar aggressive surgical approach. This review presents the current management of retroperitoneal and mesenteric liposarcomas.

Undifferentiated pleomorphic sarcoma (UPS) and myxofibrosarcoma
(MFS) are genomically complex tumors commonly diagnosed in the extremities or trunk of elderly patients. They likely represent a spectrum of
disease differentiated by myxoid stroma and curvilinear vessels observed
in MFS but not in UPS. Limb-sparing surgery is the standard of care
although the infiltrative nature of MFS mandates wider resection margins
than are necessary for UPS. UPS are conversely associated with high risks
of distal recurrence, often prompting recommendations for adjuvant
chemotherapy. In both histologies, anthracycline-based therapies or gemcitabine and docetaxel are used to manage advanced disease; immunotherapy may be of benefit in a subset of patients.

Over the past 20 years, gastrointestinal stromal tumor (GIST) has evolved
into an increasingly complex clinical entity with ever more challenges.
While surgical resection is the gold standard, advancements in genetic
testing, therapeutic options, immunotherapy, and management of metastatic disease necessitate a comprehensive, multimodal approach for
these tumors. This chapter highlights the importance of genomic testing
of GIST, the use of neoadjuvant and adjuvant therapy for localized disease,
surgical principles for GIST, as well as current and new approaches for addressing metastatic disease.

The management of desmoid tumors (DT) is shifting toward conservative
and patient-tailored strategies. Active surveillance is currently considered
the first line of treatment for most DT patients, according to international
guidelines. When active treatment is required, several systemic and local
treatments are considered. The choice of the first-line systemic therapy
and the management of recurrence still represent a therapeutic challenge,
for which well-defined and shared guidelines are lacking. Such issues
represent the next challenge for The Desmoid Tumor Working Group.

Solitary fibrous tumor (SFT) comprises a histologic spectrum of soft tissue
neoplasms that are characterized by the unique NAB2-STAT6 gene fusion.
Changes in diagnostic terminology and site-specific classification over the
past few decades have resulted in a disjointed literature. Complete surgical excision with preservation of function remains the mainstay of treatment. New risk stratification systems including risk factors such as
mitotic rate, age, tumor size, and presence of necrosis, among others,
can be used to predict risk of recurrence or metastasis. Long-term

follow-up after surgical resection is recommended. The clinical manifestations, diagnosis, management, and prognosis of SFT are reviewed here.

Vascular sarcomas encompass 3 well-defined sarcoma types: hemangioendothelioma, Kaposi sarcoma, and angiosarcoma. These distinct types are exceedingly rare and very different in terms of clinical behavior, biological features, and treatment approach. Because of this rarity and heterogeneity, it is crucial that vascular sarcomas are treated in sarcoma reference centers or networks, in order to ensure optimal management. The diversity of vascular sarcomas also needs to be taken into account in the design of clinical trials, in order to produce meaningful results that can be consistently translated into everyday clinical practice.

Skin sarcomas are tumors that are superficial and small in size in comparison with other sarcomas arising in intramuscular or intrabdominal sites. Skin sarcomas are often underrecognized and misdiagnosed. A high level of suspicion is needed, as early recognition and appropriate management including initial surgery is important for oncologic outcomes. Here, the epidemiology, clinical presentation, management, and surveillance of 4 common cutaneous sarcomas are reviewed.

Leiomyosarcomas are soft tissue tumors that are derived from smooth muscle mainly in the pelvis and retroperitoneum. Percutaneous biopsy is paramount to confirm diagnosis. Imaging is necessary to complete clinical staging. Multimodal treatment should be directed by expert sarcoma multidisciplinary teams that see a critical volume of these rare tumors. Surgery is the mainstay of curative intent treatment; however due to its high metastatic progression, there may be a benefit for neoadjuvant systemic treatment. Adjuvant systemic treatment has no proven disease-free survival, and its main role is in the palliative setting to potentially prolong overall survival.

Synovial sarcoma and myxoid liposarcoma are translocation-related sarcomas, with a high risk of developing distant metastasis, which often affect young patients and which are sensitive to chemo and radiotherapy. Surgery is the mainstay of therapy in localized disease. In these entities, perioperative radiotherapy is frequently administered, and chemotherapy is evaluated in patients with high-risk limb/trunk wall tumors in which an advantage in overall survival has been shown in the latest clinical trials. In the advanced setting, new strategies, such as cellular therapy are being developed in these histologic types, with promising, although still preliminary, results.

The Cancer Genome Atlas: Impact and Future Directions in Sarcoma

Jessica Burns, Jeffrey M. Brown, Kevin B. Jones, and Paul H. Huang

Sarcomas are rare and heterogeneous malignancies. Owing to their low prevalence and limited capacity to conduct large-scale clinical trials, understanding the molecular mechanisms of sarcomagenesis has become important in determining appropriate treatment. The Cancer Genome Atlas soft tissue sarcoma (STS) project (TCGA-SARC) was the largest and most comprehensive attempt to profile the genomics of multiple STS subtypes. TCGA-SARC made huge contributions to disease understanding. Since the publication of TCGA-SARC, numerous studies have used molecular profiling to assess STS biology. Herein molecular profiling studies in STS are reviewed and future directions with regard to omics profiling in STS research are discussed.

SURGICAL ONCOLOGY CLINICS OF NORTH AMERICA

SERIES OF RELATED INTEREST

Surgical Clinics of North America
http://www.surgical.theclinics.com
Thoracic Surgery Clinics
http://www.thoracic.theclinics.com
Advances in Surgery
http://www.advancessurgery.com

THE CLINICS ARE AVAILABLE ONLINE!
Access your subscription at:
www.theclinics.com

Foreword

The Ever-Evolving Landscape of Sarcomas: A 2022 Update on This Complex Family of Diseases

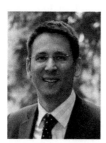

Timothy M. Pawlik, MD, PhD, MPH,
MTS, MBA, FACS, FRACS (Hon)
Consulting Editor

This issue of the *Surgical Oncology Clinics of North America* focuses on the management of sarcoma. As the title of the issue implies, sarcoma involves a wide array of heterogeneous mesenchymal neoplasms, including malignant fibrous histiocytoma, liposarcoma, leiomyosarcoma, synovial sarcoma, dermatofibrosarcoma protuberans, angiosarcoma, and rhabdomyosarcoma, among others. Typically classified on the basis of genetic alterations and light-microscopic examination of hematoxylin-eosin–stained tissue, the different histological and morphological characteristics serve to help identify the different sarcoma subtypes. In addition to histology, the prognosis of patients with sarcomas is also associated with grade, size, and location of the primary tumor. Over the last several decades, there has been increased understanding about the genetic mutations and specific cytogenetic changes associated with the various sarcoma subtypes. Treatment approaches to sarcoma have similarly evolved and are often complex and multidisciplinary in nature. In particular, approaches to the treatment of sarcoma may depend on multiple factors, including histological subtype, location, size, as well as whether the disease is primary/recurrent and/or local/distant in extent. Specifically, chemotherapy, radiotherapy, surgical resection, as well as targeted therapy may all have a role in the management of sarcoma. Given the complex and ever-evolving landscape of sarcoma treatment, I believe this current issue of *Surgical Oncology Clinics of North America* is very timely and will provide a much needed update on the topic. We have two internationally renowned experts in the field of sarcoma as our guest editors for this important issue. Dr Chandrajit P. Raut is Professor of Surgery at Harvard Medical School and Chief of the Division of Surgical Oncology at Brigham and Women's Hospital. Dr Raut also serves as the Surgical

Surg Oncol Clin N Am 31 (2022) xv–xvi
https://doi.org/10.1016/j.soc.2022.05.002
1055-3207/22/© 2022 Published by Elsevier Inc.

surgonc.theclinics.com

Director of the Dana-Farber/Brigham Cancer Center Sarcoma and Bone Oncology Programs. Dr Raut has published extensively on the topic of sarcoma with a research focus on the multidisciplinary management of sarcomas. Specifically, Dr Raut is a leader in the integration of novel targeted therapies into the treatment schema of specific tumors in an effort to improve survival. Serving as coeditor, Dr Alessandro Gronchi is similarly an international leader in the management of sarcoma. Dr Gronchi is the Chair of the Sarcoma Service in the Department of Surgery at Fondazione IRCCS Istituto Nazionale dei Tumori in Milan, Italy. Dr Gronchi serves as chairman of the soft tissue sarcoma committee of the Italian Sarcoma Group, chair of the EORTC Soft Tissue and Bone Sarcoma Group, past-president of the Connective Tissue Oncology Society, as well as a member of the Board of Directors of the Italian Society of Surgical Oncology. Dr Gronchi has authored more than 230 scientific publications and serves as Associate Editor of *The Sarcoma Journal*. Of note, both Dr Raut and Dr Gronchi help lead a transatlantic collaborative effort on retroperitoneal sarcoma (Transatlantic Retroperitoneal Sarcoma Working Group), which involves over 35 institutions worldwide.

The issue covers a number of important topics, including the treatment and surgical management of patients with a wide range of different sarcoma tumors. In addition, other important topics, such as relevant trial updates, immunotherapy in sarcoma, as well as new drug approvals in the last 5 years for sarcoma, are covered. Furthermore, The Cancer Genome Atlas and its impact and implications on the future directions in the care of sarcoma are also discussed in detail.

I owe Dr Raut and Dr Gronchi a great debt of gratitude for their work in putting together such a fantastic team of sarcoma leaders to contribute to this issue of *Surgical Oncology Clinics of North America*. These authors have done a masterful job highlighting the important and state-of-the art elements of caring for patients with sarcoma. I know that this issue of *Surgical Oncology Clinics of North America* will serve trainees and faculty well in familiarizing them with the evolving management of sarcoma. Once again, thank you to Dr Raut, Dr Gronchi, and all the contributing authors.

Timothy M. Pawlik, MD, PhD, MPH, MTS, MBA, FACS, FRACS (Hon)
Department of Surgery
The Urban Meyer III and Shelley Meyer Chair for Cancer Research
Departments of Surgery, Oncology, and Health Services Management and Policy
The Ohio State University Wexner Medical Center
395 West 12th Avenue, Suite 670
Columbus, OH 43210, USA

E-mail address:
tim.pawlik@osumc.edu

Preface

The Ever-Evolving Landscape of Sarcomas: A 2022 Update on This Complex Family of Diseases

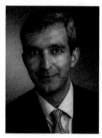   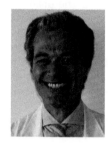

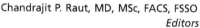

Chandrajit P. Raut, MD, MSc, FACS, FSSO   Alessandro Gronchi, MD, FSSO

Editors

Sarcomas are a heterogeneous family of rare neoplasms comprising over 100 histologies. They arise in virtually every part of the body and every type of tissue. As such, management strategies must be tailored to the specific histologic type and adapted to the site of origin. The scope of surgery and efficacy of radiation therapy, chemotherapy, targeted therapy, and immunotherapy vary considerably for each sarcoma. Incremental progress has been made broadly, warranting this updated primer. Herein, we highlight recent advances in sarcoma care with attention to details relevant to surgical oncologists. To reflect the global collaborative efforts required to make the progress featured here, we have invited a panel of international experts to work together for a balanced discussion about treatment options.

This series starts with an overview on changes in histopathologic classification by Schaefer and Gronchi. In particular, new types of lipomatous tumors and undifferentiated round cell sarcomas of bone and soft tissue are discussed. In addition, new translocation-based classifications are described, which emphasize that different morphologic phenotypes may harbor similar molecular alterations, which in turn lead to similar treatment options neurotrophic tyrosine kinase receptor (NTRK). Other novel molecular classifications are identifying subsets of histologic types with varying prognoses (CIC-rearranged, BCL-6 transcriptional corepressor [BCOR]).

Contemporary clinical trials for localized disease are summarized for gastrointestinal stromal tumors (GIST) and for sarcomas arising in the extremities and retroperitoneum in a review by Callegaro and colleagues. These trials cover neoadjuvant chemotherapy, neoadjuvant immunotherapy, neoadjuvant radiation therapy, and adjuvant targeted therapy.

Surg Oncol Clin N Am 31 (2022) xvii–xix
https://doi.org/10.1016/j.soc.2022.05.001
1055-3207/22/© 2022 Published by Elsevier Inc.

surgonc.theclinics.com

Similarly, Thirasastr and colleagues describe newly approved drugs for advanced disease. These include new targeted agents for both fourth line and beyond for GIST and GIST with mutations insensitive to prior tyrosine kinase inhibitors (TKIs), new agents approved for a variety of histologic types (eribulin), and newly approved targeted molecular inhibitors (larotrectinib, tazemetostat, sorafenib, nab-sirolimus).

Moreno Tellez and colleagues authored a comprehensive overview of immune-oncology for sarcomas. While immune checkpoint inhibition has not had the extent of success in sarcomas as noted in other malignancies, the authors focus on areas of success, including its combination with chemotherapy as a means to change the tumor microenvironment. The utility of adoptive cell therapies in selected histologic types is reviewed. Possible predictive biomarkers are identified.

Siew and colleagues describe newer information in the management of primary retroperitoneal and mesenteric liposarcoma. This includes liposarcoma-specific data drawn from the STRASS phase 3 trial and nomograms, which enable better prognostication. Importantly, the authors emphasize the differences in outcomes for well-differentiated and dedifferentiated liposarcoma (including different grades of the latter entity).

Crago and colleagues shed light on the overlap and differences between myxofibrosarcoma and undifferentiated pleomorphic sarcoma. Sensitivity to chemotherapy is discussed.

Sharma and colleagues provide an update on GIST molecular profiling and provide a detailed overview on surgical management of primary and advanced GIST. They also discuss the current state of targeted therapy for localized and advanced disease, including new drug approvals and future directions.

Spolverato and colleagues recapitulate recent evidence about spontaneous regression of desmoids on active surveillance and discuss various active management strategies, including new drugs and cryoablation. Management of desmoids is constantly evolving, and this article is a must-read for anyone who cares for individuals with desmoid.

Kazazian and colleagues review solitary fibrous tumors, with emphasis on differences based on site of origin (head/neck, central nervous system, thoracic, abdominal/pelvic/retroperitoneum, and extremity/trunk), radiation and chemotherapy options, molecular data, and recent studies on risk stratification.

Subramaniam and colleagues provide an overview of the broad spectrum of rare vascular sarcomas, including the well-described types hemangioendothelioma and angiosarcoma. Importantly, they also address a third distinct type, Kaposi sarcoma, which is often not discussed in general studies or reviews of sarcoma.

Messina and colleagues describe the four most common skin sarcomas: dermatofibrosarcoma protuberans, cutaneous angiosarcoma, pleomorphic dermal sarcoma, and cutaneous leiomyosarcoma.

Devaud and colleagues focus on leiomyosarcomas, highlighting new studies that have distinguished different molecular subtypes. Surgical management of localized disease for leiomyosarcoma of retroperitoneal and uterine origin is discussed as are standard and emerging systemic therapy options.

Hindi and Haas discuss localized and systemic therapy for both synovial sarcoma and myxoid liposarcoma. One important highlight is the neoadjuvant radiation therapy dose reduction trial for the latter, with a unique endpoint of pathologic response.

Finally, The Cancer Genome Atlas sarcoma project is detailed in an article by Burns and colleagues.

The rarity of sarcomas means identifying efficacious treatments can be challenging. Nonetheless, the authors for each of these sections, together with other investigators around the globe, have made remarkable progress over the last 5+ years.

Chandrajit P. Raut, MD, MSc, FACS, FSSO
Division of Surgical Oncology
Department of Surgery
Brigham and Women's Hospital
Center for Sarcoma and Bone Oncology
Dana-Farber Cancer Institute
Harvard Medical School
75 Francis Street
Boston, MA 02115, USA

Alessandro Gronchi, MD, FSSO
Sarcoma Service–Department of Surgery
Fondazione IRCCS Istituto Nazionale dei Tumori
Via Venezian, 1
20133 Milano, Italy

E-mail addresses:
craut@bwh.harvard.edu (C.P. Raut)
alessandro.gronchi@istitutotumori.mi.it (A. Gronchi)

WHO Pathology
Highlights of the 2020 Sarcoma Update

Inga-Marie Schaefer, MD[a],*, Alessandro Gronchi, MD[b]

KEYWORDS

- WHO classification • Sarcoma • Liposarcoma • Leiomyosarcoma
- Round cell sarcoma • Rearrangement • Risk stratification • Marker

KEY POINTS

- The 2020 WHO Classification of Soft Tissue and Bone Tumors has incorporated a number of changes to reflect recent advances made in the histopathologic and molecular diagnostic workup of soft tissue tumors.
- New entities have been added to the categories of adipocytic tumors, fibroblastic and myofibroblastic tumors, smooth muscle tumors, vascular tumors, and tumors of uncertain differentiation.
- A new category has been introduced for "undifferentiated round cell sarcomas of bone and soft tissue", which includes Ewing sarcoma, round cell sarcoma with *EWSR1-non-ETS* gene fusion, *CIC*-rearranged sarcoma, and sarcoma with *BCOR* genetic alterations.
- *EWSR1-SMAD3*-positive fibroblastic tumor and *NTRK*-rearranged spindle cell sarcoma have been included as emerging entities.
- Revisions to nomenclature, grading, and risk stratification have been made for malignant melanotic nerve sheath tumor, dedifferentiated liposarcoma, and solitary fibrous tumor.

INTRODUCTION

Soft tissue tumors comprise a wide range of entities, each with distinct diagnostic and biologic features with relevance for clinical management, which can make their diagnostic workup challenging. Recent advances in the molecular diagnostics workup of many benign and malignant mesenchymal neoplasms and the discovery of recurrent genetic aberrations have expanded the diagnostic spectrum and led to the discovery of new tumor types. The 5th edition of WHO Classification of Soft Tissue and Bone Tumors was published in early 2020,[1] 7 years after the 4th edition,[2] and features a number of revisions to existing classification and risk stratification schemes. The update reflects a consensus among an international expert panel

[a] Department of Pathology, Brigham and Women's Hospital, Harvard Medical School, 75 Francis Street, Boston, MA 02115, USA; [b] Department of Surgery, Fondazione IRCCS Istituto Nazionale dei Tumori, via Giacomo Venezian, 1, Milan 20133, Italy
* Corresponding author.
E-mail address: ischaefer@bwh.harvard.edu

Surg Oncol Clin N Am 31 (2022) 321–340
https://doi.org/10.1016/j.soc.2022.03.001

surgonc.theclinics.com

including pathologists, geneticists, a medical oncologist, surgeon, and radiologist.[3] We here highlight the most relevant changes to the soft tissue article in the 2020 World Health Organization Classification by diagnostic category and provide an update on modifications to diagnostic criteria and classification schemes. We further discuss challenging aspects in the diagnosis and/or prognostication of select well-established entities.

UPDATES TO THE 2020 WHO CLASSIFICATION
Adipocytic Tumors

Atypical spindle cell lipomatous tumor/atypical pleomorphic lipomatous tumor
Atypical spindle cell lipomatous tumor/atypical pleomorphic lipomatous tumor (ASCLT/APLT) is a benign adipocytic neoplasm and mostly affects middle-aged adults with a slight male predominance with a predilection for limbs and limb girdle.[4,5] ASCLT/APLT is characterized by ill-defined margins (**Fig. 1**) and nodular to multinodular growth and can show a range of histologic appearances with varying proportions of atypical spindle cells, adipocytes, lipoblasts, and pleomorphic/multinucleated cells within collagenous and/or myxoid matrix (**Fig. 2**A, B). The tumor cells express CD34 (**Fig. 2**C), S100, and desmin to varying extent but are generally negative for MDM2 (see **Fig. 2**C, inset) and CDK4 given the absence of *MDM2* or *CDK4* amplification.[4–6] ASCLT/APLT shows loss of RB1 expression in 50% to 70% of cases (**Fig. 2**D) resulting from deletions at 13q14 inactivating *RB1* and adjacent genes in a significant subset of cases (**Table 1**).[4,5,7] ASCLT/APLT has an excellent prognosis when completely excised and distant metastases have not been described.

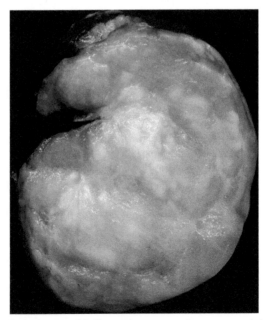

Fig. 1. Grossly, atypical pleomorphic lipomatous tumor is unencapsulated with ill-defined tumor margins and nodular growth displaying an admixture of fatty and myxoid to collagenous features.

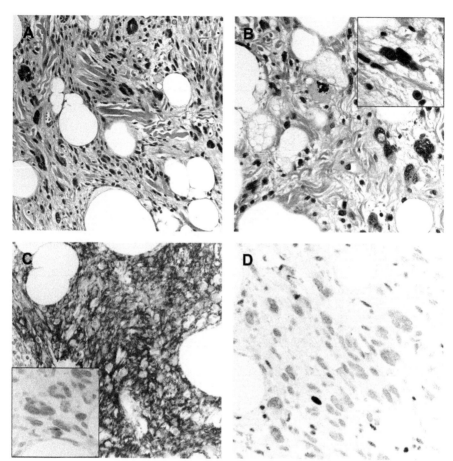

Fig. 2. Atypical pleomorphic lipomatous tumor comprised of spindle cells, adipocytic cells, pleomorphic giant cells, and scattered lipoblasts embedded in a myxoid and collagenous extracellular matrix (*A*, hematoxylin-eosin (HE), 200x; *B*, HE, x400) with occasional hyperchromatic nuclei (*B*, inset). The tumor cells express CD34 (*C*, x400), lack MDM2 expression (*C*, inset, x400), and show RB1 loss (*D*, x400).

Key Features: Atypical Spindle Cell Lipomatous Tumor/Atypical Pleomorphic Lipomatous Tumor
• Limbs and limb girdle
• Middle-aged adults, M ≥ F
• Mild-to-moderate atypia of spindle cells, adipocytes, lipoblasts, pleomorphic/multinucleated cells; myxoid to collagenous matrix
• Loss of RB1; variable expression of CD34, S100, and desmin
• Benign; local recurrence in 10% to 15% if incompletely excised

Table 1
Summary of diagnostic and prognostic features of select adipocytic neoplasms

Tumor Type	Useful Diagnostic IHC Markers	Characteristic Genomic Aberrations	Behavior
Spindle cell/ pleomorphic lipoma	RB1 loss; variable expression of CD34, desmin, S100	13q14 deletion (*RB1*)	Benign
Atypical spindle cell/ pleomorphic lipomatous tumor (ASCLT/APLT)	RB1 loss (50%–70%); variable expression of CD34, desmin, S100	13q14 deletion (*RB1*)	Benign; local recurrence in 10%–15% if incompletely excised
Atypical lipomatous tumor (ALT)/Well-differentiated liposarcoma (WDLPS)	Expression of MDM2 and/or CDK4	12q13–15 high-level amplification (*MDM2, CDK4*)	Locally aggressive; risk of dedifferentiation
Dedifferentiated liposarcoma	Expression of MDM2 and/or CDK4	12q13–15 high-level amplification (*MDM2, CDK4*)	Malignant
Myxoid liposarcoma	DDIT3 expression in high-grade cases	*FUS-DDIT3* gene fusion	Malignant
Pleomorphic liposarcoma	None	None	Malignant
Myxoid pleomorphic liposarcoma	RB1 loss (subset)	Complex chromosomal alterations	Highly malignant

Myxoid Pleomorphic Liposarcoma

Myxoid pleomorphic liposarcoma (MPLPS) is exceptionally rare and extremely aggressive, mostly arising in the mediastinum of children and young adults with female predominance as a large, deep-seated mass with ill-defined margins.[8–11] MPLPS combines histologic features of conventional myxoid liposarcoma (**Fig. 3**A) and pleomorphic liposarcoma (**Fig. 3**B). MPLPS lacks both the *FUS-DDIT3* gene fusion characteristic of myxoid liposarcoma and *MDM2* and/or *CDK4* amplification found in dedifferentiated liposarcoma (see **Table 1**) and instead shows complex chromosomal alterations with occasional losses at 13q14 involving *RB1*.[12,13] MPLPS is extremely aggressive with frequent local recurrences and distant metastases associated with poor survival.[8,9]

Key Features: Myxoid Pleomorphic Liposarcoma

- Mediastinum
- Children and young adults, F > M
- Admixture of areas resembling conventional myxoid liposarcoma and high-grade pleomorphic liposarcoma like
- RB1 loss in a subset of cases
- Complex chromosomal alterations
- Extremely aggressive

FIBROBLASTIC AND MYOFIBROBLASTIC TUMORS
EWSR1-SMAD3-Positive Fibroblastic Tumor

EWSR1-SMAD3-positive fibroblastic tumor is a recently discovered benign neoplasm, which has been included in the 2020 WHO classification as emerging entity under a provisional name.[1] These tumors show a predilection for acral and superficial location, occur over a wide age range with female predominance and are composed of a centrally located hypocellular hyalinized area (**Fig. 4**A) and more cellular areas at the periphery containing overlapping fibroblastic spindle cells without atypical features (**Fig. 4**B).[14–17] Diffuse nuclear expression of ERG is characteristic (**Fig. 4**C), whereas other markers such as CD34 and smooth-muscle actin (SMA) are negative. *EWSR1-SMAD3*-positive fibroblastic tumor is characterized by a fusion of *EWSR1* exon 7 and *SMAD3* exon 5 (**Fig. 4**D).[14,15] Their behavior is benign, but local recurrence has been observed if incompletely excised.[14,17]

Key Features: *EWSR1-SMAD3*-Positive Fibroblastic Tumor

- Acral location, superficial
- Wide age range, F > M
- Hypocellular center, hypercellular periphery
- Expression of ERG
- *EWSR1-SMAD3* gene fusion
- Benign behavior

Angiofibroma of Soft Tissue

Angiofibroma of soft tissue is a benign tumor composed of uniform bland spindle cells embedded in a network of prominent branching thin-walled blood vessels and fibromyxoid stroma with a predilection for the lower extremities of middle-aged adults with slight female predominance.[18–20] Expression of CD34 and EMA is variable.[18,20] Angiofibroma of soft tissue is characterized by recurrent t(5;8) (p15;q13) resulting in *AHRR-NCOA2* gene fusion found in 60% to 80% of cases.[19–21] These tumors behave in a benign fashion with rare local recurrences and no risk of distant metastases.

Key Features: Angiofibroma of Soft Tissue

- Lower extremities
- Middle-aged adults, F ≥ M
- Bland spindle cells, network of branching blood vessels, fibromyxoid stroma
- Variable expression of CD34 and EMA
- *AHRR-NCOA2* gene fusion
- Benign behavior

Superficial CD34-Positive Fibroblastic Tumor

This distinctive low-grade neoplasm most frequently occurs in the skin and subcutis of the lower extremities, especially the thigh, of middle-aged adults.[22,23] Superficial CD34-positive fibroblastic tumor is well circumscribed and composed of large spindle cells with abundant eosinophilic cytoplasm (**Fig. 5**A), marked nuclear pleomorphism (**Fig. 5**B), but a low mitotic rate.[20,23] They typically show strong, diffuse expression of CD34 (**Fig. 5**C) and focal cytokeratin in about two-thirds of cases.[20,23] Morphologic overlap exists with tumors described at *PRDM10*-rearranged soft tissue tumors.[24] Superficial CD34-positive fibroblastic tumor has an excellent prognosis with no local recurrences reported and only one case with distant metastasis.[22]

Key Features: Superficial CD34-Positive Fibroblastic Tumor

- Lower extremities, superficial
- Middle-aged adults, M $\geq$ F
- Eosinophilic tumor cells with granular-to-glassy cytoplasm; marked pleomorphism, few mitoses
- Expression of CD34, focal cytokeratin
- Low-grade behavior, no local recurrences, and very low risk of distant metastasis

---

SMOOTH MUSCLE TUMORS
Inflammatory Leiomyosarcoma

Inflammatory leiomyosarcoma is very rare and most frequently arises in the lower extremity of adults with male predominance.[1,25–27] Inflammatory leiomyosarcoma is characterized by eosinophilic spindle cells with blunt-ended elongated nuclei surrounded by a prominent inflammatory infiltrate, consisting mostly of small lymphocytes and occasionally admixed plasma cells or histiocytes with xanthomatous appearance (**Fig. 6**A, B). The tumor cells express SMA, desmin (**Fig. 6**C), and/or caldesmon. Inflammatory leiomyosarcoma shows a distinct near-haploid karyotype, with or without subsequent chromosome doubling.[26–28] The prognosis appears to be very good, with metastases being documented in only a subset of cases, although long-term follow-up data are limited.[27,29]

Key Features: Inflammatory Leiomyosarcoma

- Lower extremity, trunk, retroperitoneum; deep-seated
- Mostly adults, M > F
- Eosinophilic spindle cells with blunt-ended elongated nuclei; fascicular or storiform growth; mostly low grade
- Prominent inflammatory infiltrate
- Expression of SMA, desmin and/or caldesmon
- Near-haploid karyotype
- Good prognosis (data limited)

VASCULAR TUMORS
Anastomosing Hemangioma

Anastomosing hemangioma is most commonly found in the kidney and retroperitoneal adipose tissue, ovary, liver, and other anatomic locations affecting mostly adults and rarely children, without sex predilection.[30–33] Anastomosing hemangioma is characterized by a hemorrhagic mahogany spongy appearance, loosely lobulated architecture, and can be associated with a medium-caliber vessel.[32] Sinusoidal capillary-sized vessels (**Fig. 7**A) with scattered hobnail endothelial cells and a framework of nonendothelial supporting cells are characteristic.[32] Although mild cytologic atypia can be found, mitoses are usually rare or absent and multilayering is not seen, helping in the distinction from angiosarcoma.[32,34] Vascular thrombi are frequent (**Fig. 7**B); extramedullary

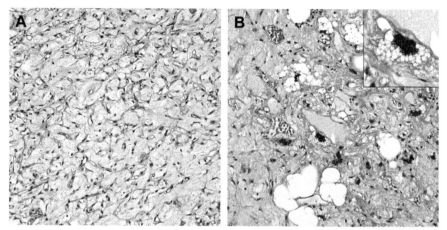

Fig. 3. Myxoid pleomorphic liposarcoma combining morphologic features of conventional myxoid liposarcoma (*A*, HE, x200) and pleomorphic liposarcoma (*B*, HE, x200; inset, HE, x400).

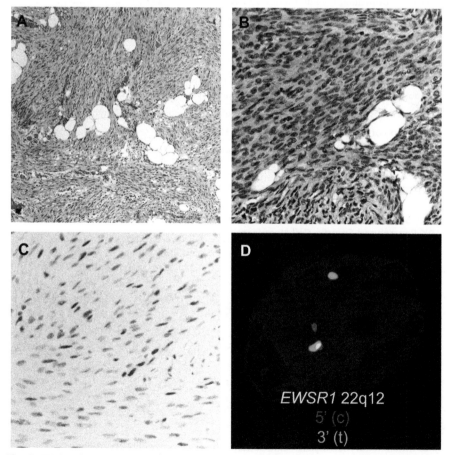

Fig. 4. EWSR1-SMAD3-positive fibroblastic tumor with hypocellular hyalinized area (*A*, HE, x200) and more cellular areas containing fibroblastic spindle cells (*B*, HE, x400) with expression of ERG (*C*, x200) and presence of EWSR1 gene rearrangement detected by FISH (*D*).

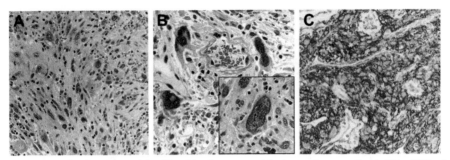

Fig. 5. Superficial CD34-positive fibroblastic tumor with sheet-like growth (*A*, HE, x200) of large eosinophilic tumor cells with marked nuclear pleomorphism (*B*, HE, x400; inset) and strong, diffuse expression of CD34 (*C*, x400).

hematopoiesis and striking hyaline globules are found in a subset of cases.[32] The endothelial tumor cells express CD34, CD31, and ERG.[32] Recurrent *GNAQ*[34,35] or *GNA14*[34,36] activating mutations are characteristic of anastomosing hemangioma.

Key Features: Anastomosing Hemangioma

- Mostly kidney, retroperitoneum
- Adults, F = M
- Lobulated growth, anastomosing sinusoidal capillary-sized vessels with hobnailing endothelium; extramedullary hematopoiesis and hyaline globules in a subset of cases
- No/rare mitoses, no endothelial multilayering; mild cytologic atypia in some cases
- Expression of vascular markers (CD34, CD31, ERG)
- Recurrent *GNAQ* or *GNA14* activating mutations
- Benign

TUMORS OF UNCERTAIN DIFFERENTIATION
NTRK-Rearranged Spindle Cell Neoplasm (Emerging)

NTRK-rearranged spindle cell neoplasm is a molecularly defined category of tumors (outside of infantile fibrosarcoma), which includes the recently described

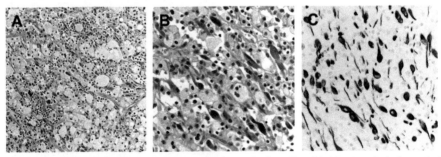

Fig. 6. Inflammatory leiomyosarcoma containing spindle cells with blunt-ended elongated nuclei surrounded by a prominent inflammatory infiltrate, consisting of histiocytes with xanthomatous appearance (*A*, HE, x200; *B*, HE, x400). The tumor cells are highlighted by strong expression of desmin (*C*, x400).

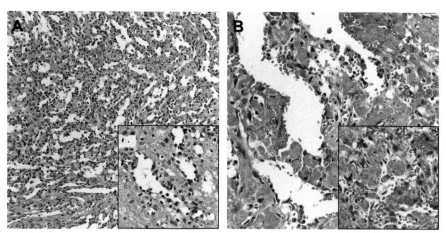

Fig. 7. Anastomosing hemangioma consisting of anastomosing sinusoidal capillary-sized vessels (*A*, HE, x200) with scattered hobnail endothelial cells (*A*, inset, HE, x400) and vascular thrombi (*B*, HE, x200; inset, HE, x400).

lipofibromatosis-like neural tumor and tumors that closely mimic peripheral nerve sheath tumor.[37,38] Most cases harbor *NTRK1* gene fusions with various partners (eg, *LMNA*, *PTR*, *TPM3*), and rarely *NTRK2* or *NRTK3* gene rearrangements represent potential treatment targets for inhibitors of the TRK family of kinases.[39] *NTRK*-rearranged spindle cell neoplasm includes a wide range of morphologic appearances, usually consisting of a population of haphazardly arranged monomorphic spindle cell, distinctive stromal and perivascular keloidal collagen, and infiltration into adipose tissue (**Fig. 8**).[1] The tumor cells frequently express S100, CD34, and pan-TRK (see **Fig. 8**C) but not SOX10.[40–42] The prognosis appears to depend on histologic grade. Benign lipofibromatosis-like neural tumor shows infiltrative growth and has a propensity for local recurrence if incompletely excised but does not metastasize.[1,40] Distant metastases may be observed in tumors with high-grade morphologic features.[1]

Key Features: *NTRK*-Rearranged Spindle Cell Neoplasm
• Molecularly defined category of tumors
• Mostly children and young adults
• Extremities and trunk, superficial, or deep location
• Wide morphologic range; monomorphic spindle cell, stromal/perivascular keloidal collagen, infiltrating fat
• Expression of S100, CD34, and pan-TRK; SOX10-negative
• *NTRK1*, *NTRK2*, or *NTRK3* gene fusion
• Wide prognostic range depending on the tumor grade

NEW CATEGORY: UNDIFFERENTIATED ROUND CELL SARCOMAS OF BONE AND SOFT TISSUE

A new category has been introduced for "undifferentiated small round cell sarcomas of bone and soft tissue," which includes Ewing sarcoma, sarcoma with *EWSR1*-non-ETS

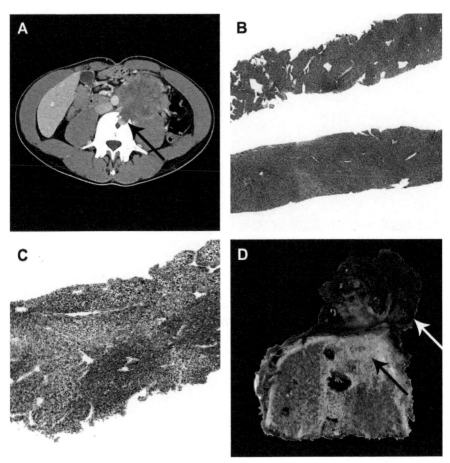

Fig. 8. NTRK-rearranged spindle cell neoplasm arising in the retroperitoneum on CT-imaging (*A*) showing infiltration into adjacent vertebral bone (*A, arrow*). This tumor consisted of a population of haphazardly arranged monomorphic spindle cells (*B*, HE, x40) with positive staining for pan-TRK in tumor cells (*C*, x40) on a pre-treatment biopsy. The patient received neoadjuvant NTRK-inhibitor therapy for 4 months resulting in partial response, before the tumor was surgically resected. The post-treatment specimen (*D*) reveals residual tumor (*white arrow*) invading vertebral bone (*black arrow*).

fusions, *CIC*-rearranged sarcoma, and sarcoma with *BCOR* genetic alterations (**Table 2**).

Sarcoma with EWSR1-non-ETS Fusions

This group of round and spindle cell sarcomas includes those with fusions of *EWSR1* or *FUS* and fusion partners not belonging to the ETS gene family, specifically *EWSR1-NFATC2* and *EWSR1-PATZ-1*. *EWSR1-NFATC2* and *FUS-NFATC2* sarcomas have a predilection for long bones, and rare cases of *EWSR1-NFATC2* sarcoma have also been reported in somatic soft tissue sites (see **Table 2**).[43–45] *NFATC2*-rearranged sarcomas occur in children and adults with male predominance.[44,45] *EWSR1-PATZ1* sarcomas arise in deep somatic soft tissue, are most common in the chest wall and abdomen, and occur over a wide age range without sex predilection[1,46,47] In addition

Table 2
Clinico-pathologic features of novel round cell sarcoma subtypes

Differential Diagnosis		
EWSR1-NFATC2 and *FUS-NFATC2* Sarcoma • Mostly long bones • Children and adults, M > F • Round/spindle cells in hyaline background • Variable expression of CD99, PAX7, NKX2.2, AE1/AE3 • Local recurrence and distant metastasis *EWSR1-PATZ1* Sarcoma • Mostly chest wall • Wide age range, F = M • Small round/spindled cells, fibrous stroma • Variable expression of myogenic and neurogenic markers, CD34 • Local recurrence and distant metastasis	*CIC*-Rearranged Sarcoma • Trunk and extremities • Young adults, M > F • Diffuse sheets of undifferentiated round to ovoid cells, intervening fibrous stroma; common necrosis, high mitotic rate • Expression of WT1 and ETV4; limited CD99 • T(4;19) (q35;q13) or t(10;19) (q26;q13) resulting in *CIC-DUX4* fusion • Very aggressive, poor prognosis	*BCOR*-Rearranged Sarcoma • Bone and soft tissue • Children, M > F • Primitive small round to ovoid cells solid sheets or nested; variable mitotic rate, rare necrosis • Expression of BCOR and/or CCNB3; variable CD99 • Inv(X) (p11) resulting in *BCOR-CCNB3* fusion • Aggressive, poor prognosis

to the *EWSR1-PATZ1* gene fusion, frequent inactivation of *CDKN2A* has been observed.[47] *NFATC2*-rearranged sarcomas are composed of round cell and/or spindle cells with little cytoplasm in a fibrohyaline to myxohyaline background with an expression of CD99 in about half of cases, PAX7, NKX2.2, and/or focal dot-like AE1/AE3 in a subset of cases.[1] *EWSR1-PATZ1* sarcomas consist of small round and/or spindled cells often with fibrous stroma (**Fig. 9**), can express myogenic and neurogenic markers and CD34 to varying extent.[1] *NFATC2*-rearranged sarcomas,

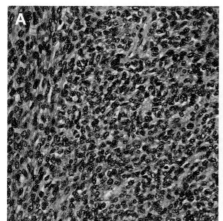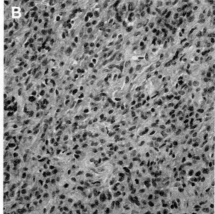

Fig. 9. Examples of EWSR1-PATZ1 sarcoma (*A* and *B*, HE, x400) consisting of small round to spindled cells with varying extent of fibrous stroma.

and *EWSR1-PATZ1* sarcomas show variable clinical behavior and may recur locally and/or develop distant metastases,[43,46–48] but long-term follow up data are limited. Both entities respond poorly to systemic chemotherapies.[1]

CIC-rearranged sarcoma

CIC-rearranged sarcoma mostly affects young male adults with a predilection for the somatic soft tissue of trunk and extremities and behaves more aggressively than Ewing sarcoma (see **Table 2**).[49] *CIC*-rearranged sarcomas contain moderately pleomorphic round to ovoid cells with frequent mitoses, apoptoses, and necrosis (**Fig. 10**A) and show expression of WT1 (**Fig. 10**B) and ETV4 in most cases, whereas CD99 staining is usually limited.[50,51] These tumors harbor characteristic *CIC-DUX4* fusion resulting from t(4;19) (q35;q13) or t(10;19) (q26;q13) and rarely alternate *CIC-FOXO4* fusion (**Fig. 10**C).[52,53] *CIC*-rearranged sarcomas are highly aggressive with frequent distant metastases and a poor prognosis.

Sarcoma with BCOR Genetic Alterations

This group of primitive round cell sarcomas includes *BCOR*-rearranged sarcoma and tumors with BCOR internal tandem duplication as described in infantile undifferentiated round cell sarcoma and primitive myxoid mesenchymal tumors of infancy. *BCOR*-rearranged sarcoma shows a predilection for bone and soft tissue of male children[54,55] and is characterized by *BCOR-CCNB3* rearrangement resulting from inv(X) (p11) (see **Table 2**) or rare, alternate rearrangement of *BCOR* with *MAML3* or *ZC3H7B*.[56] *BCOR*-rearranged sarcomas contain a uniform population of primitive small round to ovoid cells in solid sheets or nested, surrounded by a capillary network (**Fig. 11**A).[55] Expression of BCOR and/or CCNB3 (**Fig. 11**B, C) can be helpful in the differential diagnostic workup but is not entirely specific.[54,55,57] *BCOR*-rearranged sarcomas are less aggressive than *CIC*-rearranged sarcoma and have 5-year-overall survival rates of ~75%, comparable to Ewing sarcoma.[55,58]

REVISIONS TO NOMENCLATURE, GRADING, AND RISK STRATIFICATION

Select updates to concepts in nomenclature, grading, and risk stratification for malignant melanotic nerve sheath tumor, dedifferentiated liposarcoma, and solitary fibrous tumor (SFT) are summarized in **Box 1**. The 2020 WHO Classification discourages the terminology benign/malignant SFT and one of the (several) validated risk models is preferred. Please refer to Kazazian and colleagues' article, "Towards Better

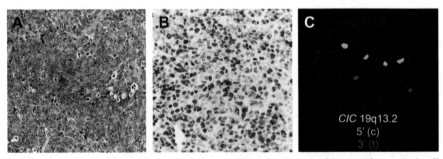

Fig. 10. CIC-rearranged sarcoma containing moderately pleomorphic round to ovoid cells with frequent mitoses, apoptoses, and necrosis (*A*, HE, x400) with expression of WT1 (*B*, x400) and detection of CIC rearrangement by FISH (*C*).

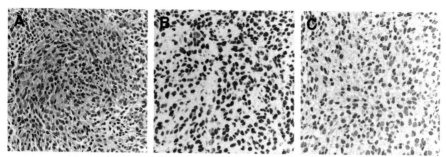

Fig. 11. BCOR-rearranged sarcoma consisting of a uniform population of primitive small round to ovoid cells (*A*, HE, x400) with expression of BCOR (*B*, x400) and CCNB3 (*C*, x400).

Understanding and Management of Solitary Fibrous Tumor," in this issue for details on risk stratification for solitary fibrous tumor.

CHALLENGES IN THE CLASSIFICATION OF WELL-ESTABLISHED ENTITIES
Atypical Lipomatous Tumor/Well-Differentiated Liposarcoma

Atypical lipomatous tumor (ALT)/well-differentiated liposarcoma (WDLPS) is a locally aggressive adipocytic neoplasm consisting either partly of entirely of an adipocytic component with at least focal nuclear atypia in adipocytes and stromal cells.[1] ALT and WDLPS describe the same entity. However, by convention, the term ALT is used when referring to tumors arising at anatomic sites amenable to complete surgical resection, such as the extremities or superficial locations. In contrast, WDLPS is used for lesions occurring at deep-seated, central body sites such as the retroperitoneum, for which radical multivisceral surgery is considered appropriate and where the risk of disease progression due to either local spread or dedifferentiation causing systemic spread tends to be higher.[1,59] The overall risk of local recurrence for ALT/WDLPS ranges at 30% to 50%, but distant metastases virtually never occur (unless dedifferentiation develops). Anatomic location of ALT/WDLPS is the major prognostic factor: the 10-year to 20-year overall mortality rates vary by anatomic site and have been estimated as less than 2% for ALT arising in the extremities and greater than 20% for WDLPS arising in the retroperitoneum.[1]

Box 1
Select updates to concepts in nomenclature, grading, and risk stratification[3]

Key Revision to Nomenclature, Grading, and Risk Stratification

Malignant Melanotic Nerve Sheath Tumor (MPNST):
- *Formerly "melanotic schwannoma"; change in nomenclature to reflect aggressive clinical behavior*

Dedifferentiated Liposarcoma (DDLPS):
- *Recognition of adverse prognostic impact of high FNCLCC grade and myogenic (specifically rhabdomyoblastic) differentiation*

Solitary fibrous tumor (SFT):
- *New prognostic model predicting metastatic risk based on patient age, mitotic rate, tumor size, and necrosis*

Modified from: Kallen ME, Hornick JL. The 2020 WHO Classification: What's New in Soft Tissue Tumor Pathology? Am J Surg Pathol. 2021;45(1):e1-e23.

PROGNOSTIC IMPACT OF DIFFERENTIATION IN DEDIFFERENTIATED LIPOSARCOMA

Dedifferentiated liposarcoma (DDLPS) describes ALT/WDLPS that progressed to a nonlipogenic sarcoma.[60] The nonlipogenic component is generally high grade and may exhibit a broad spectrum of histologic grades. Morphologically low-grade nonlipogenic components consisting of areas with relatively bland-appearing spindle cells with intermediate cellularity have been recognized and are described as "low-grade dedifferentiation" to emphasize the morphologic difference from conventional "high-grade" components.[1,61] Of note, "low grade" here represents a morphologic description (and not, for instance, to FNCLCC grading). The range of histologic appearances of high-grade nonlipogenic components in DDLPS is wide, and occasionally, lipoblastic differentiation can be found in otherwise high-grade nonlipogenic areas that are termed "homologous" lipoblastic (pleomorphic liposarcoma like) differentiation in analogy to the heterologous differentiation frequently observed in DDLPS.[62] In addition, it has been demonstrated that myogenic, in particular rhabdomyoblastic, differentiation in DDLPS is associated with worse outcome, as is higher FNCLCC grade.[63]

RISK STRATIFICATION IN MYXOID LIPOSARCOMA

Myxoid liposarcoma is a malignant adipocytic neoplasm composed of uniform, round to ovoid cells with admixed small lipoblasts, prominent branching capillary vessels surrounded by a myxoid stroma, and characteristic *FUS-DDIT3* (or rarely, *EWSR1-DDIT3*) gene fusion.[1] As defined by the WHO Classification of Soft Tissue and Bone Tumors, myxoid liposarcoma is considered high grade if greater than 5% of the tumor consists of areas of hypercellularity often displaying round cell morphology, with reduced myxoid matrix, less prominent capillary vasculature, increased nuclear grade, increased mitotic activity, frequently with a chorded or trabecular architecture and round cell morphology. Although high-grade liposarcoma can histologically mimic other round cell neoplasms and was therefore in the past termed "round-cell liposarcoma", "high-grade" myxoid liposarcoma is now the widely accepted terminology and significantly hypercellular tumors behave as aggressively as those with round cell morphology. However, a morphologic spectrum exists without easily defined or reproducible cut-offs. The presence of high-grade features is associated with significantly poorer prognosis[1] and presence and extent of hypercellularity should therefore be reported. As recently demonstrated, nuclear expression of DDIT3 can be observed in 96% of high-grade liposarcomas and may be helpful in the distinction from other round cell sarcoma.[64]

DIAGNOSTIC DISTINCTION OF MYXOFIBROSARCOMA AND UNDIFFERENTIATED PLEOMORPHIC SARCOMA

Although myxofibrosarcoma and undifferentiated pleomorphic sarcoma may share certain overlapping features, their diagnostic distinction is generally made based on clinic-pathologic features (eg, anatomic site and depth) and histomorphologic criteria summarized in **Table 3**.

Myxofibrosarcoma is a malignant fibroblastic neoplasm characterized by multinodular growth, myxoid stroma, pleomorphism, and distinctive curvilinear blood vessels occurring mostly in the lower extremity of adults with slight male predominance.[1,65] More than half of the cases arise in dermal/subcutaneous soft tissue, whereas the remainder arises in fascia or deep skeletal muscle.[1,65] The histomorphologic spectrum is wide, but all cases share the features listed above and the diagnosis is generally based on histologic criteria as specific immunohistochemical markers or genetic

Table 3
Clinico-pathologic features helpful in the distinction of myxofibrosarcoma and undifferentiated pleomorphic sarcoma

Differential Diagnosis	
Myxofibrosarcoma	Undifferentiated pleomorphic sarcoma
• Mostly limbs and limb girdle (lower > upper extremities)	• Wide anatomic distribution (extremities > trunk)
• Adults (usually 50–70 y), M ≥ F	• Mostly adults (50–70 y)
• Multinodular architecture, infiltrative margins	• Diagnosis of exclusion, that is, absence of specific morphologic, immunohistochemical or molecular genetic features
• Myxoid stroma, pleomorphism, characteristic curvilinear blood vessel, increased cellularity in higher-risk cases	• Pleomorphic morphology with frequent bizarre multinucleated giant cells, often patternless
• Highly complex karyotypes	• Highly complex karyotypes
• Local/repeated recurrences in 30%–50% of cases; metastases in up to 35% of cases	• Local recurrence/distant metastases (limited data)

markers are absent.[1] Myxofibrosarcoma demonstrates highly complex karyotypes with intratumor heterogeneity and triploid or triploid chromosome numbers.[1] Given their infiltrative growth, local recurrence occurs in 30% to 50% of cases, and distant metastases develop in 20% to 35% of cases.[1,65]

In contrast, undifferentiated pleomorphic sarcoma, belonging to the group of "undifferentiated sarcomas", represents a diagnosis of exclusion given the absence of an identifiable line of differentiation as determined by histologic examination and available ancillary techniques.[1,66] Undifferentiated pleomorphic sarcoma usually affects adults, being most common between 50 and 70 years of age, and is usually deep seated.[66] These sarcomas closely resemble other types of pleomorphic sarcomas and often show a patternless appearance with frequent bizarre multinucleated giant cells. Their karyotypes are complex without distinctive recurrent genetic aberrations. Although long-term follow-up data are relatively limited, the 5-year metastasis-free survival for patients with undifferentiated sarcomas arising in limbs or trunk among the group of pleomorphic sarcomas in adults has been reported as 83%.[67]

SUMMARY

The 2020 WHO Classification of Soft Tissue and Bone Tumors includes several novel and emerging entities and features a number of revisions to existing classification and risk stratification schemes to incorporate recent advances in the diagnostic workup of these tumors. This update integrates a morphology-based approach combined with evaluation for characteristics of cytogenetic/molecular genetic alterations and associated immunohistochemical markers to improve diagnostic precision, reproducibility, and prognostication for state-of-the-art clinical management.

CONFLICT OF INTEREST DISCLOSURE

The authors have nothing to disclose.

ACKNOWLEDGMENTS

This work was supported by the National Institutes of Health (NIH)/National Cancer Institute (NCI) K08 CA241085 grant (I.-M. Schaefer) and SARC (Sarcoma Alliance for Research through Collaboration) (I.-M. Schaefer). The authors thank Dr. Christopher D. M. Fletcher, Dr. Esther Baranov, and the Division for Cytogenetics, Department of Pathology, Brigham and Women's Hospital, Harvard Medical School, for contributing to some of the cases illustrated.

REFERENCES

1. WHO Classification of Tumours Editorial Board. 5th ed. WHO classification of tumours: soft tissue and bone tumours, 3. Lyon: IARC Press; 2020. World Health Organization.
2. Fletcher C, Bridge JA, Hogendoorn PCW, et al. WHO classification of tumours of soft tissue and bone. Lyon: IARC Press; 2013.
3. Kallen ME, Hornick JL. The 2020 WHO classification: what's new in soft tissue tumor pathology? Am J Surg Pathol 2021;45(1):e1–23.
4. Marino-Enriquez A, Nascimento AF, Ligon AH, et al. Atypical spindle cell lipomatous tumor: clinicopathologic characterization of 232 cases demonstrating a morphologic spectrum. Am J Surg Pathol 2017;41(2):234–44.
5. Creytens D, van Gorp J, Savola S, et al. Atypical spindle cell lipoma: a clinicopathologic, immunohistochemical, and molecular study emphasizing its relationship to classical spindle cell lipoma. Virchows Arch 2014;465(1):97–108.
6. Mentzel T, Palmedo G, Kuhnen C. Well-differentiated spindle cell liposarcoma ('atypical spindle cell lipomatous tumor') does not belong to the spectrum of atypical lipomatous tumor but has a close relationship to spindle cell lipoma: clinicopathologic, immunohistochemical, and molecular analysis of six cases. Mod Pathol 2010;23(5):729–36.
7. Bahadir B, Behzatoglu K, Hacihasanoglu E, et al. Atypical spindle cell/pleomorphic lipomatous tumor: a clinicopathologic, immunohistochemical, and molecular study of 20 cases. Pathol Int 2018;68(10):550–6.
8. Alaggio R, Coffin CM, Weiss SW, et al. Liposarcomas in young patients: a study of 82 cases occurring in patients younger than 22 years of age. Am J Surg Pathol 2009;33(5):645–58.
9. Coffin CM, Alaggio R. Adipose and myxoid tumors of childhood and adolescence. Pediatr Dev Pathol 2012;15(1 Suppl):239–54.
10. Boland JM, Colby TV, Folpe AL. Liposarcomas of the mediastinum and thorax: a clinicopathologic and molecular cytogenetic study of 24 cases, emphasizing unusual and diverse histologic features. Am J Surg Pathol 2012;36(9):1395–403.
11. Creytens D, van Gorp J, Ferdinande L, et al. Array-based comparative genomic hybridization analysis of a pleomorphic myxoid liposarcoma. J Clin Pathol 2014; 67(9):834–5.
12. Hofvander J, Jo VY, Ghanei I, et al. Comprehensive genetic analysis of a paediatric pleomorphic myxoid liposarcoma reveals near-haploidization and loss of the RB1 gene. Histopathology 2016;69(1):141–7.
13. Creytens D, Folpe AL, Koelsche C, et al. Myxoid pleomorphic liposarcoma-a clinicopathologic, immunohistochemical, molecular genetic and epigenetic study of 12 cases, suggesting a possible relationship with conventional pleomorphic liposarcoma. Mod Pathol 2021;34(11):2043–9.
14. Kao YC, Flucke U, Eijkelenboom A, et al. Novel EWSR1-SMAD3 gene fusions in a group of acral fibroblastic spindle cell neoplasms. Am J Surg Pathol 2018;42(4): 522–8.

15. Michal M, Berry RS, Rubin BP, et al. EWSR1-SMAD3-rearranged fibroblastic tumor: an emerging entity in an increasingly more complex group of fibroblastic/myofibroblastic neoplasms. Am J Surg Pathol 2018;42(10):1325–33.

16. Habeeb O, Korty KE, Azzato EM, et al. EWSR1-SMAD3 rearranged fibroblastic tumor: case series and review. J Cutan Pathol 2021;48(2):255–62.

17. Foot O, Hallin M, Jones RL, et al. EWSR1-SMAD3-positive fibroblastic tumor. Int J Surg Pathol 2021;29(2):179–81.

18. Marino-Enriquez A, Fletcher CD. Angiofibroma of soft tissue: clinicopathologic characterization of a distinctive benign fibrovascular neoplasm in a series of 37 cases. Am J Surg Pathol 2012;36(4):500–8.

19. Yamada Y, Yamamoto H, Kohashi K, et al. Histological spectrum of angiofibroma of soft tissue: histological and genetic analysis of 13 cases. Histopathology 2016; 69(3):459–69.

20. Bekers EM, Groenen P, Verdijk MAJ, et al. Soft tissue angiofibroma: clinicopathologic, immunohistochemical and molecular analysis of 14 cases. Genes Chromosomes Cancer 2017;56(10):750–7.

21. Jin Y, Moller E, Nord KH, et al. Fusion of the AHRR and NCOA2 genes through a recurrent translocation t(5;8)(p15;q13) in soft tissue angiofibroma results in upregulation of aryl hydrocarbon receptor target genes. Genes Chromosomes Cancer 2012;51(5):510–20.

22. Carter JM, Weiss SW, Linos K, et al. Superficial CD34-positive fibroblastic tumor: report of 18 cases of a distinctive low-grade mesenchymal neoplasm of intermediate (borderline) malignancy. Mod Pathol 2014;27(2):294–302.

23. Lao IW, Yu L, Wang J. Superficial CD34-positive fibroblastic tumour: a clinicopathological and immunohistochemical study of an additional series. Histopathology 2017;70(3):394–401.

24. Puls F, Pillay N, Fagman H, et al. PRDM10-rearranged Soft tissue tumor: a clinicopathologic study of 9 cases. Am J Surg Pathol 2019;43(4):504–13.

25. Merchant W, Calonje E, Fletcher CD. Inflammatory leiomyosarcoma: a morphological subgroup within the heterogeneous family of so-called inflammatory malignant fibrous histiocytoma. Histopathology 1995;27(6):525–32.

26. Chang A, Schuetze SM, Conrad EU 3rd, et al. So-called "inflammatory leiomyosarcoma": a series of 3 cases providing additional insights into a rare entity. Int J Surg Pathol 2005;13(2):185–95.

27. Arbajian E, Koster J, Vult von Steyern F, et al. Inflammatory leiomyosarcoma is a distinct tumor characterized by near-haploidization, few somatic mutations, and a primitive myogenic gene expression signature. Mod Pathol 2018;31(1): 93–100.

28. Nord KH, Paulsson K, Veerla S, et al. Retained heterodisomy is associated with high gene expression in hyperhaploid inflammatory leiomyosarcoma. Neoplasia 2012;14(9):807–12.

29. Michal M, Rubin BP, Kazakov DV, et al. Inflammatory leiomyosarcoma shows frequent co-expression of smooth and skeletal muscle markers supporting a primitive myogenic phenotype: a report of 9 cases with a proposal for reclassification as low-grade inflammatory myogenic tumor. Virchows Arch 2020;477(2): 219–30.

30. O'Neill AC, Craig JW, Silverman SG, et al. Anastomosing hemangiomas: locations of occurrence, imaging features, and diagnosis with percutaneous biopsy. Abdom Radiol (NY) 2016;41(7):1325–32.

31. Brown JG, Folpe AL, Rao P, et al. Primary vascular tumors and tumor-like lesions of the kidney: a clinicopathologic analysis of 25 cases. Am J Surg Pathol 2010; 34(7):942–9.

32. Montgomery E, Epstein JI. Anastomosing hemangioma of the genitourinary tract: a lesion mimicking angiosarcoma. Am J Surg Pathol 2009;33(9):1364–9.

33. Caballes AB, Abelardo AD, Farolan MJ, et al. Pediatric anastomosing hemangioma: case report and review of renal vascular tumors in children. Pediatr Dev Pathol 2019;22(3):269–75.

34. Joseph NM, Brunt EM, Marginean C, et al. Frequent GNAQ and GNA14 mutations in hepatic small vessel neoplasm. Am J Surg Pathol 2018;42(9):1201 7.

35. Bean GR, Joseph NM, Gill RM, et al. Recurrent GNAQ mutations in anastomosing hemangiomas. Mod Pathol 2017;30(5):722–7.

36. Bean GR, Joseph NM, Folpe AL, et al. Recurrent GNA14 mutations in anastomosing haemangiomas. Histopathology 2018;73(2):354–7.

37. Suurmeijer AJH, Dickson BC, Swanson D, et al. A novel group of spindle cell tumors defined by S100 and CD34 co-expression shows recurrent fusions involving RAF1, BRAF, and NTRK1/2 genes. Genes Chromosomes Cancer 2018;57(12): 611–21.

38. Kao YC, Suurmeijer AJH, Argani P, et al. Soft tissue tumors characterized by a wide spectrum of kinase fusions share a lipofibromatosis-like neural tumor pattern. Genes Chromosomes Cancer 2020;59(10):575–83.

39. Drilon A. TRK inhibitors in TRK fusion-positive cancers. Ann Oncol 2019; 30(Supplement_8):viii23–30.

40. Agaram NP, Zhang L, Sung YS, et al. Recurrent NTRK1 Gene Fusions Define a Novel Subset of Locally Aggressive Lipofibromatosis-like Neural Tumors. Am J Surg Pathol 2016;40(10):1407–16.

41. Davis JL, Lockwood CM, Stohr B, et al. Expanding the Spectrum of Pediatric NTRK-rearranged Mesenchymal Tumors. Am J Surg Pathol 2019;43(4):435–45.

42. Hung YP, Fletcher CDM, Hornick JL. Evaluation of pan-TRK immunohistochemistry in infantile fibrosarcoma, lipofibromatosis-like neural tumour and histological mimics. Histopathology 2018;73(4):634–44.

43. Diaz-Perez JA, Nielsen GP, Antonescu C, et al. EWSR1/FUS-NFATc2 rearranged round cell sarcoma: clinicopathological series of 4 cases and literature review. Hum Pathol 2019;90:45–53.

44. Bode-Lesniewska B, Fritz C, Exner GU, et al. EWSR1-NFATC2 and FUS-NFATC2 Gene Fusion-Associated Mesenchymal Tumors: Clinicopathologic Correlation and Literature Review. Sarcoma 2019;2019:9386390.

45. Perret R, Escuriol J, Velasco V, et al. NFATc2-rearranged sarcomas: clinicopathologic, molecular, and cytogenetic study of 7 cases with evidence of AGGRECAN as a novel diagnostic marker. Mod Pathol 2020;33(10):1930–44.

46. Chougule A, Taylor MS, Nardi V, et al. Spindle and Round Cell Sarcoma With EWSR1-PATZ1 Gene Fusion: a sarcoma with polyphenotypic differentiation. Am J Surg Pathol 2019;43(2):220–8.

47. Bridge JA, Sumegi J, Druta M, et al. Clinical, pathological, and genomic features of EWSR1-PATZ1 fusion sarcoma. Mod Pathol 2019;32(11):1593–604.

48. Wang GY, Thomas DG, Davis JL, et al. EWSR1-NFATC2 Translocation-associated Sarcoma Clinicopathologic Findings in a Rare Aggressive Primary Bone or Soft Tissue Tumor. Am J Surg Pathol 2019;43(8):1112–22.

49. Antonescu CR, Owosho AA, Zhang L, et al. Sarcomas With CIC-rearrangements are a distinct pathologic entity with aggressive outcome: a clinicopathologic and molecular study of 115 cases. Am J Surg Pathol 2017;41(7):941–9.

50. Specht K, Sung YS, Zhang L, et al. Distinct transcriptional signature and immunoprofile of CIC-DUX4 fusion-positive round cell tumors compared to EWSR1-rearranged Ewing sarcomas: further evidence toward distinct pathologic entities. Genes Chromosomes Cancer 2014;53(7):622–33.

51. Hung YP, Fletcher CD, Hornick JL. Evaluation of ETV4 and WT1 expression in CIC-rearranged sarcomas and histologic mimics. Mod Pathol 2016;29(11): 1324–34.

52. Sugita S, Arai Y, Tonooka A, et al. A novel CIC-FOXO4 gene fusion in undifferentiated small round cell sarcoma: a genetically distinct variant of Ewing-like sarcoma. Am J Surg Pathol 2014;38(11):1571–6.

53. Solomon DA, Brohl AS, Khan J, et al. Clinicopathologic features of a second patient with Ewing-like sarcoma harboring CIC-FOXO4 gene fusion. Am J Surg Pathol 2014;38(12):1724–5.

54. Pierron G, Tirode F, Lucchesi C, et al. A new subtype of bone sarcoma defined by BCOR-CCNB3 gene fusion. Nat Genet 2012;44(4):461–6.

55. Kao YC, Owosho AA, Sung YS, et al. BCOR-CCNB3 Fusion Positive Sarcomas: A Clinicopathologic and Molecular Analysis of 36 Cases With Comparison to Morphologic Spectrum and Clinical Behavior of Other Round Cell Sarcomas. Am J Surg Pathol 2018;42(5):604–15.

56. Specht K, Zhang L, Sung YS, et al. Novel BCOR-MAML3 and ZC3H7B-BCOR Gene Fusions in Undifferentiated Small Blue Round Cell Sarcomas. Am J Surg Pathol 2016;40(4):433–42.

57. Kao YC, Sung YS, Zhang L, et al. BCOR Overexpression Is a Highly Sensitive Marker in Round Cell Sarcomas With BCOR Genetic Abnormalities. Am J Surg Pathol 2016;40(12):1670–8.

58. Cohen-Gogo S, Cellier C, Coindre JM, et al. Ewing-like sarcomas with BCOR-CCNB3 fusion transcript: a clinical, radiological and pathological retrospective study from the Societe Francaise des Cancers de L'Enfant. Pediatr Blood Cancer 2014;61(12):2191–8.

59. Gronchi A, Lo Vullo S, Fiore M, et al. Aggressive surgical policies in a retrospectively reviewed single-institution case series of retroperitoneal soft tissue sarcoma patients. J Clin Oncol 2009;27(1):24–30.

60. Evans HL. Liposarcoma: a study of 55 cases with a reassessment of its classification. Am J Surg Pathol 1979;3(6):507–23.

61. Elgar F, Goldblum JR. Well-differentiated liposarcoma of the retroperitoneum: a clinicopathologic analysis of 20 cases, with particular attention to the extent of low-grade dedifferentiation. Mod Pathol 1997;10(2):113–20.

62. Marino-Enriquez A, Fletcher CD, Dal Cin P, et al. Dedifferentiated liposarcoma with "homologous" lipoblastic (pleomorphic liposarcoma-like) differentiation: clinicopathologic and molecular analysis of a series suggesting revised diagnostic criteria. Am J Surg Pathol 2010;34(8):1122–31.

63. Gronchi A, Collini P, Miceli R, et al. Myogenic differentiation and histologic grading are major prognostic determinants in retroperitoneal liposarcoma. Am J Surg Pathol 2015;39(3):383–93.

64. Baranov E, Black MA, Fletcher CDM, et al. Nuclear expression of DDIT3 distinguishes high-grade myxoid liposarcoma from other round cell sarcomas. Mod Pathol 2021;34(7):1367–72.

65. Mentzel T, Calonje E, Wadden C, et al. Myxofibrosarcoma. Clinicopathologic analysis of 75 cases with emphasis on the low-grade variant. Am J Surg Pathol 1996;20(4):391–405.

66. Widemann BC, Italiano A. Biology and Management of Undifferentiated Pleomorphic Sarcoma, Myxofibrosarcoma, and Malignant Peripheral Nerve Sheath Tumors: State of the Art and Perspectives. J Clin Oncol 2018;36(2):160–7.

67. Fletcher CD, Gustafson P, Rydholm A, et al. Clinicopathologic re-evaluation of 100 malignant fibrous histiocytomas: prognostic relevance of subclassification. J Clin Oncol 2001;19(12):3045–50.

Relevant Trials Update in Sarcomas and Gastrointestinal Stromal Tumors

What Surgeons Should Know

Dario Callegaro, MD[a],*, Christina L. Roland, MD, MS[b],
Chandrajit P. Raut, MD, MSc, FACS, FSSO[c]

KEYWORDS

• Sarcoma • Soft tissue sarcoma • Retroperitoneal sarcoma • GIST • Clinical trial
• Surgery • Radiotherapy • Chemotherapy

KEY POINTS

- Radiotherapy (RT) improves local control in patients with high-risk soft tissue sarcoma (STS) of the extremity and superficial trunk.
- A subset of high-risk patients with STS of the extremity and superficial trunk may benefit from adjuvant/neoadjuvant chemotherapy.
- Results of the EORTC-62092 (STRASS) trial suggest a possible effect of RT in improving local control of patients with GI-GII liposarcoma.
- Adjuvant imatinib has established itself as a standard in patients with high-risk gastrointestinal stromal tumor but ongoing trials will be important to properly understand the optimal treatment duration.

INTRODUCTION

In recent years, there has been great interest in the sarcoma community for the completion of several trials in the localized setting.[1–3] Rarity of sarcomas, a plethora of different histologic types, and fragmentation of care referral have stymied trial development. However, a better understanding of disease biology, improvements in cross-center collaboration, and improved patient referral pathways have played a key role in overcoming these main obstacles to trial development in patients with soft tissue sarcoma (STS) and gastrointestinal stromal tumor (GIST). The treatment of patients with STS and GIST is, now more than ever, multidisciplinary, including in

a Department of Surgery, Fondazione IRCCS Istituto Nazionale dei Tumori, Via Venezian 1, Milan 20133, Italy; b Department of Surgery, The University of Texas MD Anderson Cancer Center, 1400 Pressler St., Unit 1484, Houston, TX 77030, USA; c Department of Surgery, Brigham and Women's Hospital, Dana-Farber Cancer Institute, Harvard Medical School, 75 Francis Street, Boston, MA 02115, USA
* Corresponding author.
E-mail address: dario.callegaro@istitutotumori.mi.it

Surg Oncol Clin N Am 31 (2022) 341–360
https://doi.org/10.1016/j.soc.2022.03.002

the localized setting. Therefore, surgical oncologists need to be familiar with trials of medical and radiation therapies. In the current review, we will discuss recent trials and trials update in patients with extremity and trunk wall STS, retroperitoneal sarcoma (RPS), and GIST. We will focus mainly on the latest trials in the localized setting while summarizing historical trials in tables.

SOFT TISSUE SARCOMA OF THE EXTREMITY AND TRUNK WALL

Most STS occur in the extremity and trunk wall. Compared with other locations, STS in these sites are characterized by a broad histologic variety. After wide resection, the risk of local recurrence (LR) and distant metastasis (DM) at 10 years are in the 5% to 10% range and 25% to 30% range, respectively. DM is the main cause of tumor-related death in this population.[4]

Early generation trials focusing on improving local outcome after limb-sparing surgery showed a benefit of perioperative radiotherapy (RT) in reducing the risk of LR, with no effect on survival (**Table 1**). More recent trials that aimed to improve local control focused on the use of radioenhancers and on RT dose de-escalation in specific histologies to decrease the RT-associated morbidity, which can be up to 40%. Both the dose reduction of preoperative radiotherapy in myxoid liposarcoma (DOREMY) trial and the Act.In.Sarc trial are discussed in detail below.[2,5]

Numerous adjuvant/neoadjuvant chemotherapy trials focusing on reducing DM in localized resected STS have been controversial, with marginal benefit at 10 years in meta-analysis.[6,7] More recently, reappraisal of old and new studies in light of risk-stratified analysis showed that only high-risk patients (defined as patients with a "Sarculator" nomogram-predicted 10-year overall survival [OS]<60%) benefited from adjuvant/neoadjuvant chemotherapy, and that lack of homogeneity in trials population might strongly affect the results from trials.[8,9] Patient selection in chemotherapy trials is key, and the use of nomogram-based criteria might help identify a subset of patients most likely to benefit from chemotherapy. Here, we discuss the results of a standard chemotherapy versus histology-tailored chemotherapy randomized controlled trial (RCT) and review them in light of a risk-stratified analysis.[9]

Neoadjuvant Chemotherapy in High-Risk Soft Tissue Sarcomas: Final Results of a Randomized Trial from Italian (ISG), Spanish (GEIS), French (FSG), and Polish (PSG) Sarcoma Groups[3,9,10]

Purpose and rationale
The aim of this study was to investigate whether neoadjuvant histotype-tailored chemotherapy is superior to standard anthracycline plus ifosfamide chemotherapy in 5 high-risk sarcoma subtypes of the extremity or trunk.

Study design and endpoints
This open label, phase 3 RCT included patients with localized, greater than 5 cm, deeply seated and high-grade (grade 3 FNCLCC) STS with one of the following 5 histologic subtypes: myxoid liposarcoma (MLPS), undifferentiated pleomorphic sarcoma (UPS), leiomyosarcoma (LMS), synovial sarcoma (SS), and malignant peripheral nerve sheath tumors (MPNST). Patients were randomized to receive either 3 cycles of epirubicin/ifosfamide or the following regimens per subtype: trabectedin for MLPS, gemcitabine and docetaxel for UPS, gemcitabine and dacarbazine for LMS, high-dose ifosfamide for SS, and etoposide with ifosfamide for MPNST. The primary endpoint was disease-free survival (DFS), and safety was a secondary endpoint. The study was terminated early because of the third prespecified futility interim analysis.

Table 1
Localized extremity and superficial trunk STS clinical trials

Year and Authors	Study Design	Cohort(s) and Eligibility	Major Finding	Impact on Practice
Rosenberg and colleagues,[15] 1982	Phase 3 RCT	Amputation (n = 16) vs limb-sparing resection + postoperative RT (n = 27)	No difference in DFS or OS. Increased LR in limb-sparing group (0 vs 15%, P = .06)	Limb-sparing surgery standard of care
Pisters and colleagues,[16] 1996	Phase 3 RCT	Adjuvant brachytherapy (n = 78) vs no brachytherapy (n = 86) in patients with low-grade and high-grade extremity or superficial trunk STS	Improved 5-y local control in brachytherapy group (89%) compared with no brachytherapy (66%) in high-grade tumors, with no difference in OS. No difference in local control for low-grade tumors	Brachytherapy improved local control after complete resection of high-grade STS
Yang and colleagues,[17] 1998 Beane and colleagues,[18] 2014	Phase 3 RCT	Postoperative adjuvant RT (n = 70) vs surgery alone (n = 71)	Decreased 10-y LR with RT (0 vs 22%, P = .003) with no difference in DM or OS	Adjuvant RT improved local control after limb-sparing surgery in patients with STS
O'Sullivan and colleagues,[14] 2002 Davis and colleagues,[19] 2005	Phase 3 RCT	Preoperative 50 Gy vs postoperative 66 Gy external beam RT	No difference in LR Increased acute wound complications in preoperative RT group (35% vs 17%). Increased late toxicity on postoperative RT group (48.2% vs 31.5%)	Preoperative or postoperative RT acceptable as adjuvant therapy for localized STS. Increased acute toxicity with preoperative RT, increased late toxicity with postoperative RT
Kraybill and colleagues,[20] 2005; Kraybill and colleagues,[21] 2010 RTOG 9514	Phase 2, single arm	3 cycles mesna, doxorubicin, ifosfamide and dacarbazine (MAID) + XRT preoperatively + 3 cycles postoperative chemotherapy	97% grade 3 toxicity, 5% grade 5 toxicity. At 7.7 y f/u, 5-y DM rate 28%, favorable compared with historical controls	Combination MAID-RT feasible but with high toxicity
Sarcoma Meta-analysis collaboration (SMAC),[6] 1997	Meta-analysis	1568 patients from 14 trials of doxorubicin-based adjuvant chemotherapy	10% (5%–15%) absolute risk-reduction for distant metastases at 10 y in chemotherapy group compared with placebo	Adjuvant doxorubicin-based chemotherapy should be considered for patients with localized resectable STS

(continued on next page)

Table 1
(continued)

Year and Authors	Study Design	Cohort(s) and Eligibility	Major Finding	Impact on Practice
Pervaiz and colleagues,[7] 2008	Meta-analysis	Added 4 trials to SMAC-1998: 1953 patients from 18 trials	11% (3%–19%) absolute risk reduction for survival in doxorubicin + ifosfamide compared with placebo	Combination doxorubicin + ifosfamide potentially more efficacious than doxorubicin alone
Woll and colleagues, 2012 EORTC 62931[22] Pasquali and colleagues,[8] 2019	Phase 3 RCT	Adjuvant doxorubicin + ifosfamide (5 cycles) vs observation in resected grade II–III STS	Overall: no difference in OS Post hoc Sarculator-based risk-stratification analysis showed higher OS (HR 0.50) and DFS (HR 0.49) in chemotherapy arm	High-risk patients (Sarculator predicted-OS<60%) should be considered for adjuvant chemotherapy
Gronchi and colleagues,[23] 2016	Phase 3 RCT	Epirubicin + ifosfamide: 3 cycles preoperative vs 3 cycles preoperative + 2 cycles postoperative (ie, 3 vs 5)	No difference in survival (3 cycles were not inferior to 5 cycles). 25% in pregroup/ postgroup did not complete postoperative chemotherapy	Consideration of short-course preoperative chemotherapy
Gronchi and colleagues,[3] 2020; Gronchi and colleagues,[10] 2017	Phase 3 RCT	A 3-cycle preoperative standard chemotherapy (epirubicin + ifosfamide) vs histotype-tailored chemotherapy	Reduced DFS in histotype-tailored chemotherapy group (38%) vs standard chemotherapy (62%)	No benefit of histotype-tailored chemotherapy over standard chemotherapy for localized extremity/trunk STS
Bonvalot and colleagues,[2] 2019	Phase 2/3 RCT	Nanoparticle NBTXR3 + RT vs RT alone	Improved pCR with NBTXR3 + RT (16%) vs RT (8%)	Validates improved pCR with radioenhancer in sarcoma
Lansu and colleagues,[5] 2020	Phase 2, single arm	Reduced dose preoperative XRT (36 Gy) in MLPS	Extensive pathologic response in the surgical specimens of 91% of patients. Local control rate of 100% at a median follow-up of 25 mo	Deintensification of preoperative RT should be considered in MLPS

Abbreviations: DFS, disease free-survival; DM, distant metastases; OS, overall survival; RCT, randomized controlled trial; RT, radiotherapy; STS, soft tissue sarcoma.

Results: primary and secondary endpoints

At a median follow-up of 52 months, the final analysis of 287 randomized patient demonstrated a trend in 5-year DFS (0.55 v 0.47; P = .32) and a statistically significant difference in OS (0.76 v 0.66; P = .02) in favor of epirubicin plus ifosfamide over histology-tailored chemotherapy.

Conclusions

There was no benefit of histotype-tailored chemotherapy over standard chemotherapy in the 5 subtypes of localized STS included in the study.

Commentary

Although histologic type is one of the most important prognostic factors for determining outcomes for STS, current available histology-specific regimens are not superior to anthracycline-based regimens, supporting the continued use of combination, doxorubicin-based chemotherapy for selected high-risk patients. However, our ability to identify those most likely to benefit remains challenging. Predictive nomograms, such as Sarculator[11] may help identify those who most likely to achieve maximum benefit. In particular, a post hoc Sarculator-based risk stratification analysis showed that high-risk patients treated with anthracyclin-based chemotherapy fared much better than predicted by the nomogram.[9] Conversely, this did not happen to high-risk patients treated with histology-tailored chemotherapy. This might further support the use of doxorubin/ifosfamide in high-risk patients and underlines the importance of patient selection in STS clinical trial.

NBTXR3, a First in Class Radioenhancer Hhafnium Oxide Nanoparticle, plus Radiotherapy versus Radiotherapy Alone in Patients with Locally Advanced Soft-Tissue Sarcoma (Act.In.Sarc): a Multicentre, Phase 2-3,Rrandomized, Clinical Trial[2]

Purpose and rationale

Pathologic complete response (pCR) after preoperative therapy is increasingly identified as a significant prognostic marker but occurs in less than 20% of patients with STS. NBTXR3 is an intratumorally administered 50nm nanoparticle composed of crystalline hafnium oxide, which is activated by ionizing radiation, resulting in cell-localized high-energy cell death, without added toxicity to the surrounding tissues, as shown in earlier clinical trials.[12] The RCT was designed to evaluate pathologic response of combination NBTXR3 plus external beam radiation versus radiation alone in patients with locally advanced STS of the extremity or trunk wall.

Study design and endpoints

Between 2015 and 2017, 180 treatment-naïve patients with primary extremity or trunk STS (tumor volume <3000 mL) treated at 32 international sites were randomized 1:1 to receive either a single dose of preoperative NBTXR3 (volume equivalent to 10% tumor volume) plus 50 Gy external beam RT or RT alone in 25 fractions during 5 weeks and underwent resection 4 to 8 weeks after completion of RT. Patients were stratified based on histology type (MLPS vs others). pCR was defined as less than 5% residual malignant cells as assessed using the EORTC-STBSG recommendations.[13]

Results: primary and secondary endpoints

pCR was significantly higher in patients treated with NBTXR3 + XRT compared with XRT alone (16% vs 8%; P = .044), most notable in patients with grade 2 to 3 STS. In addition, more patients in the NBTXR3 + XRT group underwent an R0 resection (81% vs 62%, P = .04). There was no difference in RECIST response. Serious adverse events occurred in 39% of NBTXR3 + XRT patients compared with 30% XRT alone and included hypotension following NBTXR3 injection and postoperative wound complications. No treatment-related deaths occurred.

Conclusions
The Act.In.Sarc trial met its primary endpoint, with a greater proportion of NBTXR3 + XRT patients achieving pCR compared with XRT alone, without increased toxicity.

Commentary
Pathologic response is increasingly becoming a standard measure to evaluate biological efficacy in STS and other tumor types. This trial demonstrates the safety and efficacy of first-in-class radioenhancer for the treatment of extremity or trunk STS to potentiate RT response. Although these data are encouraging, further follow-up is needed to evaluate whether this translates into improved oncologic outcomes.

Dose Reduction of Preoperative Radiotherapy in Myxoid Liposarcoma (DOREMY)[5]

Purpose and rationale
Treatment of localized extremity sarcoma is surgery. As shown by O'Sullivan and colleagues, preoperative RT and postoperative RT are both effective in reducing the risk of LR.[14] Preoperative RT is associated with increased wound complications, whereas postoperative RT is associated with increased long-term toxicity. Retrospective data suggest that MLPS is more sensitive to RT than other histologic types, suggesting that lower doses may be safe with reduced short-term and long-term toxicities. The aim of this study was to evaluate the oncologic safety of decreasing the preoperative RT dose from 50 to 36 Gy for MLPS.

Study design and endpoints
DOREMY was a phase 2, nonrandomized trial conducted from 2010 to 2020 in 9 tertiary sarcoma centers in Europe and the United States where 79 patients with non-metastatic MLPS of the extremity or trunk underwent preoperative RT of 36 Gy, given in once daily fractions of 2 Gy, 5 fractions per week followed by standard surgical resection. The primary endpoint was defined as extensive treatment response (<50% viable tumor on surgical pathology) and the dose reduction was regarded as a success if 70% or more of the patient achieved an extensive treatment response.

Results: primary and secondary endpoints
Overall, 70 of 77 (91%) patients showed extensive pathologic response, meeting the primary endpoint. Patients with larger tumors were less likely to achieve treatment response. In addition, wound complications occurred in 22% of patients, significantly lower than historical controls.

Conclusions
The findings of the DOREMY nonrandomized clinical trial suggest that deintensification of preoperative RT is effective in MLPS with reduced short-term morbidity.

Commentary
Data from DOREMY support the emergence of histology-based sarcoma management. Future studies evaluating de-escalation of care including reduced-dose radiation (as shown in DOREMY), histology-tailored chemotherapy and risk-based surveillance strategies will result in improvements in long-term quality of life for patients with localized STS.

GASTROINTESTINAL STROMAL TUMOR

GISTs are rare mesenchymal tumors accounting for less than 1% of all gastrointestinal malignancies but are the most common sarcoma histology. Identification of constitutively active mutations in the *KIT* and *PDGFRA* protooncogenes encoding receptor tyrosine kinases revolutionized management of this disease. The use of tyrosine kinase inhibitors (TKIs), including imatinib, sunitinib, regorafenib, ripretinib, and avapritinib, dramatically improved outcomes for patients with metastatic GIST.[24–28]

Surgery remains the principal and only potentially curative treatment of patients with resectable, primary GIST. However, despite ostensibly macroscopically complete resection, rates of recurrence are high, and 5-year OS was reported as low as 54%.[29] The success of TKIs in the metastatic setting spurred the investigation of the utility of imatinib, the first approved TKI in GIST, in the adjuvant setting after resection of primary GIST (**Table 2**).

In addition, because GISTs may be large at diagnosis, imatinib was also studied in the neoadjuvant setting to determine if tumors may respond with important consequences on subsequent surgery and outcome. Hereunder, we will review recent trials on adjuvant/neoadjuvant imatinib. A trial attempting surgery in metastatic GIST is summarized in **Table 2**.

One Versus 3 Years of Adjuvant Imatinib for Operable Gastrointestinal Stromal Tumor: a Randomized Trial (Scandinavian Sarcoma Group XVIII/Arbeitsgemeinschaft Internistische Onkologie, SSGXVIII/AIO)[30,31]

Purpose and rationale
One year of adjuvant imatinib was known to improve recurrence-free survival (RFS) in patients with primary, localized GIST when compared with placebo.[32] This study investigated the role of duration adjuvant imatinib in preventing recurrence and improving survival after surgery in patients with GIST at high risk of recurrence.

Study design and endpoints
This randomized, open-label phase 3 trial compared 3 years versus 1 year of 400 mg adjuvant imatinib in patients with high-risk features (size >10 cm, mitotic count >10/50 HPF, size >5 cm and mitotic count >5/50 HPF, or tumor rupture).

Primary endpoint was RFS (measured from date of randomization to date of first documented radiographic or pathologic recurrence or death, whichever occurred first). Secondary endpoints were safety, OS (measured from date of randomization to date of death, any cause), and GIST-specific survival (measured from date of randomization to date of death considered to be secondary to GIST).

Results: primary and secondary endpoints
With 200 patients in each arm, the study confirmed improved RFS and OS with 3 years of adjuvant imatinib over 1 year. Specifically, the 5-year and 10-year RFS rates were 71% and 53% in the 3-year cohort and 52% and 42% in the 1-year cohort. The 5-year and 10-year OS rates were 92% and 79% in the 3-year cohort and 82% and 65% in the 1-year cohort.

Imatinib was generally well tolerated but discontinuation rates were high, 26% in the 3-year arm and 13% in the 1-year arm.

Conclusions
Three years of adjuvant imatinib is superior in efficacy compared with 1 year.

Table 2
GIST—adjuvant and neoadjuvant imatinib trials and attempted trial on surgery in metastatic GIST

Year and Authors	Study Design	Cohort(s) and Eligibility	Endpoints and Major Findings	Impact on Practice
Dematteo and colleagues,[37] 2013 ACOSOG Z9000	Single-arm, multicenter, phase 2	Adjuvant imatinib 400 mg/d × 1 y (n = 106) Eligibility: Complete resection Tumor ≥10 cm, intraperitoneal rupture, or up to 4 peritoneal implants	Primary endpoint: OS 1-y 99%, 3-y 97%, 5-y 83% Secondary endpoint: RFS 1-y 96%, 3-y 60%, 5-y 40% 83% completed 1 y of therapy	Adjuvant imatinib was well tolerated and safe. Tumor mutation had an impact on efficacy of adjuvant imatinib on RFS
Dematteo and colleagues,[32] 2009 Corless and colleagues,[38] 2014 ACOSOG Z9001	Randomized, placebo-controlled, multicenter phase 3	Adjuvant imatinib 400 mg/d × 1 y (n = 359) vs placebo × 1 y (n = 354) Eligibility: Complete resection Tumor ≥3 cm	Primary endpoint: RFS 1 y RFS 98% (imatinib) vs 83% (placebo) No difference in OS (cross-over design)	Adjuvant imatinib was associated with improved RFS compared with placebo. Based on this, US Food and Drug Administration approved imatinib for postoperative treatment of adult patients after resection of KIT-positive GIST
Joensuu and colleagues,[31] 2020; Joensuu and colleagues,[39] 2016 SSG XVIII/AIO	Randomized, multicenter phase 3	Adjuvant imatinib 400 mg/d × 3 y (n = 200) vs × 1 y (n = 200) Eligibility: Complete resection High risk—tumor >10 cm, mitotic count >10/50 HPF, tumor >5 cm and mitotic count >5/50 HPF, or tumor rupture	Primary endpoint: RFS 3-y arm—5-y 71%, 10-y 53% 1-y arm—5-y 52%, 10-y 42% Secondary endpoint: OS 3 y arm—5-y 92%, 10-y 79% 1 y arm—5-y 82%, 10-y 65% Discontinuation 26% (3-y arm), 13% (1-y arm)	Longer duration adjuvant imatinib improved not only RFS but also importantly OS. This established the new standard of care—3 y of adjuvant imatinib for patients with high-risk primary GIST

Study	Trial design	Treatment/Eligibility	Results	Comments
Casali and colleagues, 2015 EORTC 62024[40]	Randomized, open-label, multicenter phase 3	Adjuvant imatinib 400 mg/d × 2 y (n = 417) vs observation (n = 454) Eligibility: Complete resection High-risk—tumor >10 cm, mitotic count >10/50 HPF, or tumor >5 cm and mitotic count >5/50 HPF Intermediate risk—tumor ≤5 cm and mitotic count 6–10/50 HPF or tumor >5–10 cm and mitotic count ≤5/50 HPF	Primary endpoint: IFFS 2-y arm—5-y 87% (89% in high-risk cohort). Observation—5-y 84% (73% in high-risk cohort). Secondary endpoints: RFS, OS 2-y arm—3-y RFS 84%, 5-y RFS 69% 5-y OS 100% Observation—3-y RFS 66%, 5-y RFS 63% 5-y OS 99%	This study again confirmed that adjuvant imatinib delayed recurrence. However, in the initial analysis, there was no difference in IFFS at 5 y
Eisenberg and colleagues,[34] 2009 Wang and colleagues,[35] 2012 RTOG 0132/ACRIN 665	Single-arm, multicenter, phase 2	Neoadjuvant imatinib 600 mg/d × 8–12 wk + adjuvant imatinib 600 mg/d × 2 y Eligibility: Primary GIST ≥ 5 cm (Group A, n = 31) Resectable metastatic/recurrent GIST ≥2 cm (Group B, n = 22)	Radiographic response: Group A Partial 7%, stable 83%, unknown 10% Group B Partial 5%, stable 91%, progression 5% 5-y PFS, DSS, OS: Group A 57%, 77%, 77% Group B 30%, 77%, 68%	Neoadjuvant imatinib was safe, and risk of progression during neoadjuvant therapy was low
McAuliffe and colleagues,[41] 2009	Single-institution, randomized phase 2	Neoadjuvant imatinib 600 mg/d × 3 (n = 7), 5 (n = 6), or 7 (n = 6) days and adjuvant imatinib 600 mg/d × 2 y Eligibility: Primary GIST ≥1 cm (n = 19)	Primary endpoint: 5-y OS 87% 5-y DSS 95% Secondary endpoint: 5-y DFS 65	This study confirmed that preoperative imatinib was safe and well tolerated. Radiographic response could be observed within 1 wk of initiation of therapy by 18-FDG-PET and histologically

(continued on next page)

Table 2
(continued)

Year and Authors	Study Design	Cohort(s) and Eligibility	Endpoints and Major Findings	Impact on Practice
Du and colleagues,[42] 2014	Phase 3 RCT	Imatinib alone (n = 22) vs imatinib + surgery (n = 19) in patients with metastatic GIST. Study closed early due to poor accrual (target accrual: n = 210)	Nonsignificant trend toward better PFS in surgery arm (primary endpoint, 88% vs 58%, p0.09)	Selected metastatic patients may benefit from surgery. Decision should be made at expert centers following multidisciplinary discussion

Abbreviations: DSS, disease-specific survival; IFFS, imatinib failure-free survival; OS, overall survival; PFS, progression-free survival; RFS, recurrence-free survival.

Commentary

This study established the current baseline standard of care of 3 years of adjuvant therapy for patients following a macroscopically complete resection of high-risk GISTs. The authors did not report the disease-specific survival (DSS) but did mention that 82% (1 year) and 83% (3 years) of patients who died in both arms had confirmed metastatic disease. The study did include patients who are now known to be less sensitive to the dose of 400 mg/d imatinib (*KIT* exon 9 mutation) and who are likely insensitive to imatinib ("wild-type," *PDGFRA* D842 V mutation); subsequent analysis found that patients with those mutations derived no additional benefit with additional duration therapy at the 400 mg/d dose. Thus, the magnitude of benefit in those with sensitive mutations may be underestimated in the overall results.

Efficacy and Tolerability of 5-Year Adjuvant Imatinib Treatment for Patients with Resected Intermediate-Risk or High-Risk Primary Gastrointestinal Stromal Tumor: the PERSIST-5 Clinical Trial[33]

Purpose and rationale

Three years of adjuvant imatinib is associated with lower recurrence rates and higher OS rates in patients with primary GIST at high risk of recurrence compared with 1 year. However, the impact of longer duration therapy (5 years) on efficacy and tolerability is uncertain.

Study design and endpoints

This single-arm, multi-institutional, phase 2 trial included patients with resected primary, KIT-positive GIST at intermediate or high risk of recurrence (any site $\geq$2 cm with $\geq$5 mitoses per 50 HPF or any nongastric GIST $\geq$5 cm). All patients were treated with 400 mg/d for 5 years or until discontinuation of drug due to progression or intolerance.

Results: primary and secondary endpoints

Of 91 patients, only 51% completed the full 5 years of imatinib therapy planned. Estimated 5-year RFS was 90% and OS was 95%. Of 7 patients who recurred, 6 recurred after discontinuation of imatinib and only one patient, who had an imatinib-insensitive *PDGFRA* exon 18 D842 V mutation, recurred on drug. The most common reason for discontinuation was patient choice rather than adverse effects.

Conclusions

No patients with sensitive mutations recurred while on imatinib. Recurrences in patients following discontinuation of therapy were observed within 2 years of stopping imatinib.

Commentary

This study confirmed that 5-year of adjuvant imatinib is effective at reducing the risk of recurrence in patients with resected primary GISTs harboring sensitive mutations while on drug. Once patients stop imatinib, they should be followed closely for the next 2 years to monitor for recurrence. Importantly, each successive adjuvant imatinib study found that progressively longer duration of therapy resulted in progressively higher rates of drug discontinuation. Future trials should consider this to maintain enrollment.

Phase II Trial of Neoadjuvant/Adjuvant Imatinib Mesylate (IM) for Advanced Primary and Metastatic/Recurrent Operable Gastrointestinal Stromal Tumor (GIST): Early Results of RTOG 0132/ACRIN 6665[34,35]

Purpose and rationale

This was the first multi-institutional trial evaluating the utility of neoadjuvant imatinib. Long-term analysis evaluated duration of impact.

Study design and endpoints

This phase 2 trial include 2 separate cohorts, those with primary GIST of 5 cm or greater (Group A) and those with resectable metastatic/recurrent GIST of 2 cm or greater (Group B), both treated with imatinib 600 mg/d for 8 to 12 weeks followed by postoperative imatinib for 2 years.

Endpoints included drug-related toxicity, surgical complication assessment, tumor response to preoperative therapy, time-to-progression, and progression-free survival (PFS), DSS, OS.

Results: primary and secondary endpoints

There were 31 patients in Group A and 22 in group B. Imatinib therapy was well tolerated. Complications were believed to be consistent with complex and, in some cases, reoperative abdominal surgery. Radiographic response (RECIST) to neoadjuvant therapy was partial in 7% (Group A) and 5% (Group B), stable in 83% and 91%, progression in 5% (Group B), and unknown in 10% (Group A). In Group A, the 5-year PFS, DSS, and OS rates were 57%, 77%, and 77%, respectively. In Group B, the 5-year PFS, DSS, and OS rates were 30%, 77%, and 68%, respectively. In both groups, most of those who progressed did so after discontinuing imatinib following the planned course.

Conclusions

A high percentage of patients experienced disease progression after discontinuation of 2-year adjuvant therapy.

Commentary

Preoperative imatinib for 8 to 12 weeks was found to be safe and well tolerated, with limited risk of progression. Radiographic response as measured by RECIST criteria based on tumor size demonstrated that most patients had stable disease. However, duration of *preoperative* therapy was shorter than what is generally recommended nowadays (6 months or until best response), and tumor dimensions rather than tumor density (Choi criteria) formed the basis for assessing response.[36]

Future Trials in Patients with Gastrointestinal Stromal Tumor

Two adjuvant trials are exploring longer duration of adjuvant imatinib. The SSG XXIII/NCT02413736 open-label, phase 3 trial randomized GIST patients with high risk of recurrence after resection (gastric GIST with mitotic count >10/50 HPFs, nongastric GIST with mitotic count >5/50 HPFs, or tumor rupture) to 3 or 5 years of adjuvant imatinib 400 mg/d. Primary endpoint is RFS. The ImadGIST/NCT02260505 open-label, phase 3 trial randomized GIST patients with at least a 35% of recurrence based on NCCN criteria to 3 or 6 years of imatinib at doses 300 to 400 mg/d. Primary endpoint is DFS. These 2 studies will help confirm whether even longer duration imatinib therapy in the adjuvant setting is better than 3 years.

RETROPERITONEAL SARCOMA

RPS represents about 15% of all STS. Their natural history is mainly determined by histologic type and grade. Complete surgical resection is the mainstay of treatment of localized RPS. In consideration of their rarity, there is little prospective evidence and treatment choices are guided also by retrospective studies and expert consensus articles.

The first prospective studies in patients with RPS have focused on treatments that could potentially reduce the risk of LR, as this is the main cause of failure of patients with liposarcoma. The role of adjuvant/neoadjuvant RT with or without radioenhancer, with different timing and delivering modalities, has been investigated since the 1990s (**Table 3**), intending to determine if preoperative RT decreases the risk of LR. From a methodological perspective, the early studies in patients with RPS had major limitations. First, they were not collaborative, and each included a limited number of patients thereby inhibiting a meaningful analysis of this research question. Second, because the histology-specific behavior of RPS was not fully appreciated, these studies treated RPS as a single disease. The varied mix of histologies in the trial arms may have affected the study results. Another confounding factor in these studies was that both primary and recurrent RPS were usually included despite the second having a much worse outcome after surgery.

Keeping in mind these limitations, those studies were very important to understand that (1) preoperative RT was feasible and well tolerated, both with and without radio-enhancer, (2) brachytherapy was associated with intolerable toxicity, (3) there was no clear benefit associated with intraoperative radiotherapy (IORT) while it was associated with neurologic toxicity when administered at high dose, and (4) postoperative RT was burdened by a high risk of gastrointestinal toxicity with a little chance to deliver a proper dose to the tumor bed due to dose constraints to the surrounding organs. These considerations were key to developing the next generation trials.

Over the years, the creation of a strong multicontinent collaborative network (Transatlantic Australasian Retroperitoneal Sarcoma Working Group, TARPSWG) overcame, at least in part, the constraints related to the rarity of RPS and drove the successful completion of the first large RCT in patients with RPS (STRASS trial).

The US-based ACOSOG-Z9031 trial (NCT00091351) was the first organic attempt of addressing the role of preoperative RT in patients with primary localized RPS. This multicentric phase 3 RCT randomized patients to preoperative RT versus surgery alone. The trial opened in 2004 but it was prematurely closed after 2 years due to lack of accrual, with less than 20 patients enrolled.

From the evidence provided by the first-generation trials, of the growing international collaboration and of a strong drive toward centralizing patients with RPS in sarcoma referral centers, especially in Europe and Canada, a trial with similar design and inclusion criteria was developed by EORTC in 2010: the EORTC 62092 (STRASS) trial.[1] This is the first large RCT completed in patients with RPS, and it is discussed in detail below.

Preoperative Radiotherapy plus Surgery Versus Surgery Alone for Patients with Primary Retroperitoneal Sarcoma (EORTC-62092: STRASS): a Multicenter, Open-Label, Randomized, Phase 3 Trial[1]

Purpose and rationale

Intra-abdominal recurrence is the main cause of tumor-related death in patients with RPS. In first-generation trials, preoperative RT proved to be feasible and well tolerated in patients with RPS and, from the experience with ESTS, RT has the potential to decrease abdominal recurrence rate.

Study design and endpoints

This phase 3 RCT compared preoperative RT (50.4 Gy) +surgery versus surgery alone in patients with primary (nonrecurrent, nonmetastatic) localized RPS suitable for both complete resection and preoperative RT.

The primary endpoint was abdominal recurrence free survival (ARFS): a composite endpoint defined by LR, peritoneal sarcomatosis found at surgery, macroscopically incomplete (R2) resection, local or distant progression while on preoperative RT, and tumor becoming inoperable after randomization. Progression during RT, which

Table 3
Localized RPS trials

Year and Authors	Study Type	RCT Arms or Study Group	Major Finding	Impact on Practice
Sindelar and colleagues,[43] 1993	Phase III RCT (primary or recurrent RPS)	Experimental arm: 20 Gy IORT + postoperative low-dose (35–40 Gy) external-beam RT (n = 15) Control arm: postoperative high-dose (50–55-Gy) external-beam RT alone (n = 20)	Similar median survival (45 mo IORT group vs 52 mo control group) and DFI (19 mo IORT group vs 38 mo control group) Fewer radiation-related enteritis (2/15 vs 10/20) but more radiation-related peripheral neuropathy (9/15 vs 1/20) in IORT group	Postoperative RT is burdened by high gastrointestinal toxicity and currently it is not recommended. IORT did not impact survival or DFI and, at this dose, it was associated with significant neurologic toxicity
Robertson and colleagues,[44] 1995	Phase I, one arm	Iododeoxyuridine (IdUrd) + RT (n = 16, 11/16 resected) + surgery. IdUrd + RT: 5 cycles preoperative or 3 cycles preoperative + 2 cycles postoperative (total RT dose: 63.5 Gy)	Encouraging local control with combination + resection (24 mo local progression free survival 45%), treatment overall well tolerated	The combination of preoperative RT + radiosensitizer is feasible in patients with RPS
Jones and colleagues,[45] 2002 Smith and colleagues,[46] 2014	Phase II, one-arm (primary or recurrent RPS)	Preoperative RT (45–50 Gy, n = 40) + surgery + postoperative brachytherapy (20–25 Gy, n = 19)	No difference in 10-y RFS (56% vs 69%) or OS (52% vs 76%) among patients who received brachytherapy and those who did not. Brachytherapy was associated with increased acute and early postoperative morbidity and mortality	Preoperative RT is well tolerated. Postoperative brachytherapy is not recommended for treatment of patients with RPS
Pisters,[47] 2003	Phase I (primary or recurrent RPS)	Preoperative RT (18–50.4 Gy) + concurrent continuous infusion doxorubicin + surgery + IORT (15 Gy). N = 35	Toxicity: at 50.4 Gy 18% grade 3–4 nausea. 86% completed preoperative chemoradiation as planned. 83% were resected. 76% of patients who had surgery received IORT	The combination of preoperative RT + low-dose infusional doxorubicin is feasible and safe up to a total dose of 50.4 Gy

Roeder,[48] 2014	Phase I/II, one arm (primary or recurrent RPS)—unplanned interim analysis due to slow accrual	Neoadjuvant IMRT (50–56 Gy) + surgery + IORT (10–12 Gy). N = 27	Good results in terms of local control (5-y local control rate 72%) and OS (5-y OS 74%)	Combination of preoperative RT + surgery + IORT is feasible with acceptable toxicity
Gronchi and colleagues,[49] 2014	Phase I/II, one arm	High-dose long-infusion ifosfamide (HLI) 3 cycles + concomitant preoperative RT (50.4 Gy) followed by surgery. N = 83	Combined chemoradiation completed in 72% of patients. Preoperative RT completed in 88%. 95% were resected. RECIST PR: 8%. Five-year RFS 44%, 5-y OS 59%	Combination of HLI + RT feasible in about 2/3 of the patients and safe
Bonvalot and colleagues,[1] 2020 EORTC 62092 (STRASS)	Phase III RCT	Preoperative RT (50.4 Gy) + surgery vs surgery alone. N = 266	Overall: no difference in ARFS in the 2 groups An unplanned post hoc sensitivity analysis on patients with liposarcoma showed signal of better ARFS in RT arm (HR 0.62)	Results of STRASS suggest a possible effect of preoperative RT on ARFS in patients with G1–G2 liposarcoma

Abbreviations: DFI, disease-free interval; IORT, intraoperative radiotherapy; PR, partial response; RCT, randomized controlled trial; RFS, relapse-free survival; RT, radiotherapy.

occurred in 14% of patients, was not considered as an event in a sensitivity analysis, considering that 79% of the patients who progressed during RT could still proceed to a macroscopically complete resection.

Results: primary and secondary endpoints

A total of 266 patients were randomized in 5 years. At a median FU of 43 months, ARFS was similar in the 2 arms (about 60% at 3 years). An unplanned post hoc sensitivity analysis showed a strong signal in favor of preoperative RT in patients with low-grade liposarcoma, with a 10% absolute gain in ARFS at 3 years (HR 0·62, 95% CI 0·38–1·02). In the subgroup analyses, patients with LMS and high-grade DDLPS did not seem to benefit from preoperative RT. Metastasis free-survival and OS did not differ in the 2 arms.

In terms of safety, RT was very well tolerated (of note, 95% of patients received intensity-modulated RT). The most common grade 3 to 4 side effect was lymphopenia in 77% of the patients in the experimental arm. There was no difference in reoperation rate (10%–11%) and postoperative mortality (1.6%) between the 2 arms.

Commentary

STRASS was the first large multicentric RCT completed in patients with primary RPS. The trial included all histologic types and was designed expecting a large benefit from preoperative RT. These 2 choices reflect, on one hand, the poor understanding of histology-specific outcomes in 2010, at time of trial design, and on the other hand, the fear of not being able to complete the trial in a reasonable timeframe considering the rarity of the disease and the failure of the ACOSOG-Z9031 trial. The trial was overall negative but a post hoc sensitivity analysis showed a strong signal of efficacy of RT on ARFS in patients with liposarcoma, although without any impact on OS at the current follow-up. STRASS was a negative trial but it has been very informative about the role of preoperative RT in patients with RPS. The trial results discourage the use of preoperative RT in patients with LMS and HG DDLPS. On the contrary, preoperative RT can be considered in patients with WDLPS and G1-2 DDLPS.

Ongoing Trials in Retroperitoneal Sarcoma

STRASS-2 is a multicentric phase 3 RCT that is comparing preoperative chemotherapy + surgery versus surgery alone in patients with primary (nonrecurrent, nonmetastatic) resectable high-risk DDLPS and LMS of the retroperitoneum. In the experimental arm, patients with DDLPS are treated with 3 cycles of doxorubicin 75 mg/m^2 and ifosfamide 9 g/m^2, whereas patients with LMS are treated with 3 cycles of doxorubicin 60 mg/m^2 and dacarbazine with a minimal threshold of 900 mg/m^2 per cycle. The primary endpoint of the study is DFS. The expected accrual is 250 patients in 7 years, with the first patient enrolled in 2021.

STRASS-2 is focusing on those histology types with a higher risk of distant recurrence, which did not gain benefit from RT in STRASS. Given the recent observation that high-risk ESTS are more likely to benefit from adjuvant/neoadjuvant chemotherapy, it is of particular importance to test this hypothesis specifically in patients with RPS. Indeed, although retroperitoneal LMS may mimic the biological behavior of extremity high-risk STS (with a high risk of distant metastases and a low risk of LR), high-grade DDLPS of the retroperitoneum carry a significant risk of both local and distant recurrence. Results of STRASS-2 will inform on the role of neoadjuvant chemotherapy in this specific location.

SUMMARY

Despite surgery remaining the cornerstone of treatment of patients with localized STS and GIST, recent trials and trial updates have shed light on the role of adjuvant/ neoadjuvant-targeted therapy, chemotherapy, and RT. Patients with high-risk STS of the extremity and superficial trunk benefit from RT in terms of better local control. The adoption of risk-based criteria to select patients for adjuvant/neoadjuvant chemotherapy may be the key to developing new and reevaluating old chemotherapy trials. In addition, the role of immunotherapy in specific types of sarcoma, including metastatic UPS, alveolar soft parts sarcoma and angiosarcoma, are being established and potentially extended into the localized setting. In patients with RPS, results of the STRASS trial point in the direction of a possible effect of RT in improving local control of patients with GI–GII liposarcoma. Adjuvant imatinib has established itself as a standard in patients with high-risk GIST but ongoing trials will be important to properly understand the optimal treatment duration. Continued development of collaborative, histology-specific trials is critical to advancing multimodality care in sarcoma.

DISCLOSURE

The authors have nothing to disclose.

REFERENCES

1. Bonvalot S, Gronchi A, Le Péchoux C, et al. Preoperative radiotherapy plus surgery versus surgery alone for patients with primary retroperitoneal sarcoma (EORTC-62092: STRASS): A multicentre, open-label, randomised, phase 3 trial. Lancet Oncol 2020;21(10):1366–77.

2. Bonvalot S, Rutkowski PL, Thariat J, et al. NBTXR3, a first-in-class radioenhancer hafnium oxide nanoparticle, plus radiotherapy versus radiotherapy alone in patients with locally advanced soft-tissue sarcoma (act.in.sarc): A multicentre, phase 2-3, randomised, controlled trial. Lancet Oncol 2019;20(8):1148–59.

3. Gronchi A, Palmerini E, Quagliuolo V, et al. Neoadjuvant chemotherapy in high-risk soft tissue sarcomas: Final results of a randomized trial from italian (ISG), spanish (GEIS), french (FSG), and polish (PSG) sarcoma groups. J Clin Oncol 2020;38(19):2178–86.

4. Callegaro D, Miceli R, Bonvalot S, et al. Impact of perioperative chemotherapy and radiotherapy in patients with primary extremity soft tissue sarcoma: Retrospective analysis across major histological subtypes and major reference centres. Eur J Cancer 2018;105:19–27.

5. Lansu J, Bovée JVMG, Braam P, et al. Dose reduction of preoperative radiotherapy in myxoid liposarcoma: A nonrandomized controlled trial. JAMA Oncol 2021;7(1):e205865.

6. Sarcoma Meta-analysis Collaboration (SMAC). Adjuvant chemotherapy for localised resectable soft tissue sarcoma in adults. Cochrane Database Syst Rev 2000; 4:CD001419.

7. Pervaiz N, Colterjohn N, Farrokhyar F, et al. A systematic meta-analysis of randomized controlled trials of adjuvant chemotherapy for localized resectable soft-tissue sarcoma. Cancer 2008;113(3):573–81.

8. Pasquali S, Pizzamiglio S, Touati N, et al. The impact of chemotherapy on survival of patients with extremity and trunk wall soft tissue sarcoma: Revisiting the results of the EORTC-STBSG 62931 randomised trial. Eur J Cancer 2019;109:51–60.

9. Pasquali S, Palmerini E, Quagliuolo V, et al. Neoadjuvant chemotherapy in high-risk soft tissue sarcomas: A sarculator-based risk stratification analysis of the ISG-STS 1001 randomized trial. Cancer 2022;128(1):85–93.

10. Gronchi A, Ferrari S, Quagliuolo V, et al. Histotype-tailored neoadjuvant chemotherapy versus standard chemotherapy in patients with high-risk soft-tissue sarcomas (ISG-STS 1001): An international, open-label, randomised, controlled, phase 3, multicentre trial. Lancet Oncol 2017;18(6):812–22.

11. DIGITAL FOREST srl. Applestore. 2020. Available at: https://geo.itunes.apple.com/us/app/sarculator/id1052119173?mt=8google play; https://play.google.com/store/apps/details?id=it.digitalforest.sarculator. Accessed February 18, 2022.

12. Bonvalot S, Le Pechoux C, De Baere T, et al. First-in-human study testing a new radioenhancer using nanoparticles (NBTXR3) activated by radiation therapy in patients with locally advanced soft tissue sarcomas. Clin Cancer Res 2017; 23(4):908–17.

13. Wardelmann E, Haas RL, Bovée JV, et al. Evaluation of response after neoadjuvant treatment in soft tissue sarcomas; the european organization for research and treatment of cancer-soft tissue and bone sarcoma group (EORTC-STBSG) recommendations for pathological examination and reporting. Eur J Cancer 2016;53:84–95.

14. O'Sullivan B, Davis AM, Turcotte R, et al. Preoperative versus postoperative radiotherapy in soft-tissue sarcoma of the limbs: A randomised trial. Lancet 2002;359(9325):2235–41.

15. Rosenberg SA, Tepper J, Glatstein E, et al. The treatment of soft-tissue sarcomas of the extremities: Prospective randomized evaluations of (1) limb-sparing surgery plus radiation therapy compared with amputation and (2) the role of adjuvant chemotherapy. Ann Surg 1982;196(3):305–15.

16. Pisters PW, Harrison LB, Leung DH, et al. Long-term results of a prospective randomized trial of adjuvant brachytherapy in soft tissue sarcoma. J Clin Oncol 1996;14(3):859–68.

17. Yang JC, Chang AE, Baker AR, et al. Randomized prospective study of the benefit of adjuvant radiation therapy in the treatment of soft tissue sarcomas of the extremity. J Clin Oncol 1998;16(1):197–203.

18. Beane JD, Yang JC, White D, et al. Efficacy of adjuvant radiation therapy in the treatment of soft tissue sarcoma of the extremity: 20-year follow-up of a randomized prospective trial. Ann Surg Oncol 2014;21(8):2484–9.

19. Davis AM, O'Sullivan B, Turcotte R, et al. Late radiation morbidity following randomization to preoperative versus postoperative radiotherapy in extremity soft tissue sarcoma. Radiother Oncol 2005;75(1):48–53.

20. Kraybill WG, Harris J, Spiro IJ, et al. Phase II study of neoadjuvant chemotherapy and radiation therapy in the management of high-risk, high-grade, soft tissue sarcomas of the extremities and body wall: Radiation therapy oncology group trial 9514. J Clin Oncol 2006;24(4):619–25.

21. Kraybill WG, Harris J, Spiro IJ, et al. Long-term results of a phase 2 study of neoadjuvant chemotherapy and radiotherapy in the management of high-risk, high-grade, soft tissue sarcomas of the extremities and body wall: Radiation therapy oncology group trial 9514. Cancer 2010;116(19):4613–21.

22. Woll PJ, Reichardt P, Le Cesne A, et al. Adjuvant chemotherapy with doxorubicin, ifosfamide, and lenograstim for resected soft-tissue sarcoma (EORTC 62931): A multicentre randomised controlled trial. Lancet Oncol 2012;13(10):1045–54.

23. Gronchi A, Stacchiotti S, Verderio P, et al. Short, full-dose adjuvant chemotherapy (CT) in high-risk adult soft tissue sarcomas (STS): Long-term follow-up of a randomized clinical trial from the italian sarcoma group and the spanish sarcoma group. Ann Oncol 2016;27(12):2283–8.

24. Blanke CD, Demetri GD, von Mehren M, et al. Long-term results from a randomized phase II trial of standard- versus higher-dose imatinib mesylate for patients with unresectable or metastatic gastrointestinal stromal tumors expressing KIT. J Clin Oncol 2008;26(4):620–5.

25. Demetri GD, van Oosterom AT, Garrett CR, et al. Efficacy and safety of sunitinib in patients with advanced gastrointestinal stromal tumour after failure of imatinib: A randomised controlled trial. Lancet 2006;368(9544):1329–38.

26. Demetri GD, Reichardt P, Kang YK, et al. Efficacy and safety of regorafenib for advanced gastrointestinal stromal tumours after failure of imatinib and sunitinib (GRID): An international, multicentre, randomised, placebo-controlled, phase 3 trial. Lancet 2013;381(9863):295–302.

27. Blay JY, Serrano C, Heinrich MC, et al. Ripretinib in patients with advanced gastrointestinal stromal tumours (INVICTUS): A double-blind, randomised, placebo-controlled, phase 3 trial. Lancet Oncol 2020;21(7):923–34.

28. Kang YK, George S, Jones RL, et al. Avapritinib versus regorafenib in locally advanced unresectable or metastatic GI stromal tumor: A randomized, open-label phase III study. J Clin Oncol 2021;39(28):3128–39.

29. DeMatteo RP, Lewis JJ, Leung D, et al. Two hundred gastrointestinal stromal tumors: Recurrence patterns and prognostic factors for survival. Ann Surg 2000; 231(1):51–8.

30. Joensuu H, Eriksson M, Sundby Hall K, et al. One vs three years of adjuvant imatinib for operable gastrointestinal stromal tumor: A randomized trial. JAMA 2012; 307(12):1265–72.

31. Joensuu H, Eriksson M, Sundby Hall K, et al. Survival outcomes associated with 3 years vs 1 year of adjuvant imatinib for patients with high-risk gastrointestinal stromal tumors: An analysis of a randomized clinical trial after 10-year follow-up. JAMA Oncol 2020;6(8):1241–6.

32. Dematteo RP, Ballman KV, Antonescu CR, et al. Adjuvant imatinib mesylate after resection of localised, primary gastrointestinal stromal tumour: A randomised, double-blind, placebo-controlled trial. Lancet 2009;373(9669):1097–104.

33. Raut CP, Espat NJ, Maki RG, et al. Efficacy and tolerability of 5-year adjuvant imatinib treatment for patients with resected intermediate- or high-risk primary gastrointestinal stromal tumor: The PERSIST-5 clinical trial. JAMA Oncol 2018; 4(12):e184060.

34. Eisenberg BL, Harris J, Blanke CD, et al. Phase II trial of neoadjuvant/adjuvant imatinib mesylate (IM) for advanced primary and metastatic/recurrent operable gastrointestinal stromal tumor (GIST): Early results of RTOG 0132/ACRIN 6665. J Surg Oncol 2009;99(1):42–7.

35. Wang D, Zhang Q, Blanke CD, et al. Phase II trial of neoadjuvant/adjuvant imatinib mesylate for advanced primary and metastatic/recurrent operable gastrointestinal stromal tumors: Long-term follow-up results of radiation therapy oncology group 0132. Ann Surg Oncol 2012;19(4):1074–80.

36. Choi H, Charnsangavej C, Faria SC, et al. Correlation of computed tomography and positron emission tomography in patients with metastatic gastrointestinal stromal tumor treated at a single institution with imatinib mesylate: Proposal of new computed tomography response criteria. J Clin Oncol 2007;25(13):1753–9.

37. DeMatteo RP, Ballman KV, Antonescu CR, et al. Long-term results of adjuvant imatinib mesylate in localized, high-risk, primary gastrointestinal stromal tumor: ACOSOG Z9000 (alliance) intergroup phase 2 trial. Ann Surg 2013;258(3):422–9.

38. Corless CL, Ballman KV, Antonescu CR, et al. Pathologic and molecular features correlate with long-term outcome after adjuvant therapy of resected primary GI stromal tumor: The ACOSOG Z9001 trial. J Clin Oncol 2014;32(15):1563–70.

39. Joensuu H, Eriksson M, Sundby Hall K, et al. Adjuvant imatinib for high-risk GI stromal tumor: Analysis of a randomized trial. J Clin Oncol 2016;34(3):244–50.

40. Casali PG, Le Cesne A, Poveda Velasco A, et al. Time to definitive failure to the first tyrosine kinase inhibitor in localized GI stromal tumors treated with imatinib as an adjuvant: A european organisation for research and treatment of cancer soft tissue and bone sarcoma group intergroup randomized trial in collaboration with the australasian gastro-intestinal trials group, UNICANCER, french sarcoma group, italian sarcoma group, and spanish group for research on sarcomas. J Clin Oncol 2015;33(36):4276–83.

41. McAuliffe JC, Hunt KK, Lazar AJ, et al. A randomized, phase II study of preoperative plus postoperative imatinib in GIST: Evidence of rapid radiographic response and temporal induction of tumor cell apoptosis. Ann Surg Oncol 2009;16(4):910–9.

42. Du CY, Zhou Y, Song C, et al. Is there a role of surgery in patients with recurrent or metastatic gastrointestinal stromal tumours responding to imatinib: A prospective randomised trial in china. Eur J Cancer 2014;50(10):1772–8.

43. Sindelar WF, Kinsella TJ, Chen PW, et al. Intraoperative radiotherapy in retroperitoneal sarcomas. final results of a prospective, randomized, clinical trial. Arch Surg 1993;128(4):402–10.

44. Robertson JM, Sondak VK, Weiss SA, et al. Preoperative radiation therapy and iododeoxyuridine for large retroperitoneal sarcomas. Int J Radiat Oncol Biol Phys 1995;31(1):87–92.

45. Jones JJ, Catton CN, O'Sullivan B, et al. Initial results of a trial of preoperative external-beam radiation therapy and postoperative brachytherapy for retroperitoneal sarcoma. Ann Surg Oncol 2002;9(4):346–54.

46. Smith MJ, Ridgway PF, Catton CN, et al. Combined management of retroperitoneal sarcoma with dose intensification radiotherapy and resection: Long-term results of a prospective trial. Radiother Oncol 2014;110(1):165–71.

47. Pisters PW, Ballo MT, Fenstermacher MJ, et al. Phase I trial of preoperative concurrent doxorubicin and radiation therapy, surgical resection, and intraoperative electron-beam radiation therapy for patients with localized retroperitoneal sarcoma. J Clin Oncol 2003;21(16):3092–7.

48. Roeder F, Ulrich A, Habl G, et al. Clinical phase I/II trial to investigate preoperative dose-escalated intensity-modulated radiation therapy (IMRT) and intraoperative radiation therapy (IORT) in patients with retroperitoneal soft tissue sarcoma: Interim analysis. BMC Cancer 2014;14. 617-2407-14-617.

49. Gronchi A, De Paoli A, Dani C, et al. Preoperative chemo-radiation therapy for localised retroperitoneal sarcoma: A phase I-II study from the italian sarcoma group. Eur J Cancer 2014;50(4):784–92.

New Drug Approvals for Sarcoma in the Last 5 Years

Prapassorn Thirasastr, MD[a], Mehdi Brahmi, MD, PhD[b], Armelle Dufresne, MD, PhD[b],
Neeta Somaiah, MD[a],*, Jean-Yves Blay, MD, PhD[b],*

KEYWORDS

- Sarcoma • Connective tissue tumors • Gastrointestinal stromal tumors
- Precision medicine • Targeted treatments

KEY POINTS

- New generations of tyrosine kinase inhibitors blocking KIT and PDGFRA primary and resistance mutations are now availableImmunotherapy of sarcomas using PDL1, PD1, or CTLA-4 Ab has limited activity in unselected populations of advanced sarcoma sarcomas.
- Several histotypes, such as, ASPS, chordoma respond to ICP. New biomarkers are now identified, such as the presence of tertiary lymphoid structures.
- New tyrosine and serine threonine kinases are demonstrated active in sarcomas with somatic molecular alterations on genes encoding oncoprotein driver of specific sarcoma histotypes.

RIPRETINIB AND AVAPRITINIB IN GASTROINTESTINAL STROMAL TUMOR

During the past few years, treatment focused on primary and secondary driver mutations in *KIT*-mutated or *PDGFR*-mutated gastrointestinal stromal tumors (GISTs) have seen some advances. The main driver mutations in GIST include *KIT* (75%–80%) and platelet-derived growth factor receptor-α (*PDGFRA*; 8%–10%), with a small subset negative for *KIT* and *PDGFRA* mutations (10%–15%) that harbor other molecular alterations such as succinate dehydrogenase (SDH) deficiency (majority), *BRAF* and neurofibromatosis type 1 (*NF1)* mutations.[1] Imatinib, sunitinib, and regorafenib were the 3 approved agents in unresectable/metastatic GIST patients in first, second, and third lines, respectively, based on previous randomized studies[2,3](**Fig. 1**). Recently, the regulatory bodies granted approval to ripretinib in fourth-line GIST and to avapritinib for *PDGFR* exon 18 (D842 V)-mutated GISTs.

Resistance to imatinib can be grouped as primary or secondary resistance. The major cause of primary resistance is the D842 V *PDGFRA* mutation, which constitutes

[a] University of Texas M D Anderson Cancer Center, 1400 Holcombe Blvd., Unit 450, Houston, TX-77030, USA; [b] CLCC Léon Bérard, 28 Rue Laënnec, 69373 LYON CEDEX 8, FRANCE
* Corresponding authors.
E-mail addresses: nsomaiah@mdanderson.org (N.S.); jean-yves.blay@lyon.unicancer.fr (J.-Y.B.)

Surg Oncol Clin N Am 31 (2022) 361–380
https://doi.org/10.1016/j.soc.2022.03.003
surgonc.theclinics.com

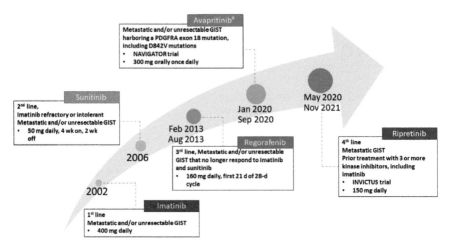

Fig. 1. The FDA and EMA approval timeline and indication(s) of drugs in metastatic GISTs. [a] Avapritinib received conditional authorization in EU in metastatic and/or unresectable GIST with a D842V PDGFRA mutation.

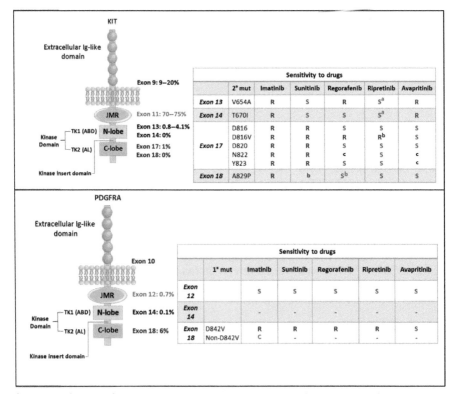

Fig. 2. Distribution of KIT and PDGFRA mutations in GISTs and sensitivity to drugs. JMR, juxtamembrane region; PDGFRA, platelet-derived growth factor receptor α. [a] Decreased response. [b] Presence of conflicting data. [c] Response depend on amino acid change.

about 5% of overall GIST cases. This mutation is located in the exon 18 of *PDGFRA*, which affects the activation loop inside the C-terminal of the tyrosine kinase domain (**Fig. 2**). The modification at D842 residue interferes with the swinging movement of the activation loop, leading to conformational shift of the adenosine triphosphate (ATP)-binding pocket, thereby preventing imatinib binding.[4] Some subsets within non-*KIT* and non-*PDGFR* mutated GISTs can also confer primary resistance.

In clinic, secondary resistance is defined by progression of disease after 6 months of initial benefit on imatinib.[5] Secondary resistance usually occurs after 20 to 24 months of imatinib treatment due to secondary mutations in a subpopulation of cancer cells. The hotspots for secondary mutations are the ATP-binding pocket (exon 13, 14 of *KIT*) and the activation loop (exon 17, 18 of *KIT*) accounting for 85% to 90% of mutations.[1,6]

Sunitinib is the second-line treatment approved in metastatic GIST and has activity against secondary mutations in the ATP-binding pocket (exon 13, 14 of *KIT*), whereas regorafenib, approved in third line, has activity against activation-loop (exon 17 of *KIT*) mutations, except D816 V substitution and has poor activity against the *KIT* exon 13 V654 A mutation.[7] The efficacy of sunitinib and regorafenib in second and third lines are greatly decreased compared with first-line imatinib. This is owing to the heterogeneity of secondary KIT mutations after imatinib and emerging cross-resistant subpopulations on therapy.

RIPRETINIB

Ripretinib, similar to imatinib, sunitinib, and regorafenib, is a type 2 receptor tyrosine kinase (RTK) inhibitor. It binds the inactive form of RTKs and demonstrated broader inhibition of *KIT/PDGFRA* mutants than previously approved tyrosine kinase inhibitors (TKIs) in preclinical studies.[8] Ripretinib exerts its potent activity by binding to both switch pocket and activation loop preventing conformation change into active form.

In a phase 1 study, ripretinib had activity across all lines of treatment.[9] The overall response rate (ORR) in the study was 21% in second-line and third-line patients and 9% in fourth line and greater. These data led to the phase 3 double-blind study (INVICTUS) in the fourth line and beyond setting, randomizing patients to ripretinib 150 mg daily or placebo. It conferred a median progression free survival (PFS) of 6.3 months compared with only 1 month in the placebo arm (HR, 0.15; 95% CI, 0.09–0.25; $P < .0001$).[10] Furthermore, ripretinib also improved median OS from 6.6 months in the placebo arm to 15.1 months (HR, 0.36; 95% CI, 0.20–0.63; $P = .0004$) with ORR of 9.4%. Longer follow-up revealed median PFS of 6.3 months and 1.0 month in the ripretinib and placebo group, respectively, with updated ORR of 11.8% in ripretinib group.[11] Currently, ripretinib 150 mg once daily is approved for fourth and later lines of treatment in GIST based on data from this phase 3 INVICTUS trial.

The recommended dose of 150 mg oral once daily was determined by the phase 1 study.[9] No relation or interaction with food was noted. In the phase 1 dose escalation/expansion study, most of the side effects were grade 1 to 2, with grade 3 to 4 treatment emergent adverse events (TEAE) in ≥5% patients of asymptomatic lipase elevation (11%), anemia (7%), hypertension (6%), and abdominal pain (5%).

In the dose-expansion phase of phase 1 and the phase 3 studies, patients who progressed on ripretinib 150 mg once daily dose as determined by response evaluation criteria in solid tumors (RECIST)1.1 were given option to increase dose to 150 mg twice daily (BID).[12] PFS on ripretinib 150 mg once daily was defined as PFS1, and after dose escalation, PFS on ripretinib 150 mg BID from the date of escalation to progression or death was defined as PFS2. In the phase 1 study, PFS2 was 5.6 months for second-line therapy, 3.3 months for third-line, and 4.6 months for fourth-line or

Table 1
Treatment-related treatment-emergent adverse events on ripretinib 150 mg once daily dose (left column) and 150 mg BID dose (right column)

TEAEs, n (%)	Ripretinib 150 mg QD[a] (n = 85)		Ripretinib 150 mg BID[a] (n = 67)	
	All Grades	Grade 3/4	All Grades	Grade 3/4
Abdominal pain	-[b]	-	18 (26.9)	7 (10.4)
Anemia	3 (3)	1 (1)	15 (22.4)	4 (6.0)
Fatigue	22 (26)	2 (2)	14 (20.9)	2 (3.0)
Dyspnea	-	-	9 (13.4)	2 (3.0)
Diarrhea	18 (21)	1(1)	19 (28.4)	1 (1.5)
Headache	-	-	7 (10.4)	1 (1.5)
Peripheral edema	-	-	7 (10.4)	1 (1.5)
Decreased appetite	13 (15)	1 (1)	16 (23.9)	1 (1.5)
PPES	18 (21)	0	12 (17.9)	0
Alopecia	42 (49)	0	11 (16.4)	0
Vomiting	-	-	11 (16.4)	0
Nausea	22 (26)	1 (1)	17 (25.4)	0
Weight decreased	13 (15)	0	11 (16.4)	0
Muscle spasms	10 (12)	0	10 (14.9)	0
Myalgia	24 (28)	1 (1)	-	-
Hypertension	7(9)	3 (4)	-	-
Constipation	13 (15)	0	-	-
Blood bilirubin increased	12 (14)	0	-	-

Abbreviations: QD, once daily; BID, twice daily; PPES, Palmar-plantar erythrodysesthesia syndrome; TEAE, Treatment-related adverse events.
[a] List of TEAE with incidence greater than 10% and/or grade 3/4.
[b] Not recorded in the trial or recorded with other terms.
Data from Blay J-Y, Serrano C, Heinrich MC, et al. The Lancet Oncology 2020(10) and George S, Chi P, Heinrich MC, et al. Eur J Cancer 2021(12).

greater. The ratio of median PFS2/PFS1 was 51%, 40%, and 84% in each line, respectively. However, dose escalation led to some worsening side effects including abdominal pain, anemia, dyspnea, fatigue, peripheral edema, decrease appetite, and diarrhea. **Table 1** details side effects of standard dosing and dose escalation from the phase 1 and phase 3 studies. Rare but serious side effects included skin cancer (cutaneous squamous cell carcinoma 4.7%, melanoma 2.4%) and congestive heart failure (1.2%).

Ripretinib was also recently evaluated in a phase 3 study (INTRIGUE) in the second-line setting in comparison to sunitinib. The preliminary results were reported at the American Association for Cancer Research; ripretinib in second line failed to show superior outcomes compared with sunitinib.[13] The ORR was 21.7% and 17.6% while median PFS was 8 and 8.3 months, for ripretinib and sunitinib, respectively. This difference was not statistically significant.

AVAPRITINIB

Avapritinib is a type I inhibitor with selective inhibition of KIT/PDGFR activation loop mutations such as PDGFRA exon 18 D842 V and KIT D816 V.[14,15] Strong preclinical data led to a phase 1 (NAVIGATOR) trial of Avapritinib in advanced GISTs divided into groups based on the presence or absence of a PDGFR exon 18 mutation.[16] *PDGFR* exon 18 (D842 V)-mutated GIST, previously resistant to all the available TKIs, demonstrated an ORR of 88% (49/56) with, complete response (CR) in 9% (5/56) and progression free rate of 81% at 12 months. In patients who received 300 mg starting dose, ORR was 93%. Based on this dramatic response, avapritinib 300 mg once daily was approved for patients with *PDGFR* exon 18 mutations in any line of treatment.

In non-D842 V patients in fourth or later lines, the ORR was 17% (17/103) with median PFS 3.7 months (95%CI: 2.8–4.6), whereas ORR in third or fourth line regorafenib-naïve patients was 26% (6/23). Median PFS was 8.6 months (95%CI:5.6–14.7).[17–19] No responses were seen in patients with V654 A or T670I *KIT* secondary mutations (0/25), whereas ORR in the group negative for these mutations was 26% (22/84). Following up on these results, a phase 3 (VOYAGER) study in third line or beyond was conducted randomizing unresectable/metastatic GIST patients between avapritinib and regorafenib. The study unfortunately did not meet its primary end point as the PFS for avapritinib was not superior to regorafenib (4.2 vs 5.6 months, HR 1.25, 95%CI 0.99–1.57, $P = .055$). The ORR was 17.1% and 7.2% for avapritinib and regorafenib, respectively. Around 14% of patients included on the study had a *KIT* V654 A or T670I mutation (exon 13/14) that we now know are resistant to avapritinib (see **Fig. 2**).

In the phase 1 dose escalation and expansion study, avapritinib showed a reasonable tolerability profile with only a few patients discontinuing due to side effects.[16] Most common adverse events are edema, nausea, fatigue, decreased appetite, diarrhea, constipation, hair color change, and cognitive impairment (**Table 2**). Avapritinib had less events associated with vascular endothelial growth factor receptor activation such as hypertension and hand-foot syndrome compared with sunitinib and regorafenib. Cognitive effects were seen more frequently with avapritinib and seemed as frequently as 40% (33/82) and were classified as memory impairment (30%), cognitive disorder (10%), confusion (9%), and encephalopathy (2%). Most cases were reported as grade 1 and managed with dose modifications or interruptions with treatment discontinuation reported in 2% (2/82).

The starting dose of avapritinib in the phase 1 dose-expansion was 400 mg daily but later reduced to 300 mg daily due to the concern regarding higher grade cognitive adverse events and no significant difference in ORR.[16] The approved dose is 300 mg daily with dose reduction to 200 mg or 100 mg daily recommended for side effect management. Avapritinib has to be taken on an empty stomach, 2 hours after or 1 hour before a meal.

ERIBULIN IN LIPOSARCOMA

Liposarcomas (LPS) are one of the most common soft tissue sarcomas (STS) believed to originate from an adipocytic lineage. Three main subtypes of LPS are well-differentiated/dedifferentiated (WDLPS/DDLPS), myxoid/round-cell (MRCLS), and pleomorphic (PLPS). WDLPS and DDLPS account for most LPS and have poorer response to chemotherapy compared with MRCLS. PLPS tend to have the worse prognosis but account for only about 10% of all LPS cases.[20]

Despite the poorer response, current standard systemic treatment in DDLPS is anthracycline-based chemotherapy recommended as a first-line treatment in advanced/metastatic disease based on studies in STS. No standard systemic options are available for pure WDLPS. In a pivotal phase 3, EORTC 62012 trial, combination doxorubicin–ifosfamide had superior ORR and median PFS compared with a single

Table 2
Treatment-related adverse effects of Avapritinib at different starting doses

TRAEs, n (%)	<300 mg (n = 30)		300 mg (n = 32)		400 mg (n = 17)	
	Grade1-2	Grade 3–4	Grade1-2	Grade 3–4	Grade1-2	Grade 3–4
Nausea	13(43)	1(3)	22(69)	0	12(71)	0
Fatigue	18(60)	1(3)	12(38)	1(3)	8(47)	3(18)
Diarrhea	11(37)	1(3)	13(41)	2(6)	6(35)	1(6)
Periorbital edema	15(50)	0	11(34)	1(3)	8(47)	0
Anemia	6(20)	5(17)	11(34)	7(22)	4(24)	1(6)
Decreased appetite	6(20)	1(3)	12(38)	0	5(29)	0
Vomiting	10(33)	1(3)	5(16)	0	8(47)	0
Memory impairment	7(23)	0	10(31)	0	7(41)	0
Hair color change	11(37)	0	8(25)	0	5(29)	0
Increased lacrimation	5(30)	0	7(22)	0	7(41)	0
Peripheral edema	10(33)	0	10(31)	0	4(24)	0
Blood bilirubin increased	3(10)	0	7(22)	1(3)	5(29)	1(6)
Face edema	3(10)	0	11(34)	0	3(18)	0
Dysgeusia	5(17)	0	7(22)	0	2(12)	0
Hypophosphatemia	3(10)	2(6)	3(9)	1(3)	4(24)	2(12)
Neutropenia	2(7)	1(3)	6(19)	3(9)	1(6)	1(6)
Dizziness	2(7)	0	6(19)	0	5(29)	0
Dyspepsia	6(20)	0	4(13)	0	2(12)	0
Alopecia	4(13)	0	4(13)	0	3(18)	0
Eyelid edema	3(10)	0	5(16)	0	3(18)	0
Headache	3(10)	0	4(13)	0	1(6)	0
Pleural effusion	2(7)	1(3)	3(9)	1(3)	0	1(6)
Cognitive disorder	1(3)	1(3)	4(13)	0	0	1(6)
Hypomagnesemia	2(7)	1(3)	3(9)	1(3)	0	1(6)

Abbreviation: TRAEs, Treatment related adverse events.
The table lists treatment-related adverse events occurring in 10% or more in 300 mg dose.
Data from Heinrich MC, Jones RL, von Mehren M, et al. The Lancet Oncology 2020(16).

agent doxorubicin (ORR 26% vs 14%, mPFS 7.4 vs 4.6 months, HR 0.74, 95%CI 0.60–0.90) but no significant benefit in OS (14.3 vs 12.8 months, 95%CI 10.5–14.3).[21] The study involved 14% and 11% of LPS patients in the combination and doxorubicin alone arm, respectively. Chemotherapy response specifically in WDLPS/DDLPS has been evaluated in retrospective studies revealing an ORR of 12% to 21%, varying based on WDLPS percentage and use of combination versus single agent therapy.[22,23] The commonly used second-line regimen in DDLPS is gemcitabine-docetaxel primarily based on the SARC002 study in STS.[23–25]

Options for later lines in DDLPS include trabectedin approved on the basis of a phase 3 randomized trial comparing trabectedin and dacarbazine in advanced LPS or leiomyosarcoma (LMS) after prior anthracycline and one additional systemic regimen (3rd line setting).[26] Trabectedin demonstrated a superior PFS of 4.2 months compared with 1.5 months in dacarbazine (HR 0.55, $P < .001$), though there was no difference in OS (12.4 vs 12.9 months, HR 0.87, $P = .37$). In the DDLPS subgroup, median PFS was 2.2 months with trabectedin compared with 1.9 months in dacarbazine

(95%CI 0.37–1.25, HR 0.68) but in MRCLS, the median PFS was 5.6 months with trabectedin compared with 1.5 months with dacarbazine (HR 0.41, 95%CI 0.17–0.98).[26]

Shortly thereafter, eribulin was added to the therapeutic armamentarium for previously treated advanced/metastatic LPS.

Eribulin mesylate is a derivative of Halichondrin B, a natural substance originally isolated from a rare marine Japanese sponge, *Halichondria okadai* but also present in more common sponges.[27] Eribulin belongs to the group of antitubulin drugs and has an inhibitory effect on microtubule polymerization leading to mitotic block and cell arrest in the G2–M phase of the cell cycle. Preclinical studies showed antitumor activity of eribulin against many established cancer cell lines including breast cancer, colon cancer, non-small cell lung cancer, and uterine sarcoma.

In a nonrandomized phase 2 study in progressive high-grade STS, patients who had received 1 or more prior combination chemotherapy or 2 or more prior single drugs for advanced disease were enrolled.[28] Of all STS patients, adipocytic sarcoma and LMS demonstrated a higher percentage of progression-free survival at 12 weeks (46.9% in adipocytic sarcoma and 21.6% in LMS). The promising results in LPS and LMS prompted a phase 3 randomized, open-label study comparing eribulin (1.4 mg/m^2 intravenously on days 1 and 8) and dacarbazine (850 mg/m^2, 1000 mg/m^2, or 1200 mg/m^2 depending on center and clinician, on day 1) every 21 days in advanced LPS or LMS patients who received 2 or greater prior systemic regimens including anthracycline (third-line setting).[29] Overall survival in eribulin group was significantly better compared with dacarbazine with a median OS of 13.5 months versus 11.5 months (HR 0.77, 95%CI 0.62–0.95, P = .0169), respectively. Median PFS was similar in eribulin and dacarbazine groups (2.6 months vs 2.6 months, HR 0.88, 95%CI 0.71–1.09, P = .23). The planned subgroup analysis revealed most of the survival benefit in the LPS group (HR 0.51, 95%CI 0.35–0.75) and not in LMS (HR 0.93, 95%CI 0.71–1.20). The PFS for the LPS group was 2.9 versus 1.7 months for eribulin versus dacarbazine, respectively (HR 0.521, 95%CI 0.35–0.78). Most of the LPS patients in this study were DDLPS (45.5%), followed by MRCLS (38.5%), and PLS (16.1%). Further analysis of the outcomes in this study revealed a statistically significant OS difference with eribulin compared with dacarbazine in DDLPS (HR 0.429, 95% CI 0.232–0.792) and PLPS (HR 0.182 95%CI 0.039–0.850) but not in MRCLS patients (HR 0.787, 95%CI 0.416–1.491) (**Table 3**).[30] Eribulin was granted Food and Drug

Table 3
Survival data in LS subgroups from the randomized phase 3 trial of eribulin compared with dacarbazine

Group/Subgroup (n)	Median OS (months)			Median PFS (months)		
	Eribulin	Dacarbazine	HR (95%CI)	Eribulin	Dacarbazine	HR (95%CI)
All LPSs (143)	15.6	8.4	0.511 (0.346–0.753)	2.9	1.7	0.521 (0.346–0.784)
Dedifferentiated[65]	18.0	8.1	0.429 (0.232–0.792)	2.0	2.1	0.691 (0.359–1.328)
Myxoid/round cell[55]	13.5	9.6	0.787 (0.416–1.491)	2.8	1.4	0.567 (0.289–1.113)
Pleomorphic[23]	22.2	6.7	0.182 (0.039–0.850)	4.4	1.4	0.337 (0.088–1.298)

Data from Demetri GD, Schöffski P, Grignani G, Blay J-Y, Maki RG, Van Tine BA, et al. Journal of Clinical Oncology. 2017 (30).

Administration (FDA) approval in unresectable/metastatic LPS patients who have received prior anthracycline-based therapy on January 28, 2016.[31]

Side effects of eribulin in LPS patients are consistent with previous studies and include alopecia, fatigue, neutropenia, and nausea.[30] In the randomized phase 3 study comparing eribulin and dacarbazine, grade 3 and greater adverse events were found in 62.9% of LPS patients in the eribulin arm, leading to drug interruption in 30%, dose reduction in 21.4%, and drug withdrawal in 7.1%. The recommended starting dose of eribulin is 1.4 mg/m^2 on days 1 and 8 of a 21-day cycle, with 2 possible dose reductions to 1.1 mg/m^2 and 0.7 mg/m^2, if needed.

SELINEXOR IN DDLS

Selinexor is a selective inhibitor of XPO1, a nuclear exportin, which can recognize nuclear export signal and export many tumor suppressor proteins including p53 and p21.[32] A preclinical study in LPS cell lines with selinexor demonstrated increasing p53 and p21 expression at the protein level leading to cell cycle arrest and apoptosis.[33] Selinexor exhibited promising activity in phase 1B study in sarcoma with response noted in the DDLPS subtype. This led to the first of its kind, phase 3 randomized double-blinded placebo-controlled crossover phase 2/3 study of selinexor in advanced unresectable DDLPS (SEAL) who were progressing and were previously treated with 1 or more systemic therapies.[34] The study met its primary end point of improved PFS of selinexor compared with placebo but the incremental numerical benefit was low (2.83 mo vs 2.07 mo, HR 0.70 [95% CI 0.52–0.95], P-value of .0228). The median OS in the selinexor arm was not significantly different from placebo but 58% of patients from the placebo crossed over to the selinexor arm. Although some DDLPS patients derived benefit, this drug is not yet approved for use in this subtype of LPS.

The recommended phase 2 dose of selinexor was 35 mg/m^2 or 60 mg fixed dose given orally twice a week, a day apart, with dose-limiting toxicities (DLTs) of grade 3 fatigue, nausea and vomiting, hyponatremia, acute cerebellar syndrome, and anorexia.[35] In the phase 2/3 study in DDLPS, the fixed dose of selinexor (60 mg twice a week, one day apart) was administered, with dose reductions allowed for toxicity. Side effects including nausea, anorexia, and fatigue of any grade were found in more than half of the patients.[34] Grades 3 to 4 adverse events noted were hyponatremia (15%), anemia (15%), and thrombocytopenia (12%). No incidence of acute cerebellar syndrome was reported at this dosing. With early institution of supportive care measures for nausea and appetite loss, the drug seems to be well tolerated with evidence of improvement in quality of life as compared with placebo in DDLPS.[36]

TAZEMETOSTAT IN EPITHELIOID SARCOMA

Epithelioid sarcoma (ES) is a rare histotype of sarcoma with an incidence close to 0.5 new cases per million per year in nationwide registries.[37] Primary tumors are observed on any anatomic sites.[37] Median age at diagnosis is 40 years with an equal gender distribution. The loss of INI1/SMARCB1 is frequently observed in ES.[38,39] INI1 is a component of the SWI/SNF complex acting as a tumor suppressor. Loss of INI1, through genetic or epigenetic mechanisms, results in the oncogenic activation of enhancer of zeste (EZH)2, which trimethylates lysine 27 of histone H3.[40,41]

The treatment of ES follows the general rules of sarcoma management in localized phase.[42,43] In advanced phase, classic cytotoxic treatments or pazopanib of advanced sarcomas have a limited activity in this disease.[44–46] Tazemetostat is a selective inhibitor of EZH2, administered orally. It provided encouraging activity in a phase 1 study, including patients with advanced solid tumors with loss of INI1/SMARCB1.[47] In the phase I study, 3 patients with ES were included: 2 achieved prolonged PFS.

A recently reported phase 2 basket study reported the activity of tazemetostat in patients with solid tumors harboring these alterations. Among the 62 patients with ES were enrolled in the study, 9 (15%) had an objective response. 16 (26%) patients had disease control at 32 weeks. Median time to response was 3·9 months (Interquartile Range (IQR) 1·9–7·4). Median progression-free survival was 5.5 months (95% CI 3·4–5·9), and median overall survival was 19.0 months. The treatment was overall well tolerated with grade 3 anemia in 4 (6%) and weight loss in 2 (3%) patients.

The treatment is approved by the FDA for the treatment of ES in advanced phase since January 2020, and under evaluation by the European Medicines Agency (EMA).

NEUROTROPHIN RECEPTOR TYROSINE KINASE (NTRK) INHIBITORS FOR NTRK FUSION POSITIVE SARCOMAS

The most recent WHO classification of soft tissue and bone neoplasms identifies the novel identity of NTRK-fusion-positive neoplasms.[48] The screening for translocation is not consistently conducted in expert sarcoma pathology laboratories. As a consequence, the exact incidence of this heterogenous entity is not precisely known. The reported incidence of infantile fibrosarcoma, fibrosarcoma, and lipofibromatosis, 3 entities where the prevalence of NTRK-fusion is high, is 0.04, 0.03, 0.1/10e6/year.[37] In an unpublished study screening 500 consecutive sarcomas with complex genomics, the exact incidence of NTRK-fusion was 1% (5/500) (personal results unreported). In GIST without canonical mutations of KIT or PDGFRA, NTRK fusions are also very rare.

Clinical trials have been published since 2017, demonstrating a high level of response rate with larotectinib and entrectinib in patients with any histologic subtypes, creating the concept of histoagnostic therapies of advanced cancers with different histologies but sharing similar actionable molecular alterations. In these studies, sarcomas represent close to 20% of included patients.[49–52] Infantile fibrosarcoma in relapse represent close to 40% of sarcomas treated with NTRK inhibitors in these trials. A specific analysis of the subgroup of patients with sarcoma treated with larotrectinib or entrectinib was presented at Connective Tissue Oncology Society (CTOS) 2019. With larotrectinib, this was a series of 71 patients, adults (n = 23, 32%) and children, all pretreated, with 29 infantile fibrosarcoma (41%), 4 GIST (6%), 2 bone sarcoma (3%), and 36 (51%) patients with more than 10 different other histologic types of sarcomas. Most rearrangements were on NTRK3 (n = 42, 59%) followed by NTRK1 (n = 26, 37%), and NTRK2 (n = 3, 5%). There were 16 (23%) CR, 45 (64%) partial responses (PR), 6 (9%) stable disease (SD), and 2 (3%) progressive disease (PD) as best response. Median duration of response was not reached. A total of 70% were still responding at the median follow-up of 16 months. Median PFS and OS were 28 and 44 months, respectively. Grade 3 and 4 side effects were limited.

With entrectinib, the series reported in CTOS 2019 included 13 adult patients, all pretreated, with 1 GIST (8%), 1 bone chondrosarcoma (8%), and 11 (84%) different other histologic subtypes of STS. Most rearrangements were on NTRK3 (n = 8, 60%) followed by NTRK1 (n = 5, 40%). There were 6 (48%) PR, 4 (32%) SD and 1 (8%) PD as best response. Median duration of response was 10 months. Median PFS and OS were 11 and 17 months, respectively. Grade 3 and 4 side effects were limited.

Given the rarity and heterogeneity of these tumors, it is considered very unlikely to be able to construct randomized clinical trials. For this reason, comparing patients as his/her own control to comparing previous PFS to PFS under NTRKi has been proposed by several studies.[53]

Larotrectinib was approved by the FDA for the treatment of tumors in advanced phase with translocation involving NTRK since November 26, 2018 and by the EMA since September 09, 2019. Entrectinib was approved by the FDA for the treatment of tumors in advanced phase with translocation involving NTRK since August 19, 2019 and by the EMA since July 31, 2020.

SORAFENIB AND NIROGACESTAT IN DESMOID TUMORS

Desmoid tumors (aka aggressive fibromatosis) are locally aggressive connective tissue tumors with an incidence close to 5/1000000/y, an F/M ratio close to 2, and a median age of diagnosis of 40 (ranging from pediatric to geriatric ages) in nationwide series.[37] Primary sites affected by these tumors include all anatomic sites, abdominal or trunk wall being common (>50%) and mesenteric sites being the most frequently life threatening although the overall mortality of these tumors remain rare. Desmoid tumors can be sporadic and harbor most often *CTNNB1* mutations in this case. About 10% of desmoid tumors are associated with germline *APC* mutations within the Gardner syndrome. The later are often intra-abdominal or thoracic and more frequently life threatening.

Symptoms vary considerably. Sometimes an asymptomatic mass, desmoid tumors can be painful, functionally impairing, compressive (occlusion, vital organs). Complications in young adults also include long-term opioid use, anxiety, depression, and interruption of education and employment.

Local treatments include watchful waiting, radiotherapy, and cryoablation, less frequently surgical removal.[54] A large number of agents have been reported to have activity against desmoid tumors, from non-steroidal anti-inflammatory drugs (NSAIDS), antiestrogens, cytotoxic chemotherapy, TKIs most often in uncontrolled studies resulting in difficulties in interpretation.[54]

Sorafenib

Gounder and colleagues reported recently an important randomized clinical trial comparing sorafenib 800 mg/d versus placebo in patients with desmoid tumors not amenable to a local treatment. A total of 87 patients were randomized, the 2-year PFS rate was 81% in the sorafenib group and 36% in the placebo group (hazard ratio 0.13; $P < .001$). Before crossover, the ORR was 33% in the sorafenib group and 20% in the placebo group demonstrating in a rigorous manner the unpredictable natural history of this disease.[55] The median time to response was 9.6 months in the sorafenib and 13.3 months in the placebo groups, respectively. A similar magnitude of activity was observed with pazopanib 800 mg/d in a randomized trial conducted against the methotrexate vinblastine (MV) combination (6-month PFS for pazopanib 83% vs 45% for MV), confirming the activity of this class of antiangiogenic agents in this rare entity.[56] Sorafenib is available in the United States since 2005.

Nirogacestat

Gamma secretase inhibitor nirogacestat given at a dose of 150 mg twice a day was reported in 2017 to be active in a limited series of patients with pretreated desmoid tumors. Seventeen patients were included in a phase II study, following a phase I study that had reported 5 out of 7 responses in desmoid tumors.[56] In this study, 5 of 17 patients (29%) responded to treatment, and 5 achieved SD. Median PFS is not reported, in the first publication, but was mentioned as not reached in a subsequent report.[57] All patient achieved a symptom improvement in these series.[57]

The FDA granted nirogacestat, with a breakthrough therapy designation for the treatment of adult patients with progressive, unresectable, recurrent, or refractory desmoid tumors, or deep fibromatosis in 2021.

PEXIDATINIB IN GIANT CELL TUMOR OF THE SOFT PARTS

Giant cell tumor of the soft parts (aka diffuse tenosynovial giant cell tumors [TGCT], pigmented villonodular synovitis [PVNS]) is a locally aggressive connective tissue tumor of the joints, affecting mostly young adults, with a predominance on the knee and ankle.[58,59] These tumors are characterized by a t(1;2) translocation in a minority of cells present in the tumor, resulting in a fusion gene colony-stimulating factor-1/collagen type VI alpha-3 (*CSF1/COL6A3*) whose protein product induces tumor growth and giant cell infiltrates.[60] Surgical resection is the standard treatment in first-line but local relapses are frequent. Clinical symptoms involve swelling, pain, and functional impairment that are characteristic of the disease in particular at relapse.[58,59] Surgery at relapse is rarely curative with less than 20% of patients free of relapse at 5 years.[58] Amputations may be required only very rarely in very large tumors. dTGCT are rarely multifocal and metastasize even more rarely.[58]

Before CSF1R antagonists, either TKIs or antibodies, the medical treatments for relapsing and inoperable tumors had limited efficacy.[58–61] The rationale for the use of CSF1R antagonists is based of the presence of the fusion gene involving CSF1, considered to be a driver of the tumor. CSF1R inhibitors, TKI or Ab, yielded tumor shrinkage and symptom relief in patients with inoperable diffuse type TCGT.[61–67] Imatinib exerts CSF1R inhibitory activity and was first reported as active in TGCT/PVNS in a case report in 2008.[61,62] The clinical efficacy of TKIs blocking CSF1R (imatinib, nilotinib, pexidartinib) and antibodies against CSF1R (emactuzumab, cabiralizumab) was confirmed after in retrospective studies and prospective clinical studies for imatinib,[62] emactuzumab,[63] nilotinib,[64] and pexidatinib.[65] Tap and colleagues reported in 2019 on the first randomized phase III study comparing placebo with pexidartinib orally 400 mg BID.[66] In this study involving 120 patients, tumor response was significantly higher (24/61, 39%) with pexidartinib versus placebo (0/59, 0%). Patient reported outcome and function improved during treatment with pexidartinib as compared with placebo.[66] Pexidartinib was approved for the treatment of dTGCT by the FDA on August 2, 2019 and is the only registered treatment of this disease.

MAMMALIAN TARGET OF RAPAMYCIN (mTOR) INHIBITORS IN PERIVASCULAR EPITHELIOID CELL TUMORS

Perivascular epithelioid cell tumors (PEComas) are rare mesenchymal neoplasms, mostly benign[37,68–70] although malignant PEComas exist and may present as locally advanced and/or metastatic diseases.[68–71] Their incidence in the nationwide NETSARC series is 0.3/1,000,000 per year.[37] The median age at diagnosis was found to be 55, with 3.7 F/M ratio and a predominance of visceral sites (especially renal, uterine, and gastrointestinal).[37] PEComas often show loss-of-function mutations of tuberous sclerosis complex (TSC)1 or TSC2 and activation of mammalian target of rapamycin complex (mTORC)1 with phosphorylation of p70S6K and ribosomal protein S6.[72,73]

Malignant PEComa in advanced phase are treated with cytotoxic chemotherapy regimens used for sarcomas with limited response rates and PFS in retrospective series.[73]A fraction of patients with PEComas benefited from treatment with mTORC1 inhibitors (sirolimus, everolimus, temsirolimus) in retrospective analyses.[72–74] Sanfilippo and colleagues reported on a 41% ORR with mTORC1 treatment, with a median PFS of 9 months, superior to that achieved with anthracyclins, gemcitabine, or pazopanib in this retrospective series of 40 patients.[73]

This prompted prospective studies of a new generation of mTORC1 inhibitors.[75] Nab-sirolimus was given at a dose of 100 mg/m^2 IV weekly for 2 weeks every 3 weeks in a phase II study involving 34 patients. The ORR was 39% (12 of 31) with 1 CR (3%) and 36% PR, 16 (52%) SD with 7 of 12 responders still treated at a median follow-up of 2.5 years, and a median PFS of 10 months and a median OS of 40 months. 8 of 9 (89%) patient with a documented TSC2 mutation were responders versus 2 of 16 (13%) without TSC2 mutation. Nab-sirolimus was approved for the treatment of advanced PEComas by the FDA on November 22, 2021 and is the only registered treatment of this disease.

POTENTIAL OPTIONS IN THE NEAR FUTURE
Cyclin-dependent kinase (CDK) 4/6 Inhibitors in Liposarcoma

Supernumerary ring chromosomes formed by a segment of chromosome 12q13-15 are found in both WDLPS and DDLPS resulting in multiple gene amplifications, with MDM2 (Mouse double minute 2) and CDK4 being the most frequent genes amplified (100% and 90%, respectively).[76] MDM2 has a major function in the regulation of p53, an important tumor suppressor involved in growth arrest, senescence, and apoptosis in response to cellular damage. MDM2 regulates p53 at both the mRNA and protein level by blocking the transactivation domain and inducing degradation via E3-ubiquitin ligase activity.[77] CDK4/CDK6, together with CDK2, play a crucial role in cell cycle progression from G1 to S phase by Rb1 phosphorylation and activation of E2F.[78]

Palbociclib, a potent oral CDK4/6 inhibitor has demonstrated activity in CDK4-amplified LPS cell lines and xenografts. Data from a phase 1 study of the drug showed 2 patients with prolonged stable disease for several years prompting a phase 2 study with palbociclib 200 mg once daily for 14 out of 21 days.[79] The primary end point was met with a 12-week PFS of 66% (90% CI, 51%−100%) and a median PFS of 18 weeks. A subsequent phase 2 trial was conducted with the dose of 125 mg daily, 21 days out of a 28 day-cycle, the same dose approved in breast cancer, and revealed a compatible median PFS of 17.9 weeks (2-sided 95% CI: 11.9–24.0 weeks) with less incidence of grade 3 to 4 neutropenia (33%) and no neutropenic fever events.[80]

Another active CDK4/6 inhibitor evaluated in LPS is abemaciclib. A phase 2 study done in DDLS revealed PFS at 12 weeks of 76% (95% CI 57%–90%), median PFS of 30.4 weeks (95% CI 28.9-NE) and ORR of 3.45% (1 partial response from 29 patients).[81]

Currently, a CDK4 inhibitor is not approved in LPS treatment but palbociclib, is included as a valid category 2A option in the National Comprehensive Cancer Network (NCCN) guidelines, and there is an ongoing randomized placebo controlled study with abemaciclib in DDLPS (NCT04967521).[82]

T-cell Therapy in Synovial Sarcoma and MRCLS

Synovial sarcoma and MRCLS are rare mesenchymal tumors responsible for around 5% to 10% of STS cases.[83] Chromosomal translocation t(X;18) (p11.2;q11.2) producing SS18-SSX fusion protein is pathognomonic of synovial sarcoma and the translocation t(12;16) (q13;p11) producing fusion protein FUS-DDIT3 is pathognomonic of MRCLS.[84–86] Both these types of sarcoma are relatively more chemosensitive than other types of STS.

Synovial sarcomas and MRCLS have low mutation burden and poor response to checkpoint blockade.[87] However, 70% to 80% of these tumors express New York esophageal squamous cell carcinoma 1 (NY-ESO-1), a well-known cancer-testis antigen (CTA), which belongs to a group of antigens that have expression restricted to certain cancers and the testis.[88,89] Although several malignancies overexpress NY-ESO-1, only MRCLS and synovial sarcoma have homogenous expression with synovial sarcoma positive in both biphasic and monophasic variants.[90] This brought about studies focused on targeting this protein through cellular immune therapy.

Adoptive cell therapy (ACT) are ways to increase immune recognition of tumors by infusing tumor cell-specific T-cells. ACT can be approached in 3 different ways; one involves harvesting, expanding, and reinfusing tumor-infiltrating lymphocytes, another uses T cell receptor (TCR) recognition of intracellular tumor proteins presented on the cell surface through major histocompatibility complex (MHC)-1, and finally, chimeric antigen receptor-modified T cells that recognize and attack tumor-cell surface receptors.[91]

A promising pilot study using autologous TCR-transduced T cells following a lympho-depleting preparative chemotherapy in human leukocyte antigen (HLA)-A*0201 (MHC class-I) patients with NY-ESO-1 positive metastatic synovial sarcoma or melanoma refractory to standard treatment was first published in 2015.[92] The study demonstrated an ORR of 61% (11/18) in synovial sarcoma patients with response lasting 3 to 18 months. Significant transient neutropenia and thrombocytopenia occurred in 100% with 1 treatment-related death. In 2018, an affinity-enhanced TCR recognizing the NY-ESO-1 derived peptide SLLMWITQC (NY-ESO-1^{c259} T cells) was tested in advanced synovial sarcoma without the use of IL-2 and was noted to be safe and feasible with a 50% (6/12) ORR.[93] This study detected circulating NY-ESO-1^{c259} T cells in all responders for at least 6 months. Although side effects from IL-2 were eliminated, adverse events caused by lympho-depleting chemotherapy were noted, with grade $\geq$3 lymphopenia (100%), neutropenia (83%), anemia (83%), thrombocytopenia (67%), and febrile neutropenia (17%). Further studies and evaluation of long-term outcome is ongoing for NY-ESO-1^{c259} T cells. In addition, an ongoing phase 2 study (NCT04044768) of afamitresgene autoleucel (previously ADP-A2M4) targeting an alternate CTA, melanoma antigen gene (MAGE) A4, with high expression in synovial sarcoma and MRCLS is showing promising results as well.

CHECKPOINT INHIBITORS IN ALVEOLAR SOFT PARTS SARCOMA

Immune-checkpoint inhibitors (CPI) have been evaluated in a few sarcoma trials. Pembrolizumab, an anti-PD-1 antibody, resulted in an ORR of 18% (7/40) in bone and STS in a phase 2 trial.[87] Among STS patients, response was noted in undifferentiated pleomorphic sarcoma (UPS) (40%), DDLS (20%), and synovial sarcoma (10%). With an expansion of the cohorts, the reported ORR dropped but remained encouraging for further study. In another study, nivolumab monotherapy resulted in an ORR of 5% (3/38) with response in alveolar soft part sarcoma (ASPS), non-uterine LMS, and an unspecified sarcoma.[94]

An open-label multicenter, phase 2 study of pembrolizumab in combination with metronomic cyclophosphamide demonstrated limited activity with an ORR of 6% in STS including LMS, UPS, other sarcomas, and GIST.[95] A combination of ipilimumab/nivolumab demonstrated an ORR of 16% (6/41) with response noted in uterine LMS, non-uterine LMS, myxofibrosarcoma, UPS, and angiosarcoma.[94] Median PFS and OS was 4.1 months and 14.3 months, respectively. Currently, the role of CPI in STS is being investigated, to try and improve outcomes, with better subtype selection, or alternate CPI combinations.

Among STS, ASPS has emerged with the highest response to anti-PD-1/PD-L1 therapy. A retrospective review of 50 advanced sarcoma patients treated with CPI revealed an ORR of 4% (2/50), whereas it was 50% among ASPS patients (2/4), with the remaining 2/4 having stable disease.[96] A phase 2 combination study of axitinib plus pembrolizumab in STS, again revealed a higher ORR in ASPS patients of 54.5% (6/11), and a 3-month PFS of 72.7%.[97] Similarly, the ASPS cohort in a phase 2 study of durvalumab and tremelimumab in various sarcoma subtypes, experienced an ORR of 50% (5/10).[98] A single-arm multicenter phase 2 study testing atezolizumab in advanced ASPS patients is now ongoing, with interim data reporting an ORR of 37.2% (16/43) with 1 CR.[99] NCCN guidelines recommend pembrolizumab as a category 2A in ASPS[82]

The last 5 years has seen an exponential increase in the number of biomarker-specific or sarcoma subtype-specific clinical trials compared with prior years. This has led to a larger number of drugs being available for certain sarcomas and leading to incremental improvements in survival. In general, the benefit seen with biomarker-targeted therapies is of higher magnitude than seen in unselected sarcoma patients. We hope this pace of development continues, to further bridge the gap of the severe unmet need in sarcoma patients. We need less toxic and more effective systemic therapies for more than 50 different sarcoma subtypes.

CONFLICT OF INTEREST (J.-Y. BLAY, M. BRAHMI, A. DUFRESNE)

Research support and honoraria from Roche, Bayer, Epizyme, Daiichi Sankyo. Conflict of Interest (N. Somaiah): Research Support and honoraria from Boehringer Ingelheim, Deciphera, Ascentage, AstraZeneca, Epizyme, and Aadi Biosciences.

ACKNOWLEDGMENTS

(J.-Y. Blay, M. Brahmi, A. Dufresne): NetSARC+ (INCA & DGOS) & LYRICAN (INCA-DGOS-INSERM 12563), and EURACAN (EC 739521). We thank Francoise Ducimetiere, and Claire Chemin for expert support in NETSARC.

REFERENCES

1. Kelly CM, Gutierrez Sainz L, Chi P. The management of metastatic GIST: current standard and investigational therapeutics. J Hematol Oncol 2021;14(1):2.

2. Shetty N, Sirohi B, Shrikhande SV. Molecular target therapy for gastrointestinal stromal tumors. Translational Gastrointest Cancer 2015;4(3):207–18.

3. Farag S, Smith MJ, Fotiadis N, et al. Revolutions in treatment options in gastrointestinal stromal tumours (GISTs): the latest updates. Curr Treat Options Oncol 2020;21(7):55.

4. Nannini M, Tarantino G, Indio V, et al. Molecular modelling evaluation of exon 18 His845_Asn848delinsPro PDGFRalpha mutation in a metastatic GIST patient responding to imatinib. Sci Rep 2019;9(1):2172.

5. Mazzocca A, Napolitano A, Silletta M, et al. New frontiers in the medical management of gastrointestinal stromal tumours. Ther Adv Med Oncol 2019;11. 1758835919841946.

6. Napolitano A, Vincenzi B. Secondary KIT mutations: the GIST of drug resistance and sensitivity. Br J Cancer 2019;120(6):577–8.

7. Bauer S, George S, von Mehren M, et al. Early and next-generation KIT/PDGFRA kinase inhibitors and the future of treatment for advanced gastrointestinal stromal tumor. Front Oncol 2021;11:672500.

8. Smith BD, Kaufman MD, Lu WP, et al. Ripretinib (DCC-2618) is a switch control kinase inhibitor of a broad spectrum of oncogenic and drug-resistant KIT and PDGFRA Variants. Cancer Cell 2019;35(5):738–751 e9.

9. George S, Heinrich M, Chi P, et al. Initial results of phase I study of DCC-2618, a broad-spectrum KIT and PDGFRa inhibitor, in patients (pts) with gastrointestinal stromal tumor (GIST) by number of prior regimens. Ann Oncol 2018;29:viii576–7.

10. Blay J-Y, Serrano C, Heinrich MC, et al. Ripretinib in patients with advanced gastrointestinal stromal tumours (INVICTUS): a double-blind, randomised, placebo-controlled, phase 3 trial. Lancet Oncol 2020;21(7):923–34.

11. Zalcberg JR. Ripretinib for the treatment of advanced gastrointestinal stromal tumor. Therap Adv Gastroenterol 2021;14. 17562848211008177.

12. George S, Chi P, Heinrich MC, et al. Ripretinib intrapatient dose escalation after disease progression provides clinically meaningful outcomes in advanced gastrointestinal stromal tumour. Eur J Cancer 2021;155:236–44.

13. News in Brief in Cancer Discovery: Testing Ripretinib against Sunitinib in GIST. Cancer Discov. 2022 Mar 1;12(3):591-592. doi: 10.1158/2159-8290.CD-NB2022-0004. PMID: 35086925.

14. Evans EK., Gardino AK., Kim JL., et al.,. A precision therapy against cancers driven by *KIT/PDGFRA* mutations. Sci Transl Med. 2017 Nov 1;9(414):eaao1690. doi: 10.1126/scitranslmed.aao1690. PMID: 29093181.

15. Gebreyohannes YK, Wozniak A, Zhai ME, et al. Robust activity of avapritinib, potent and highly selective inhibitor of mutated KIT, in patient-derived xenograft models of gastrointestinal stromal tumors. Clin Cancer Res 2019;25(2):609–18.

16. Heinrich MC, Jones RL, von Mehren M, et al. Avapritinib in advanced PDGFRA D842V-mutant gastrointestinal stromal tumour (NAVIGATOR): a multicentre, open-label, phase 1 trial. Lancet Oncol 2020;21(7):935–46.

17. Heinrich MC, Jones RL, von Mehren M, et al. Clinical activity of avapritinib in ≥ fourth-line (4L+) and PDGFRA Exon 18 gastrointestinal stromal tumors (GIST). J Clin Oncol 2019;37(15_suppl):11022.

18. George S, Jones RL, Bauer S, et al. Avapritinib in patients with advanced gastrointestinal stromal tumors following at least three prior lines of therapy. Oncologist 2021;26(4):e639–49.

19. Heinrich M vMM, Jones RL. Avapritinib is highly active and well-tolerated in patients (pts) with advanced GIST driven by diverse variety of oncogenic mutations in KIT and PDGFRA. Presented at the Connective Tissue Oncology Society Annual meeting (CTOS), Nov 14-17th 2018, Rome, Italy

20. Ghadimi MP, Liu P, Peng T, et al. Pleomorphic liposarcoma: clinical observations and molecular variables. Cancer 2011;117(23):5359–69.

21. Judson I, Verweij J, Gelderblom H, et al. Doxorubicin alone versus intensified doxorubicin plus ifosfamide for first-line treatment of advanced or metastatic soft-tissue sarcoma: a randomised controlled phase 3 trial. Lancet Oncol 2014; 15(4):415–23.

22. Italiano A, Toulmonde M, Cioffi A, et al. Advanced well-differentiated/dedifferentiated liposarcomas: role of chemotherapy and survival. Ann Oncol 2012;23(6):1601–7.

23. Livingston JA, Bugano D, Barbo A, et al. Role of chemotherapy in dedifferentiated liposarcoma of the retroperitoneum: defining the benefit and challenges of the standard. Scientific Rep 2017;7(1):11836.

24. Thirasastr P AB, Lin H, Roland C, Feig B, Keung E et al. Efficacy of Gemcitabine-Docetaxel in Dedifferentiated Liposarcoma. presented at the Connective Tissue Oncology Society (CTOS) Annual Virtual Meeting, Nov 16-19th 2021.

25. Maki RG, Wathen Jk, Fau-Patel SR, et al. Randomized phase II study of gemcitabine and docetaxel compared with gemcitabine alone in patients with metastatic soft tissue sarcomas: results of sarcoma alliance for research through collaboration study 002 [corrected]. J Clin Oncol 2007;25:1527–7755 (Electronic)).

26. Demetri GD, von Mehren M, Jones RL, et al. Efficacy and safety of trabectedin or dacarbazine for metastatic liposarcoma or leiomyosarcoma after failure of conventional chemotherapy: results of a phase III randomized multicenter clinical trial. J Clin Oncol 2016;34(8):786–93.

27. Swami U, Chaudhary I, Ghalib MH, et al. Eribulin – a review of preclinical and clinical studies. Crit Rev Oncol Hematol 2012;81(2):163–84.

28. Schöffski P, Ray-Coquard IL, Cioffi A, et al. Activity of eribulin mesylate in patients with soft-tissue sarcoma: a phase 2 study in four independent histological subtypes. Lancet Oncol 2011;12(11):1045–52.

29. Schöffski P, Chawla S, Maki RG, et al. Eribulin versus dacarbazine in previously treated patients with advanced liposarcoma or leiomyosarcoma: a randomised, open-label, multicentre, phase 3 trial. Lancet 2016;387(10028):1629–37.

30. Demetri GD, Schöffski P, Grignani G, et al. Activity of eribulin in patients with advanced liposarcoma demonstrated in a subgroup analysis from a randomized phase III Study of Eribulin Versus Dacarbazine. J Clin Oncol 2017;35(30):3433–9.

31. Osgood CL, Chuk MK, Theoret MR, et al. FDA approval summary: eribulin for patients with unresectable or metastatic liposarcoma who have received a prior anthracycline-containing regimen. Clin Cancer Res 2017;23:1557–3265 (Electronic)).

32. Kau TR, Way JC, Silver PA. Nuclear transport and cancer: from mechanism to intervention. Nat Rev Cancer 2004;4(2):106–17.

33. Garg M, Kanojia D, Mayakonda A, et al. Molecular mechanism and therapeutic implications of selinexor (KPT-330) in liposarcoma. Oncotarget 2017;8(5):7521–32.

34. Gounder MRA, Somaiah N, et al. A phase 2/3, randomized, double blind, crossover, study of selinexor versus placebo in advanced unresectable dedifferentiated liposarcoma. Presented at the Connective Tissue Oncology Society (CTOS) Annual Virtual Meeting, Nov 18-21st 2020. Abstract 20.

35. Abdul Razak AR, Mau-Soerensen M, Gabrail NY, et al. First-in-class, first-in-human phase i study of selinexor, a selective inhibitor of nuclear export, in patients with advanced solid tumors. J Clin Oncol 2016;34(34):4142–50.

36. Gounder M, Abdul Razak AR, Gilligan AM, et al. Health-related quality of life and pain with selinexor in patients with advanced dedifferentiated liposarcoma. Future Oncol 2021;17(22):2923–39.

37. de Pinieux G, Karanian M, Le Loarer F, et al. Nationwide incidence of sarcomas and connective tissue tumors of intermediate malignancy over four years using an expert pathology review network. PLoS One 1932;2021:6203 (Electronic)).

38. Modena P, Lualdi E, Facchinetti F, et al. SMARCB1/INI1 tumor suppressor gene is frequently inactivated in epithelioid sarcomas. Cancer Res 2005;65(10):4012–9 (0008-5472 (Print)).

39. Chbani L, Guillou L, Terrier P, et al. Epithelioid sarcoma: a clinicopathologic and immunohistochemical analysis of 106 cases from the French sarcoma group. Am J Clin Pathol 2009;131(2):222–7.

40. Phelan ML, Sif S, Narlikar GJ, et al. Reconstitution of a core chromatin remodeling complex from SWI/SNF subunits. Mol Cell 1999;3(2):247–53.

41. Wilson BG, Wang X, Shen X, et al. Epigenetic antagonism between polycomb and SWI/SNF complexes during oncogenic transformation. Cancer Cell 2010;1878–3686 (Electronic)).

42. Blay JY, Hindi N, Bollard J, et al. SELNET clinical practice guidelines for soft tissue sarcoma and GIST. Cancer Treat Rev 2022;102(1532-1967):102312 (Electronic)).

43. von Mehren M, Kane JM, Bui MM, et al. NCCN Guidelines Insights: Soft Tissue Sarcoma, Version 1.2021. J Natl Compr Canc Netw 2020;18(12):1604–12.

44. Frezza AM, Jones RL, Lo Vullo S, et al. Anthracycline, Gemcitabine, and Pazopanib in Epithelioid Sarcoma: A Multi-institutional Case Series. JAMA Oncol 2018; 4(9):e180219.

45. Touati N, Schoffski P, Litiere S, et al. European Organisation for Research and Treatment of Cancer Soft Tissue and Bone Sarcoma Group Experience with Advanced/Metastatic Epithelioid Sarcoma Patients Treated in Prospective Trials: Clinical Profile and Response to Systemic Therapy. Clin Oncol (R Coll Radiol) 2018;30(7):448–54.

46. Pink D, Richter S, Gerdes S, et al. Gemcitabine and docetaxel for epithelioid sarcoma: results from a retrospective, multi-institutional analysis. Oncology 2014; 87(2):95–103.

47. Italiano A, Soria JC, Toulmonde M, et al. Tazemetostat, an EZH2 inhibitor, in relapsed or refractory B-cell non-Hodgkin lymphoma and advanced solid tumours: a first-in-human, open-label, phase 1 study. Lancet Oncol 2018;19(5):649–59.

48. Davis JL, Al-Ibraheemi A, Rudzinski ER, et al. Mesenchymal neoplasms with NTRK and other kinase gene alterations. Histopathology 2022;80(1):4–18.

49. Drilon A, Siena S, Ou SI, et al. Safety and Antitumor Activity of the Multitargeted Pan-TRK, ROS1, and ALK Inhibitor Entrectinib: Combined Results from Two Phase I Trials (ALKA-372-001 and STARTRK-1). Cancer Discov 2017;7(4):400–9.

50. Laetsch TW, DuBois SG, Mascarenhas L, et al. Larotrectinib for paediatric solid tumours harbouring NTRK gene fusions: phase 1 results from a multicentre, open-label, phase 1/2 study. Lancet Oncol 2018;19(5):705–14.

51. Hong DS, DuBois SG, Kummar S, et al. Larotrectinib in patients with TRK fusion-positive solid tumours: a pooled analysis of three phase 1/2 clinical trials. Lancet Oncol 2020;21(4):531–40.

52. Paz-Ares L, Barlesi F, Siena S, et al. Patient-reported outcomes from STARTRK-2: a global phase II basket study of entrectinib for ROS1 fusion-positive non-small-cell lung cancer and NTRK fusion-positive solid tumours. ESMO Open 2021;6(3): 100113.

53. Krebs MG, Blay JY, Le Tourneau C, et al. Intrapatient comparisons of efficacy in a single-arm trial of entrectinib in tumour-agnostic indications. ESMO Open 2021; 6(2):100072 (2059-7029 (Electronic)).

54. Desmoid Tumor Working G. The management of desmoid tumours: A joint global consensus-based guideline approach for adult and paediatric patients. Eur J Cancer 2020;127:96–107 (1879-0852(Electronic)).

55. Gounder MM, Mahoney MR, Van Tine BA, et al. Sorafenib for Advanced and Refractory Desmoid Tumors. N Engl J Med 2018;379(25):2417–28.

56. Toulmonde M, Pulido M, Ray-Coquard I, et al. Pazopanib or methotrexate-vinblastine combination chemotherapy in adult patients with progressive desmoid tumours (DESMOPAZ): a non-comparative, randomised, open-label, multicentre, phase 2 study. Lancet Oncol 2019;20(9):1263–72.

57. Villalobos VM, Hall F, Jimeno A, et al. Long-Term Follow-Up of Desmoid Fibromatosis Treated with PF-03084014, an Oral Gamma Secretase Inhibitor. Ann Surg Oncol 2018;25(3):768–75.

58. Palmerini E, Staals EL, Maki RG, et al. Tenosynovial giant cell tumour/pigmented villonodular synovitis: outcome of 294 patients before the era of kinase inhibitors. Eur J Cancer 2015;51(2):210–7 (1879-0852 (Electronic)).

59. Mastboom MJL, Palmerini E, Verspoor FGM, et al. Surgical outcomes of patients with diffuse-type tenosynovial giant-cell tumours: an international, retrospective, cohort study. Lancet Oncol 2019;20(6):877–86.

60. West RB, Rubin BP, Miller MA, et al. A landscape effect in tenosynovial giant-cell tumor from activation of CSF1 expression by a translocation in a minority of tumor cells. Proc Natl Acad Sci U S A 2006;103(3):690–5.

61. Blay JY, Sayadi H, Thiesse P, Thiesse P, et al. Complete response to imatinib in relapsing pigmented villonodular synovitis/tenosynovial giant cell tumor (PVNS/TGCT). Ann Oncol 2008;19(4):821–2 (1569-8041 (Electronic)).

62. Cassier PA, Gelderblom H, Stacchiotti S, et al. Efficacy of imatinib mesylate for the treatment of locally advanced and/or metastatic tenosynovial giant cell tumor/pigmented villonodular synovitis. Cancer 2012;118(6):1649–55 (1097-0142 (Electronic)).

63. Cassier PA, Italiano A, Gomez-Roca CA, et al. CSF1R inhibition with emactuzumab in locally advanced diffuse-type tenosynovial giant cell tumours of the soft tissue: a dose-escalation and dose-expansion phase 1 study. Lancet Oncol 2015;16(8):949–56.

64. Gelderblom H, Cropet C, Chevreau C, et al. Nilotinib in locally advanced pigmented villonodular synovitis: a multicentre, open-label, single-arm, phase 2 trial. Lancet Oncol 2018;19(5):639–48.

65. Tap WD, Wainberg ZA, Anthony SP, et al. Structure-Guided Blockade of CSF1R Kinase in Tenosynovial Giant-Cell Tumor. N Engl J Med 2015;373(5):428–37.

66. Tap WD, Gelderblom H, Palmerini E, et al. Pexidartinib versus placebo for advanced tenosynovial giant cell tumour (ENLIVEN): a randomised phase 3 trial. Lancet 2019;394(10197):478–87.

67. Brahmi M, Cassier P, Dufresne A, et al. Long term term follow-up of tyrosine kinase inhibitors treatments in inoperable or relapsing diffuse type tenosynovial giant cell tumors (dTGCT). PLoS One 2020;15(5):e0233046.

68. Doyle LA, AP, Hornick JL. PEComa. In: WHO classification of tumors editorial board. Soft tissue and bone tumours. Lyon (France): International Agency for Research on Cancer; 2020. p. 312–4.

69. Folpe AL, Kwiatkowski DJ. Perivascular epithelioid cell neoplasms: pathology and pathogenesis. Hum Pathol 2010;41(1):1–15.

70. Stacchiotti S, Frezza AM, Blay JY, et al. Ultra-rare sarcomas: a consensus paper from the Connective Tissue Oncology Society community of experts on the incidence threshold and the list of entities. Cancer 2021;127(16):2934–42.

71. Kenerson H, Folpe AL, Takayama TK, et al. Activation of the mTOR pathway in sporadic angiomyolipomas and other perivascular epithelioid cell neoplasms. Hum Pathol 2007;38(9):1361–71.

72. Dufresne A, Brahmi M, Karanian M, et al. Using biology to guide the treatment of sarcomas and aggressive connective-tissue tumours. Nat Rev Clin Oncol 2018; 15(7):443–58 (1759-4782 (Electronic)).

73. Sanfilippo R, Jones RL, Blay JY, et al. Role of Chemotherapy, VEGFR Inhibitors, and mTOR Inhibitors in Advanced Perivascular Epithelioid Cell Tumors (PEComas). Clin Cancer Res 2019;25(17):5295–300.

74. Wagner AJ, Malinowska-Kolodziej I, Morgan JA, et al. Clinical activity of mTOR inhibition with sirolimus in malignant perivascular epithelioid cell tumors: targeting the pathogenic activation of mTORC1 in tumors. J Clin Oncol 2010;28(5):835–40.

75. Wagner AJ, Ravi V, Riedel RF, et al. nab-Sirolimus for patients with malignant perivascular epithelioid cell tumors. J Clin Oncol 2021;39(33):3660–70.

76. Kim YJ, Kim M, Park HK, et al. Co-expression of MDM2 and CDK4 in transformed human mesenchymal stem cells causes high-grade sarcoma with a dedifferentiated liposarcoma-like morphology. Lab Invest 2019;99(9):1309–20.

77. Marine JC, Lozano G. Mdm2-mediated ubiquitylation: p53 and beyond. Cell Death Differ 2010;17(1):93–102.

78. O'Leary B, Finn RS, Turner NC. Treating cancer with selective CDK4/6 inhibitors. Nat Rev Clin Oncol 2016;13(7):417–30.

79. Dickson MA, Tap WD, Keohan ML, et al. Phase II trial of the CDK4 inhibitor PD0332991 in patients with advanced CDK4-amplified well-differentiated or dedifferentiated liposarcoma. J Clin Oncol 2013;31(16):2024–8.

80. Dickson MA, Schwartz GK, Keohan ML, et al. Progression-free survival among patients with well-differentiated or dedifferentiated liposarcoma treated with CDK4 Inhibitor Palbociclib: A Phase 2 Clinical Trial. JAMA Oncol 2016;2(7): 937–40.

81. Dickson MA, Koff A, D'Angelo SP, et al. Phase 2 study of the CDK4 inhibitor abemaciclib in dedifferentiated liposarcoma. J Clin Oncol 2019;37(15_suppl):11004.

82. von Mehren M., Kane JM., Bui MM., et al., NCCN Guidelines Insights: Soft Tissue Sarcoma, Version 1.2021. J Natl Compr Canc Netw. 2020 Dec 2;18(12):1604-1612. doi: 10.6004/jnccn.2020.0058. PMID: 33285515.

83. Gazendam AM, Popovic S, Munir S, et al. Synovial sarcoma: a clinical review. Curr Oncol 2021;28(3):1909–20.

84. Svejstrup JQ. Synovial sarcoma mechanisms: a series of unfortunate events. Cell 2013;153(1):11–2.

85. Hostein I, Menard A, Bui BN, et al. Molecular detection of the synovial sarcoma translocation t(X;18) by real-time polymerase chain reaction in paraffin-embedded material. Diagn Mol Pathol 2002;11(1):16–21.

86. Baranov E, Black MA, Fletcher CDM, et al. Nuclear expression of DDIT3 distinguishes high-grade myxoid liposarcoma from other round cell sarcomas. Mod Pathol 2021;34(7):1367–72.

87. Tawbi HA, Burgess M, Bolejack V, et al. Pembrolizumab in advanced soft-tissue sarcoma and bone sarcoma (SARC028): a multicentre, two-cohort, single-arm, open-label, phase 2 trial. Lancet Oncol 2017;18(11):1493–501.

88. Lai JP, Robbins PF, Raffeld M, et al. NY-ESO-1 expression in synovial sarcoma and other mesenchymal tumors: significance for NY-ESO-1-based targeted therapy and differential diagnosis. Mod Pathol 2012;25(6):854–8.

89. Mitchell G, Pollack SM, Wagner MJ. Targeting cancer testis antigens in synovial sarcoma. J Immunother Cancer 2021;9(6):e002072.

90. Jungbluth AA, Antonescu CR, Busam KJ, et al. Monophasic and biphasic synovial sarcomas abundantly express cancer/testis antigen NY-ESO-1 but not MAGE-A1 or CT7. Int J Cancer 2001;94(2):252–6.

91. Rohaan MW, Wilgenhof S, Haanen J. Adoptive cellular therapies: the current landscape. Virchows Arch 2019;474(4):449–61.

92. Robbins PF, Kassim SH, Tran TL, et al. A pilot trial using lymphocytes genetically engineered with an NY-ESO-1-reactive T-cell receptor: long-term follow-up and correlates with response. Clin Cancer Res 2015;21(5):1019–27.

93. D'Angelo SP, Melchiori L, Merchant MS, et al. Antitumor Activity Associated with Prolonged Persistence of Adoptively Transferred NY-ESO-1 (c259)T Cells in Synovial Sarcoma. Cancer Discov 2018;8(8):944–57.

94. D'Angelo SP, Mahoney MR, Van Tine BA, et al. Nivolumab with or without ipilimumab treatment for metastatic sarcoma (Alliance A091401): two open-label, non-comparative, randomised, phase 2 trials. Lancet Oncol 2018;19(3):416–26.

95. Toulmonde M, Penel N, Adam J, et al. Use of PD-1 Targeting, Macrophage Infiltration, and IDO Pathway Activation in Sarcomas: A Phase 2 Clinical Trial. JAMA Oncol 2018;4(1):93–7.

96. Groisberg R, Hong DS, Behrang A, et al. Characteristics and outcomes of patients with advanced sarcoma enrolled in early phase immunotherapy trials. J Immunother Cancer 2017;5(1):100.

97. Wilky BA, Trucco MM, Subhawong TK, et al. Axitinib plus pembrolizumab in patients with advanced sarcomas including alveolar soft-part sarcoma: a single-centre, single-arm, phase 2 trial. Lancet Oncol 2019;20(6):837–48.

98. Somaiah N, Conley AP, Lin HY, et al. A phase II multi-arm study of durvalumab and tremelimumab for advanced or metastatic sarcomas. J Clin Oncol 2020; 38(15_suppl):11509.

99. Naqash AR, O'Sullivan Coyne GH, Moore N, et al. Phase II study of atezolizumab in advanced alveolar soft part sarcoma (ASPS). J Clin Oncol 2021;39(15_suppl): 11519.

Immunotherapy in Sarcoma

Where Do Things Stand?

Cristiam Moreno Tellez, MD[a], Yan Leyfman, MD[b],
Sandra P. D'Angelo, MD[c], Breelyn A. Wilky, MD[a],*,
Armelle Dufresne, MD, PhD[d]

KEYWORDS

- Soft tissue sarcoma • Immune checkpoint inhibitors • Tumor microenvironment
- Tertiary lymphoid structure • Adoptive cellular therapy • Immunotherapy

KEY POINTS

- ICIs induce responses in only about 20% of unselected sarcoma patients in clinical trials.
- Efficacy signals with checkpoint blockade may be higher in alveolar soft part sarcoma , angiosarcoma, , and dLPS.
- Current trials are exploring combination therapies with checkpoint blockade to overcome immune evasion mechanisms.
- Adoptive cellular therapies are promising, but studies have been limited to SS and myxoid/round cell liposarcomas.
- Biomarkers of efficacy are under investigation and critical to improve the selection of patients for immunotherapy clinical trials.

INTRODUCTION

The development of modern immunotherapy, including immune checkpoint inhibitors (ICIs) that block PD1/PD-L1 and CTLA-4, and adoptive cellular therapies, has created an entirely new paradigm for cancer treatment, with remarkable activity in many different solid and hematologic malignancies. Sarcomas, a rare and heterogeneous group of over 150 different bone and soft tissue cancers, have long been theorized to be susceptible to immune recognition and attack. With this explosion of therapeutic opportunities, the past 5 years have seen remarkable growth in clinical trials and laboratory efforts to explore immunotherapy for bone and soft tissue sarcomas (STSs).

C. Moreno Tellez and Y. Leyfman contributed equally to this article as co-first-authors.
[a] Department of Medicine, University of Colorado School of Medicine, 12801 E 17th Avenue, Mailstop 8117, Aurora, CO 80045, USA; [b] Department of Hematology Oncology, Icahn School of Medicine at Mount Sinai, 1468 Madison Avenue, New York, NY 10029, USA; [c] Memorial Sloan Kettering Cancer Center and Weill Cornell Medical College, 300 East 66th Street, New York, NY 10065, USA; [d] Department of Medical Oncology, Centre Leon Berard, 28 rue Laennec, Lyon 69008, France
* Corresponding author.
E-mail address: breelyn.wilky@cuanschutz.edu

Surg Oncol Clin N Am 31 (2022) 381–397
https://doi.org/10.1016/j.soc.2022.03.004
1055-3207/22/© 2022 Elsevier Inc. All rights reserved.
surgonc.theclinics.com

However, early experiences with ICIs have been disappointing in trials of unselected sarcoma subtypes, with collective responses of only about 20%. Although adoptive cellular therapies targeting cancer testis antigens (CTAs) such as NY-ESO-1 and MAGE-A4 are highly promising, these strategies are limited by human leukocyte antigen (HLA) allele frequency in the general population, and only two sarcoma subtypes reliably express these targets. The majority of sarcomas are immunologically "cold" with sparse immune infiltration, which may explain the poor response to immunotherapy. The lack of immune responses may hinge on the genetic background, with sarcomas often having low tumor mutational burden (TMB) or being driven by translocations, which may limit neoantigens for exploitation of immune responses. Finally, the small sample sizes of clinical trials, and the heterogeneity of biomarker explorations in trials or in laboratory settings challenges our ability to select optimal patients for future immunotherapy clinical trials. In this review, we will discuss the current state of immunotherapy for sarcomas, highlighting notable prior investigations of immunotherapy, reviewing ongoing clinical trials, and speculating on future directions for the field.

IMMUNE CHECKPOINT INHIBITORS

Immune checkpoint proteins serve as critical regulators of immune responses, and blocking antibodies to the PD1/PD-L1 and CTLA-4 inhibitory axes are now used as monotherapy or in combinations with chemotherapies in the first or second line in more than 50 cancer types.[1] The earliest trial of ipilimumab monotherapy in synovial sarcoma (SS) patients was terminated early due to lack of response.[2] The pivotal phase 2 trial of pembrolizumab in bone and STSs showed responses in 4 of 10 patients with undifferentiated pleomorphic sarcoma (UPS) and 2 of 10 patients with dedifferentiated liposarcoma (dLPS).[3] Minimal activity was seen in SS, leiomyosarcoma (LMS), or bone sarcomas. Shortly afterward, a phase II trial of nivolumab versus ipilimumab with nivolumab in bone sarcomas and STS confirmed low responses with nivolumab alone, but 6 of 38 patients treated with combination ipilimumab/nivolumab achieved a response, including two complete responses in myxofibrosarcoma (MFS) and uterine leiomyosarcoma (uLMS).[4] Subsequent expansion cohorts in both the pembrolizumab monotherapy and ipilimumab/nivolumab studies further explored activity in UPS and dLPS, with response rates falling to approximately 23% for UPS, and 10% overall for dLPS. The combination of nivolumab with ipilimumab led to an overall response rate (ORR) of 17% and 29% in dLPS and UPS, respectively.[5,6] Additional studies have identified strong signals of activity for alveolar soft part sarcoma (ASPS) and cutaneous angiosarcomas. More than 150 patients with ASPS have been treated in clinical trials including PD1/PD-L1 antibodies, with responses ranging from 7.1% to more than 50% (**Table 1**). For angiosarcomas, multiple retrospective case reports[7–9] and genetic profiling of patients identifying frequent UV damage signatures in cutaneous subtypes[10] formed the basis for an expansion cohort in the dual anti-CTLA-4 and anti-PD1 blockade in rare tumor (DART) study run through SWOG.[11] Of 16 evaluable patients, the ORR was 25%; however, three of five patients with primary cutaneous scalp/face angiosarcoma attained a confirmed response, with 6-month progression-free survival (PFS) rate of 38%.

Apart from the activity in ASPS, angiosarcoma, UPS and dLPS, and the occasional sporadic responses in other sarcoma types, the overall modest responses with ICI monotherapy suggest that other resistance mechanisms may be limiting the efficacy of checkpoint blockade, potentially through a suppressive immune microenvironment. Thus, combination strategies with various chemotherapies and targeted therapies are

Table 1
Responses of alveolar soft part sarcoma to regimens containing immune checkpoint inhibitors

Therapy	N	Response Rate (95% CI)	mPFS (months, 95% CI)	Reference
Nivolumab (OSCAR trial)	14	7.1% (0.2–33.9)	6.0 (3.7–9.3)	Kawai et al,[87] CTOS 2020
Retrospective multi-institutional series (monotherapy, N = 31, combination N = 29)	60	40.4% NR	13.4 (10.1–16.7)	Hindi et al,[88] ASCO 2021
Durvalumab/Tremelimumab (ASPS subset)	10	50% NR	34.23 (1.84 – NR)	Somaiah et al,[89] ASCO 2020
Atezolizumab	44	37.2% NR	NR	Naqash et al,[90] ASCO 2021
Axitinib/pembrolizumab	11	54.5% (24.6–81.9)	12.4 (2.7–22.3)	Wilky et al,[14] 2019
Geptanolimab	37	37.8% (22.5–55.2)	6.9 (5.0 – NR)	Shi et al,[91] 2020
Toripalimab, ASPS subset	12	25.0%	11.1 (NR)	Yang et al,[92] 2020

Abbreviations: ASCO, American Society of Clinical Oncology; ASPS, alveolar soft part sarcoma; CTOS, Connective Tissue Oncology Society; mPFS, median progression-free survival; NR, not reached, not reported.

increasingly being explored (**Table 2**). The next series of ICI trials for sarcomas were aimed at suppressive immune phenotypes such as T-regulatory cells or tumor-associated macrophages (TAMs) or suppressive cytokines such as vascular endothelial growth factor (VEGF). The PEMBROSARC study combined metronomic cyclophosphamide, which has been shown to suppress T-regulatory cells and augment T cell and natural killer (NK) cell function, with pembrolizumab in bone and STSs.[12] Unfortunately, only 1 of 50 STS patients achieved a response, and only three were progression free at 6 months. A later cohort of 17 osteosarcoma patients treated in this study revealed one patient achieving a response with three others experiencing tumor shrinkage; however, the median PFS was still low at only 1.4 months.[13] Additional studies have investigated tyrosine kinase inhibitors (TKIs) along with PD1 blockade. In a Phase 2 study of the pan VEGFR inhibitor axitinib with pembrolizumab, remarkable responses were observed in 6 of 11 patients with ASPS; however, only two responses in epithelioid sarcoma and soft tissue LMS were observed among the other STS patients on the study.[14] A phase 2 trial of the broader spectrum TKI sunitinib with nivolumab was also completed.[15] Of 58 evaluable patients, the ORR was 21%, with responses observed in angiosarcoma, clear cell sarcoma, ASPS, extraskeletal myxoid chondrosarcoma, and SS. The 6-month PFS rate was 48% by central assessment. Finally, a third study combined the selective VEGFR-2 TKI apatinib with the anti-PD1 antibody camrelizumab for 43 patients with osteosarcomas.[16] The ORR was 20.9%, with two long-term responders. The 6-month PFS rate was 50.9%. Ongoing studies are continuing to explore immunotherapy combinations using TKIs impacting broader kinomes and proven activity in sarcoma, such as cabozantinib (NCT04339738, angiosarcoma; NCT04551430, STS; NCT05019703, osteosarcoma). However, given the limited responses for all-comers, additional biomarkers are needed to identify the subset of patients likely to benefit from this approach.

Emerging transcriptomic data have shed light on immune classifications of sarcomas, identifying an immune-high subset that correlates with response to pembrolizumab monotherapy, and a vascular-enriched subset that has not yet been correlated with responses to TKI-containing combinations.[17] The majority of sarcomas have very

Table 2
Summary of responses to checkpoint inhibitors and combinations in various sarcoma subtypes

Sarcoma Subtypes	Checkpoint Inhibitor	Combination Partner	N	ORR	Median PFS (months)	Reference
LMS, UPS, GIST, others	Pembrolizumab	Cyclophosphamide	57	2%	1.4	Toulmonde et al[13]
STS	Pembrolizumab	Axitinib	33	25%	4.7	Wilky et al,[14] 2019
All Sarcoma	Nivolumab ± ipilimumab	None	43/42	5%/16%	1.7/4.1	D'Angelo et al,[4] 2018
All Sarcoma	Pembrolizumab	None	84	18%/5%	4.5/2	Tawbi et al,[3] 2017
STS	Ipilimumab	Dasatinib	28	0%	2.8	D'Angelo et al,[93] 2017
All Sarcoma	Durvalumab	Tremelimumab	57	14.3%	4.5	Somaiah et al,[89] 2020
GIST, UPS, DDLPS	Nivolumab ± ipilimumab	None	66	0% – 14%	1.5–5.5	Chen et al,[6] 2020
STS	Pembrolizumab	Doxorubicin	30	33%	6.9	Livingston et al,[20] 2021
STS	Ipilimumab/Nivolumab	Trabectedin	41	19.50%	6	Gordon et al,[94] 2019
STS	Nivolumab	Sunitinib	68	13%	5.6	Martin-Broto et al,[15] 2020
Bone	Nivolumab	Sunitinib	40	5%	3.7	Palmerini et al,[95] 2020
All Sarcomas	Pembrolizumab	Doxorubicin	37	22%	8.1	Pollack et al,[21] 2020

low expression of immune-related genes and suggest a failure to mount an immune response due to innate lack of immunogenicity, either from lack of neoantigens or failure of antigen presentation and recognition. Thus, the newest wave of combination ICI clinical trials for sarcomas is now focused on inducing immunogenicity that can then be perpetuated by downstream checkpoint blockade. The main strategies being explored include radiation therapy, cytotoxic chemotherapy, and other agents such as cytokines that aim to generate novel neoantigens or induce the production of danger signals from dying or injured tumor cells to draw in innate immune cells.

Radiation has been shown in numerous cancers to increase immunogenic cell death, boost antigen-presenting cell priming, and activate effector T cell responses through the formation of double-stranded DNA breaks that can activate the cGAS-STING pathway and promote inflammatory cytokine production.[18] SU2C-SARC032 is a randomized Phase 2 trial of 105 patients with high-grade stage III extremity UPS or dLPS treated with preoperative radiation therapy with or without adjuvant pembrolizumab (NCT02301039). With accrual completed, the results of this study may greatly impact the upfront management of sarcomas, leading to potential improvement in distant metastasis and pathologic response.

Cytotoxic chemotherapy, particularly doxorubicin and other anthracyclines, has been shown in a variety of cancers to induce the release of damage-associated markers and cytokines and promote type 1 interferon (IFN) production by tumor cells to improve immunogenicity.[19] Two single-arm phase 2 studies have recently been reported showing promising activity of doxorubicin with pembrolizumab for advanced/metastatic sarcomas.[20,21] The ORR was 19% in the Pollack study, which included bone and STS, and 36.7% in the Livingston study, which was all STS. Pollack reported a median PFS of 8.1 months with a 24-week PFS rate of 73%. The heterogeneous study population including a fair number of atypical sarcoma subtypes may have influenced the longer PFS; however, a subset of patients showed prolonged benefit. The median PFS in the Livingston study was 5.7 months, and 6-month PFS rate was 44% in a more selected STS population. Overall, the combination of doxorubicin with immune therapy has a solid rationale, and multiple ongoing trials are seeking to improve these outcomes by incorporating ifosfamide (NCT04356872, NCT04606108) or combination CTLA-4/PD1 blockade (NCT04028063). Other cytotoxics also have profound impacts on immune reactivity and are being explored in combination studies with ICIs, including gemcitabine (NCT04577014, NCT03123276, NCT04535713), trabectedin (NCT03138161), and eribulin (NCT03899805).

Another interesting strategy was explored in a phase 2 study combining an IL-2 pathway agonist, NKTR-214, with nivolumab for bone and STS (NCT03282344). Although some significant and durable responses were observed, unraveling the contribution of NKTR-214 to PD-1 blockade is difficult, an issue with all single-arm combination studies. Full results and correlative data from this study are upcoming and may shed light on underlying mechanisms of response and resistance. Similarly, Pollack and colleagues are conducting a Phase 2 trial of IFN-γ with pembrolizumab (NCT03063632) based on prior laboratory data showing that IFN-γ could upregulate MHC Class 1 expression and subsequent T-cell infiltration.[22] Thus, these are examples of directly targeting key cytokines instrumental to the early immune response and hopefully overcoming the innate resistance seen in so many sarcomas.

Biomarkers of Efficacy

As the results of these ongoing studies emerge, and critical correlative data from previously completed studies are released, we may have a better sense of biomarkers that can correlate with responses to various combinations to build into future trials.

To date, many investigations have queried sarcoma tissue archives to determine whether biomarkers that have predicted responses to checkpoint inhibitors in other cancers hold true in sarcomas. Overall, the results of these studies have been conflicting, confounded by histologic subtype differences, and limitations of assays used. Additionally, with many of these studies performed on small biopsies, sampling bias plays a real role, considering that many immune cells may lay on the leading edge of tumors or excluded outside the tumor in the stroma.

Tumor and tumor-infiltrating lymphocyte (TIL) PD1 and PD-L1 expression have been a reliable indicator of an established but exhausted immune response that can be rejuvenated with checkpoint blockade in other types of cancers.[23] In sarcomas, various studies have explored PD1/PD-L1 expression and how it may affect overall survival (OS) and event-free survival (EFS). Some studies suggest that elevated PD1/PD-L1 expression is associated with worse overall survival; however, others suggest it is favorable. Further confounding these results is that some studies use protein expression with various antibody clones, whereas others report genetic expression that are not interchangable. A recent comprehensive meta-analysis containing 15 independent studies and 1,451 patients showed that high PD-L1 expression was associated with worse overall survival (HR 1.27, $P = .000$) and worse EFS (HR 2.05, $P = .000$).[24] However, these retrospective analyses are not correlated with clinical outcomes and do not take into account the recent use of immunotherapy. Interestingly, correlative studies exploring PD-L1 expression in sarcomas treated with ICIs are similarly contradictory. Although the numbers of patients are small, PD-L1 tumor expression does not appear to be required for response to therapy, although responders often exhibit PD-L1 expression. A recent review of 154 patients treated on checkpoint inhibitor trials with PD-L1 expression status showed 6/20 PD-L1-positive patients achieved response (30%); however, 9 of 133 PD-L1 negative patients also showed a response to treatment.[25]

Another major biomarker that remains underexplored in sarcomas is the presence of TILs. Similarly to PD-L1, the presence of TILs has been shown to have either negative or positive prognostic significance in reported clinical trials reviewed in a study.[26] However, many of these studies do not go on to further profile these cells, and heterozygous TIL populations could include activated or suppressive T cells, including CD8+, CD4+, or T-regulatory cells, NK cells, B cells, or myeloid/macrophage cells, all with different functions and significance. Although numerous studies have retrospectively reported on the prevalence of these phenotypes and associations with OS, EFS, or metastasis-free survival in various sarcoma subtypes,[26] there is very limited data on associations with ICI response. Responding patients with pembrolizumab monotherapy had significantly higher CD8+ T-cell infiltration and PD-L1+ TAMs at baseline compared with nonresponders.[27] More recently, work from Petitprez and colleagues demonstrated that the presence of tertiary lymphoid structures (TLSs) containing DC-LAMP+ dendritic cells and CD20+ B cell aggregates in sarcomas also correlated retrospectively with response to pembrolizumab.[17] Building on these observations, an extended cohort of the PEMBROSARC trial enrolled 48 TLS positive sarcoma patients from 240 screened (20%) who were eligible to receive pembrolizumab and oral cyclophosphamide.[28] Among the 35 evaluable patients, 30% displayed objective response, 33.3% had stable disease, and PFS and OS were 4.1 and 14.5 months, respectively. These promising results contrast with the initial ORR of 2% and PFS of 1.4 months reported in the unselected PEMBROSARC population.[12] Overall, further investigation into the impact of TILs is desperately needed to further refine the selection of patients for combination studies that potentially target these other phenotypes.

A promising strategy for characterizing sarcomas and potentially predicting responses to ICI has proven to be advance in sequencing technology. TMB and microsatellite instability (MSI) are used as biomarkers to predict response to immuno-therapy in various cancers. Sarcomas generally have low TMB, with an average of 1.06 mutations/Mb reported in TCGA analysis.[29] However, hypermutated sarcomas with high levels of UV-associated mutations have recently been identified, mainly angiosar-coma (especially stemmed from face and scalp) and MPNST.[30] A comprehensive analysis of 47 angiosarcomas prospectively registered in a cohort reported a median TMB of 3.3 mutations/Mb in the full cohort, and a median TMB in the face and scalp angiosarcoma of 20.7 mutations/Mb, significantly higher than in all other angiosar-coma subclassifications (2.8 mutations/Mb; p 1.1 10^{-5}). Among 10 patients with face and scalp angiosarcoma, two patients were treated with ICI and showed excep-tional and durable responses. No clinical benefit was observed in the 3 of 26 patients with angiosarcoma with other localizations (outside face and scalp) treated with anti-PD1.[10] TMB was also demonstrated to correlate with mismatch repair-deficiency (MMR-D) in a series of 304 STS.[31] A low proportion of sarcomas (7/304%, 2.3%) was classified as MMR-D. MMR-D sarcomas showed a median TMB significantly higher than MMR-proficient sarcomas (16 vs 4.6, P <.001). Results from larger sar-coma cohorts are expected to determine whether TMB may be used as a single biomarker to predict a benefit to immunotherapy or whether the global context (MMR status, tumor type, carcinogen exposure) should be required. MSI-high signa-ture in a tissue agnostic fashion led to the approval of pembrolizumab by FDA. MSI status in sarcomas was assessed across 71 samples of various STS and remains an uncommon event.[32]

In addition to identifying the rarer cases of STS that exhibit high TMB or MSI high status, recent studies have shown that bulk transcriptomic data can be deconvoluted to extract contributions of various immune cell signatures. These techniques have allowed for the clustering of various sarcomas into immune low, moderate, or high ac-tivity signatures. Multiple studies mining available transcriptomic data have created sarcoma immune subsets; however, only the Petitprez study provides the correlation with responses to PD1 monotherapy.[17,33,34] Patients in the high immune expression SIC-E were more likely to achieve an objective response and to have a favorable PFS.

Overall, given the complexity of the immune microenvironment in sarcomas, including intertumor and intratumor heterogeneity, developing biomarkers for ICIs re-mains a critical need and an area of active exploration.

ADOPTIVE CELLULAR THERAPIES

As we have discussed, one of the fundamental immune evasion mechanisms in sar-comas may be the inability to mount an immune response due to poor neoantigens or faulty antigen recognition, leading to a failure to generate an adequate supply of tumor-specific T cells. Adoptive cellular therapies aim to bypass this step, by providing a large volume of autologous T cells that are either collected from the pri-mary tumor or collected from peripheral blood and engineered to be specific for a particular antigen and expanded. Most products require lymphodepleting chemo-therapy before administration. Adoptive cellular products can include engineered T-cell receptor (TCR), chimeric antigen receptor (CAR) T-cell therapies, TILs, and NK cells.

Engineered T-Cell Receptor Therapy Targeting Cancer Testis Antigens

New York esophageal squamous cell carcinoma 1 (NY-ESO-1) is a CTA, a protein involved in immunologic maturation that is typically restricted to human male germ cells, that exhibited increased expression in sarcomas, primarily SS and myxoid/round cell liposarcoma.[35,36] Because NY-ESO-1 is an intracellular antigen, which must be processed and presented in association with MHC, these targets are better suited for engineered TCR T cells. Compared with CAR-T, engineered TCR T cells require matched HLA allele subtypes in patients, generally HLA-A*02, which is found in roughly 30% of the population, and can be plagued with greater off-tumor target toxicity compared with CAR T cells.[37] In a Phase 1 clinical trial of NY-ESO-1 TCR T cell therapy that included 10 SS patients with HLA-A*02 positive tumors, no adverse fatal events occurred with persistence of T cells *in vivo*.[38] A Phase 2 clinical trial has recently begun to assess overall response, response duration, PFS, OS, safety, and tolerability.[39–42]

The melanoma antigen gene (MAGE) protein family is a highly conserved group of proteins that are present on the X chromosome and in reproductive tissues. However, MAGE-A4 has been found to be broadly expressed in many tumor types, including several reports showing expression of both NY-ESO-1 and MAGE-A4 in STS, especially SS where 70.6% are positive for either marker.[43,44] A Phase 2 study of 35 patients with SS who had been treated with a TCR T cell, afami-cel, showed showed a favorable safety profile with complete and durable responses in most of the patients.[45]

CAR T-Cell Therapies

CAR T-cell therapies, which combine the targeted specificity of antibodies with the effective capabilities of T cells, offer a promising therapeutic intervention based on their successes in treating CD19+ acute lymphoblastic leukemia and B-cell lymphomas. There are several generations of CAR T cells that differ based on their intracellular costimulatory domains, such as 4-1BB, CD28, and OX40, which enhance proliferation and survival.[46] Patients undergoing CAR T-cell therapy experience an increased degree of immune stimulation and inflammation resulting in systemic cytokine release syndrome (CRS) in some cases.[47] However, this complication is well managed with IL-6 inhibitors, like Tocilizumab, and steroids for neurotoxicity. Thus far, CAR-T protocols have struggled in solid tumors, mainly due to difficulties in finding conserved targets without prohibitive toxicity to normal organs carrying the same antigens.

For sarcomas, multiple targets have been explored in prior and ongoing clinical trials. Human epidermal growth factor receptor 2 (HER2) is a ligand that can activate downstream pathways of Ras/Raf/MEK/ERK1/2 and phospholipases to promote oncogenesis.[48] In a Phase I/II clinical trial in 19 patients with HER2+ osteosarcomas, Ewing sarcoma, neuroectodermal tumor, and desmoplastic small round cell tumor, HER2-CAR T-cell therapy demonstrated no adverse side effects with four patients achieving stable disease for 12 weeks to 14 months.[49] The study showed that the median overall survival was 10.3 months with a median follow-up time of 10.1 months. A Phase I study in 10 patients with refractory/metastatic HER2+ sarcoma showed that lymphodepletion chemotherapy followed by autologous HER2-CAR T cell therapy was associated with improved clinical benefit.[50] Results showed that one patient with osteosarcoma achieved complete response and two others had stable disease. In patients with rhabdomyosarcoma, two achieved complete response and the third exhibited stable disease. The patient with Ewing sarcoma also aachievechieved achieved stable disease. Although this therapy shows promise in patients with HER2+ sarcomas, additional studies are combining CAR T cells with ICIs (NCT04995003) to improve efficacy. Phase 1 clinical trials are currently ongoing using EGFR (NCT03618381) and GD2 (NCT02107963, NCT04539366, NCT03721068, NCT03635632) CAR T cells for pediatric sarcomas, including osteosarcoma, Ewing sarcoma, and rhabdomyosarcoma expressing these surface markers.

Other targets in earlier phases of development include insulin-like growth factor 1 receptor (IGF-1R), a transmembrane receptor tyrosine kinase, and promoter of tumor cell survival, which has has demonstrated prognostic significance in sarcomas where several cell lines have been sensitive to IGF-1R inhibition.[51] Tyrosine kinase orphan-like receptor 1 (ROR1), a transmembrane protein involved in cancer cell migration, invasion, and metastasis, is is overexpressed in osteosarcoma, Ewing's sarcoma, and rhabdomyosarcoma.[52] IGF-1R and ROR-targeted CAR T-cell therapies are still in early stages in humans.[53] CD44v6, a cancer cell marker of metastasis and tumor progression, is associated with poor prognosis in osteosarcoma patients.[54,55] It is expressed in 40% of STSs, including fibrosarcoma, LMS, liposarcoma, and UPS. When used as a therapeutic target, CAR-redirected cytokine-induced killer (CIK) T cells exhibited greater tumor growth delay compared with untreated and control-treated mouse cohorts.[56] Thus, CD44v6 remains a promising target for future study. Finally, NK cell activating receptor group 2-member D ligand (NKG2DL), a ligand from the NKG2D family involved in the activation of macrophages, T cells, and NK cells to promote antitumor immunity, is rarely expressed in normal tissue but overexpressed in osteosarcoma and Ewing's sarcoma.[57,58] Second-generation NKG2D-directed CAR-T cells against osteosarcoma and Ewing's sarcoma demonstrated increased cytotoxicity, lower tumor burden, and increased overall survival in murine models.[58,59]

TIL Therapies

TILs, which demonstrate antitumor activity *in vivo*, are extracted from resected or biopsied human tumors and undergo *ex vivo* expansion to be administered to patients following a lymphodepletion regimen.[60,61] Although they have demonstrated therapeutic efficacy in melanoma of at least 50%, their growth from other solid tumors has been varied.[62–64] The limited ability to expand them presents a challenge to their global application to serve large numbers of patients with cancer. Due to its personalized nature, each patient requires a unique infusion product to be produced, which will largely drive up costs.[65] Although robust and reproducible, the largest toxicities associated with TIL therapy include the lymphodepleting regimens, the use of interleukin-2 (IL-2), and the associated toxicity.[66–68] Recent work from Mullinax and colleagues has shown feasibility in establishing TIL cultures from sarcoma resections with about 25% of resected specimens yielding sufficient TILs for a clinical product ($\geq 2 \times 10^7$ cells).[69] Clinical trials using TIL technology have been ongoing through the NCI and other institutions, with Mullinax and colleagues currently conducting a dedicated Phase 1 clinical trial (NCT04052334). Phase 2 clinical trials studying the efficacy of TIL therapy are also enrolling for recurrent ovarian carcinosarcoma (NCT03610490) and STSs (NCT03935893).

Natural Killer Cell Therapies

NK cells, members of the innate lymphoid cell family, are effective defenders against cells infected with pathogens and tumors through their ability to express a diverse array of surface receptors.[70] Because they lack MHCs and possess cancer cell recognition capability, many studies are currently being carried out to use NK cells as novel therapeutic tools. However, despite their promise, they are limited by tumor immunoevasion, an inhospitable tumor microenvironment, and inadequate homing properties.[71,72] Irrespective, research is currently being performed to circumvent these limitations and unlock the potential of this therapy (NCT02890758, NCT02409576, NCT01875601, NCT03420963).[73]

Future Directions

Adoptive cellular therapies offer promising personalized therapies but are still in their infancy for solid tumors. Despite the present limitations for TILs, NK cells, and CAR T cells, they have all undergone refinements to improve efficacy and decrease toxicity. Methods are currently being investigated to enrich TILs through selection for CD137 or PD-1 in hopes of increasing their antitumor activity.[74,75] NK cells offer versatile potential, but further studies are needed to better understand their mechanisms of action, activation, and suppression within the tumor microenvironment.[76] New studies are attempting to augment NK cell anticancer properties through genetic modification and altered priming strategies to enhance cancer recognition, improve tumor homing, and reduce resistance.[77] The success of CAR T-cell therapies in hematological malignancies has expanded their utility to solid tumors, including sarcomas. Although CARs have demonstrated efficacy in *in vitro* models their biggest test will be their long-term efficacy in clinical trials. As more potent tumor-specific targets are defined, CAR T-cell constructs will be modified with new targets added to improve their efficacy especially in the solid tumor microenvironment.[78] Next-generation therapies should be more robust, safer, and better equipped to overcome the immunosuppressive microenvironment.

NOVEL THERAPIES

Talimogene laherparepvec (T-VEC) showed increased tumor-specific immune activation via augmenting antigen presentation and T-cell priming. A phase II clinical trial assessed the efficacy of the combination of T-VEC (injected in the palpable tumor site) with intravenous pembrolizumab in 20 patients with advanced or metastatic sarcoma.[79] Patients had 13 different sarcoma histotypes and 60% of them had received three lines or more of therapy before enrollment. The combination was well tolerated with 20% of them experiencing treatment-related adverse events and demonstrated interesting efficacy with 35% ORR and a duration of response of 56.1 weeks. Interestingly, two responders to the combination had disease progression while receiving immunotherapy just before study enrollment, suggesting synergism between treatments. The small sample size of ancillary studies limited the ability to draw definitive conclusions.

Vaccine efficacy is based on the stimulation of the endogenous immune system of patients, for example, through the presentation of an antigen by dendritic cells stimulating CD8+ T cells. Although various vaccine therapies have been explored for sarcomas over the past 20years, overall the efficacy has been limited likely due to the other suppressive mechanisms in the immune microenvironment. Future studies of vaccines in combination with other therapies including ICIs may help to overcome these resistance mechanisms. LV305 is an NY-ESO-1 expression third-generation lentiviral vector designed to deliver RNA tumor antigens to dendritic cells, selectively targeting DC-SIGN (CD209) on the surface of immature human dendritic cells. To increase the efficacy of LV305, it was then combined with G305, including a full-length NY-ESO1 protein and a toll-like receptor 4 (TLR4) agonist as an adjuvant.[80] This strategy of alternative targeting of the same antigen was called "CMB305 regimen" and assessed in a phase Ib trial.[81] In this study, 64 patients had sarcoma among which 69.8% had greater than 75% NY-ESO-1 expression. The treatment was well tolerated and led to a 61.9% control rate in sarcoma with 26.2-month overall survival. A randomized phase II study was conducted in 89 patients with advanced/metastatic SS or myxoid liposarcoma, known to frequently express NY-ESO-1, to assess the combination of CMB305 and atezolizumab versus atezolizumab alone.[82] The combination failed to significantly increase PFS and OS in the whole cohort even though there was evidence of benefit to a subset of patients who developed anti-NY-ESO-1 T-cell immune response. Given the overall lack of neoantigens as a resistance mechanism in sarcomas, future investigations of vaccines are warranted.

Macrophages and other myeloid cells are highly interesting targets for ongoing and future explorations. Dedicated studies with checkpoint inhibitors and CSF1R blockade aiming to repolarize M2 suppressive macrophages to M1 activated phenotypes are ongoing (NCT04242238), and there is a significant rationale for future investigation of targeting the CD47/SIRPα axis. A recent study highlighted variable expression and presence of macrophages across over 1200 specimens representing 24 sarcoma subtypes, with CD163+ M2 suppressive macrophages as the dominant phenotype, and preferentially present in nontranslocation sarcomas over other sarcomas.[83] CD47 staining was bimodal, with either absent or very high expression, which correlated with SIRPα expression. Subtypes with the highest expression of CD47/SIRPα on macrophages included angiosarcomas, chordoma, and pleomorphic liposarcomas. Interestingly, more than 50% of Ewing's sarcomas assessed had tumor positivity of SIRPα raising the question of an alternate function. Another study recently supported the importance of myeloid signatures in sarcoma,[84] again making this an area that should be prioritized in future clinical trials.

TRAIL-TNF axis—TRAIL is a cytokine member of the TNF superfamily, and TRAIL-R1 (death receptor 4) and TRAIL R2 (DR5) family have been shown to be expressed in a variety of sarcomas. Ongoing studies showed early promising outcomes with stimulatory agonists for DR5,[85] with plans for a dedicated phase 2 study in chondrosarcomas (NCT04950075). As of yet no combinations with checkpoint blockade have been planned but would have interesting rationale.

SUMMARY

In the past 5 years, we have seen tremendous growth in laboratory, translational, and clinical investigation that revitalizes the hope raised from Sir William Coley's initial observations in the 1890s that sarcomas could be susceptible to immune recognition and attack.[86] With a subset of sarcoma patients showing remarkable and durable responses to immune therapies even after the failure of numerous traditional treatments, it is tempting to imagine a future where the individual tumor and host genetic and immune factors can be assessed and treatments customized to overcome immune evasion. To reach this goal, we must continue to learn from every sarcoma patient treated on immune therapy clinical trials and increase collaboration in the laboratory and clinical research realms. By taking advantage of emerging genetic and immune datasets, and improving collaborative trial designs with novel agents and strategies, immunotherapy may well become a standard aspect of the sarcoma therapeutic armamentarium over the next years.

DISCLOSURE

All authors have no conflict of interest to declare.

REFERENCES

1. Robert C. A decade of immune-checkpoint inhibitors in cancer therapy. Nat Commun 2020;11(1):3801.
2. Maki RG, Jungbluth AA, Gnjatic S, et al. A Pilot Study of Anti-CTLA4 Antibody Ipilimumab in Patients with Synovial Sarcoma. Sarcoma 2013;2013:168145.

3. Tawbi HA, Burgess M, Bolejack V, et al. Pembrolizumab in advanced soft-tissue sarcoma and bone sarcoma (SARC028): a multicentre, two-cohort, single-arm, open-label, phase 2 trial. Lancet Oncol 2017;18(11):1493–501.

4. D'Angelo SP, Mahoney MR, Van Tine BA, et al. Nivolumab with or without ipilimumab treatment for metastatic sarcoma (Alliance A091401): two open-label, non-comparative, randomised, phase 2 trials. Lancet Oncol 2018;19(3):416–26.

5. Burgess MA, Bolejack V, Schuetze S, et al. Clinical activity of pembrolizumab (P) in undifferentiated pleomorphic sarcoma (UPS) and dedifferentiated/pleomorphic liposarcoma (LPS): Final results of SARC028 expansion cohorts. Jco 2019; 37(15_suppl):11015.

6. Chen JL, Mahoney MR, George S, et al. A multicenter phase II study of nivolumab +/- ipilimumab for patients with metastatic sarcoma (Alliance A091401): Results of expansion cohorts. Jco 2020;38(15_suppl):11511.

7. Florou V, Rosenberg AE, Wieder E, et al. Angiosarcoma patients treated with immune checkpoint inhibitors: a case series of seven patients from a single institution. J Immunother Cancer 2019;7(1):213.

8. Momen S, Fassihi H, Davies HR, et al. Dramatic response of metastatic cutaneous angiosarcoma to an immune checkpoint inhibitor in a patient with xeroderma pigmentosum: whole-genome sequencing aids treatment decision in end-stage disease. Cold Spring Harb Mol Case Stud 2019;5(5):a004408.

9. Sindhu S, Gimber LH, Cranmer L, et al. Angiosarcoma treated successfully with anti-PD-1 therapy - a case report. J Immunother Cancer 2017;5(1):58.

10. Painter CA, Jain E, Tomson BN, et al. The Angiosarcoma Project: enabling genomic and clinical discoveries in a rare cancer through patient-partnered research. Nat Med 2020;26(2):181–7.

11. Wagner MJ, Othus M, Patel SP, et al. Multicenter phase II trial (SWOG S1609, cohort 51) of ipilimumab and nivolumab in metastatic or unresectable angiosarcoma: a substudy of dual anti-CTLA-4 and anti-PD-1 blockade in rare tumors (DART). J Immunother Cancer 2021;9(8):e002990.

12. Toulmonde M, Penel N, Adam J, et al. Use of PD-1 Targeting, Macrophage Infiltration, and IDO Pathway Activation in Sarcomas: A Phase 2 Clinical Trial. JAMA Oncol 2018;4(1):93–7.

13. Le Cesne A, Marec-Berard P, Blay JY, et al. Programmed cell death 1 (PD-1) targeting in patients with advanced osteosarcomas: results from the PEMBROSARC study. Eur J Cancer 2019;119:151–7.

14. Wilky BA, Trucco MM, Subhawong TK, et al. Axitinib plus pembrolizumab in patients with advanced sarcomas including alveolar soft part sarcoma: a single-arm, phase 2 trial. Lancet Oncol 2019;20(6):837–48.

15. Martin-Broto J, Hindi N, Grignani G, et al. Nivolumab and sunitinib combination in advanced soft tissue sarcomas: a multicenter, single-arm, phase Ib/II trial. J Immunother Cancer 2020;8(2):e001561.

16. Xie L, Xu J, Sun X, et al. Apatinib plus camrelizumab (anti-PD1 therapy, SHR-1210) for advanced osteosarcoma (APFAO) progressing after chemotherapy: a single-arm, open-label, phase 2 trial. J Immunother Cancer 2020;8(1).

17. Petitprez F, de Reyniès A, Keung EZ, et al. B cells are associated with survival and immunotherapy response in sarcoma. Nature 2020;577:556–60.

18. Cytlak UM, Dyer DP, Honeychurch J, et al. Immunomodulation by radiotherapy in tumour control and normal tissue toxicity. Nat Rev Immunol 2022;22(2):124–38.

19. Wang YJ, Fletcher R, Yu J, et al. Immunogenic effects of chemotherapy-induced tumor cell death. Genes Dis 2018;5(3):194–203.

20. Livingston MB, Jagosky MH, Robinson MM, et al. Phase II study of pembrolizumab in combination with doxorubicin in metastatic and unresectable soft tissue sarcoma. Clin Cancer Res 2021;27(23):6424–31.
21. Pollack SM, Redman MW, Baker KK, et al. Assessment of Doxorubicin and Pembrolizumab in Patients With Advanced Anthracycline-Naive Sarcoma: A Phase 1/2 Nonrandomized Clinical Trial. JAMA Oncol 2020;6(11):1778–82.
22. Zhang S, Kohli K, Black RG, et al. Systemic Interferon-γ Increases MHC Class I Expression and T-cell Infiltration in Cold Tumors: Results of a Phase 0 Clinical Trial. Cancer Immunol Res 2019;7(8):1237–43.
23. Davis AA, Patel VG. The role of PD-L1 expression as a predictive biomarker: an analysis of all US Food and Drug Administration (FDA) approvals of immune checkpoint inhibitors. J Immunother Cancer 2019;7(1):278.
24. Zheng C, You W, Wan P, et al. Clinicopathological and prognostic significance of PD-L1 expression in sarcoma: A systematic review and meta-analysis. Medicine (Baltimore) 2018;97(25):e11004.
25. Italiano A, Bellera C, D'Angelo S. PD1/PD-L1 targeting in advanced soft-tissue sarcomas: a pooled analysis of phase II trials. J Hematol Oncol 2020;13(1):55.
26. Zhu MMT, Shenasa E, Nielsen TO. Sarcomas: Immune biomarker expression and checkpoint inhibitor trials. Cancer Treat Rev 2020;91:102115.
27. Keung EZ, Burgess M, Salazar R, et al. Correlative Analyses of the SARC028 Trial Reveal an Association Between Sarcoma-Associated Immune Infiltrate and Response to Pembrolizumab. Clin Cancer Res 2020;26(6):1258–66.
28. Italiano A, Bessede A, Bompas E, et al. PD1 inhibition in soft-tissue sarcomas with tertiary lymphoid structures: A multicenter phase II trial. Jco 2021;39(15_suppl):11507.
29. Comprehensive and Integrated Genomic Characterization of Adult Soft Tissue Sarcomas. Cell 2017;171(4):950.e28, e28.
30. Campbell BB, Light N, Fabrizio D, et al. Comprehensive Analysis of Hypermutation in Human Cancer. Cell 2017;171(5):1042.e10, e10.
31. Doyle LA, Nowak JA, Nathenson MJ, et al. Characteristics of mismatch repair deficiency in sarcomas. Mod Pathol 2019;32(7):977–87.
32. Campanella NC, Penna V, Ribeiro G, et al. Absence of Microsatellite Instability In Soft Tissue Sarcomas. Pathobiology 2015;82(1):36–42.
33. Dufresne A, Lesluyes T, Ménétrier-Caux C, et al. Specific immune landscapes and immune checkpoint expressions in histotypes and molecular subtypes of sarcoma. Oncoimmunology 2020;9(1):1792036.
34. Hu C, Chen B, Huang Z, et al. Comprehensive profiling of immune-related genes in soft tissue sarcoma patients. J Transl Med 2020;18(1):337.
35. Jungbluth AA, Antonescu CR, Busam KJ, et al. Monophasic and biphasic synovial sarcomas abundantly express cancer/testis antigen NY-ESO-1 but not MAGE-A1 or CT7. Int J Cancer 2001;94(2):252–6.
36. Hemminger JA, Ewart Toland A, Scharschmidt TJ, et al. The cancer-testis antigen NY-ESO-1 is highly expressed in myxoid and round cell subset of liposarcomas. Mod Pathol 2013;26(2):282–8.
37. Garrido F, Aptsiauri N, Doorduijn EM, et al. The urgent need to recover MHC class I in cancers for effective immunotherapy. Curr Opin Immunol 2016;39:44–51.
38. D'Angelo SP, Melchiori L, Merchant MS, et al. Antitumor Activity Associated with Prolonged Persistence of Adoptively Transferred NY-ESO-1 (c259)T Cells in Synovial Sarcoma. Cancer Discov 2018;8(8):944–57.
39. Hong, D.S. Phase I dose escalation and expansion trial to assess the safety and efficacy of ADP-A2M4 SPEAR T cells in advanced solid tumors. 2020. ASCO

Virtual Scientific Program: American Society of Clinical Oncology. J Clin Oncol, 38, no. 15_suppl. 2020. 102-102.

40. Rosenbaum E, Seier K, Bandlamudi C, et al. HLA Genotyping in Synovial Sarcoma: Identifying HLA-A*02 and Its Association with Clinical Outcome. Clin Cancer Res 2020;26(20):5448–55.

41. Ramachandran I, Lowther DE, Dryer-Minnerly R, et al. Systemic and local immunity following adoptive transfer of NY-ESO-1 SPEAR T cells in synovial sarcoma. J Immunother Cancer 2019;7(1):276.

42. D'Angelo SP, Noujaim JC, Thistlethwaite F, et al. IGNYTE-ESO: A master protocol to assess safety and activity of letetresgene autoleucel (lete-cel; GSK3377794) in HLA-A*02+ patients with synovial sarcoma or myxoid/round cell liposarcoma (Substudies 1 and 2). Jco 2021;39(15_suppl):TPS11582.

43. Ishihara M, Kageyama S, Miyahara Y, et al. MAGE-A4, NY-ESO-1 and SAGE mRNA expression rates and co-expression relationships in solid tumours. BMC Cancer 2020;20(1):606.

44. Kakimoto T, Matsumine A, Kageyama S, et al. Immunohistochemical expression and clinicopathological assessment of the cancer testis antigens NY-ESO-1 and MAGE-A4 in high-grade soft-tissue sarcoma. Oncol Lett 2019;17(4):3937–43.

45. D'Angelo SP, Van Tine BA, Attia S, et al. SPEARHEAD-1: A phase 2 trial of afamitresgene autoleucel (Formerly ADP-A2M4) in patients with advanced synovial sarcoma or myxoid/round cell liposarcoma. Jco 2021;39(15_suppl):11504.

46. June CH, O'Connor RS, Kawalekar OU, et al. CAR T cell immunotherapy for human cancer. Science 2018;359(6382):1361–5.

47. Brudno JN, Kochenderfer JN. Toxicities of chimeric antigen receptor T cells: recognition and management. Blood 2016;127(26):3321–30.

48. Roskoski R Jr. The ErbB/HER family of protein-tyrosine kinases and cancer. Pharmacol Res 2014;79:34–74.

49. Ahmed N, Brawley VS, Hegde M, et al. Human Epidermal Growth Factor Receptor 2 (HER2) –Specific Chimeric Antigen Receptor–Modified T Cells for the Immunotherapy of HER2-Positive Sarcoma. J Clin Oncol 2015;33(15):1688–96.

50. Navai SA, Derenzo C, Joseph S, et al. Abstract LB-147: Administration of HER2-CAR T cells after lymphodepletion safely improves T cell expansion and induces clinical responses in patients with advanced sarcomas. Cancer Res 2019;79(13 Supplement). LB-147-LB-147.

51. Duan Z, Choy E, Harmon D, et al. Insulin-like growth factor-I receptor tyrosine kinase inhibitor cyclolignan picropodophyllin inhibits proliferation and induces apoptosis in multidrug resistant osteosarcoma cell lines. Mol Cancer Ther 2009;8(8):2122–30.

52. Tzanakakis GN, Giatagana EM, Berdiaki A, et al. The Role of IGF/IGF-IR-Signaling and Extracellular Matrix Effectors in Bone Sarcoma Pathogenesis. Cancers (Basel) 2021;13(10).

53. Huang X, Park H, Greene J, et al. IGF1R- and ROR1-Specific CAR T Cells as a Potential Therapy for High Risk Sarcomas. PLoS One 2015;10(7):e0133152.

54. Wang Z, Zhao K, Hackert T, et al. CD44/CD44v6 a Reliable Companion in Cancer-Initiating Cell Maintenance and Tumor Progression. Front Cell Dev Biol 2018;6:97.

55. Zhang Y, Ding C, Wang J, et al. Prognostic significance of CD44V6 expression in osteosarcoma: a meta-analysis. J Orthop Surg Res 2015;10:187.

56. Leuci V, Casucci GM, Grignani G, et al. CD44v6 as innovative sarcoma target for CAR-redirected CIK cells. Oncoimmunology 2018;7(5):e1423167.

57. Fernandez L, Valentin J, Zalacain M, et al. Activated and expanded natural killer cells target osteosarcoma tumor initiating cells in an NKG2D-NKG2DL dependent manner. Cancer Lett 2015;368(1):54–63.

58. Lehner M, Götz G, Proff J, et al. Redirecting T cells to Ewing's sarcoma family of tumors by a chimeric NKG2D receptor expressed by lentiviral transduction or mRNA transfection. PLoS One 2012;7(2):e31210.

59. Fernandez L, Metais J-Y, Escudero A, et al. Memory T Cells Expressing an NKG2D-CAR Efficiently Target Osteosarcoma Cells. Clin Cancer Res 2017; 23(19):5824–35.

60. Rosenberg SA, Yang JC, Sherry RM, et al. Durable complete responses in heavily pretreated patients with metastatic melanoma using T-cell transfer immuno-therapy. Clin Cancer Res 2011;17(13):4550–7.

61. Andersen R, Donia M, Ellebaek E, et al. Long-Lasting Complete Responses in Pa-tients with Metastatic Melanoma after Adoptive Cell Therapy with Tumor-Infiltrating Lymphocytes and an Attenuated IL2 Regimen. Clin Cancer Res 2016;22(15):3734–45.

62. Besser MJ, Shapira-Frommer R, Itzhaki O, et al. Adoptive transfer of tumor-infiltrating lymphocytes in patients with metastatic melanoma: intent-to-treat anal-ysis and efficacy after failure to prior immunotherapies. Clin Cancer Res 2013; 19(17):4792–800.

63. Ben-Avi R, Farhi R, Ben-Nun A, et al. Establishment of adoptive cell therapy with tumor infiltrating lymphocytes for non-small cell lung cancer patients. Cancer Im-munol Immunother 2018;67(8):1221–30.

64. Lee HJ, Kim YA, Sim CK, et al. Expansion of tumor-infiltrating lymphocytes and their potential for application as adoptive cell transfer therapy in human breast cancer. Oncotarget 2017;8(69):113345–59.

65. Retèl VP, Steuten LM, Mewes JC, et al. Early Cost-Effectiveness Modeling for Tu-mor Infiltrating Lymphocytes (TIL) -Treatment Versus Ipilimumab in Metastatic Melanoma Patients. Value Health 2014;17(7):A640.

66. Rosenberg SA, Yannelli JR, Yang JC, et al. Treatment of patients with metastatic melanoma with autologous tumor-infiltrating lymphocytes and interleukin 2. J Natl Cancer Inst 1994;86(15):1159–66.

67. Marabondo S, Kaufman HL. High-dose interleukin-2 (IL-2) for the treatment of melanoma: safety considerations and future directions. Expert Opin Drug Saf 2017;16(12):1347–57.

68. Yang JC. Toxicities Associated With Adoptive T-Cell Transfer for Cancer. Cancer J 2015;21(6):506–9.

69. Mullinax JE, Hall M, Beatty M, et al. Expanded Tumor-infiltrating Lymphocytes From Soft Tissue Sarcoma Have Tumor-specific Function. J Immunother 2021; 44(2):63–70.

70. Guillerey C, Huntington ND, Smyth MJ. Targeting natural killer cells in cancer immunotherapy. Nat Immunol 2016;17(9):1025–36.

71. Domagala J, Lachota M, Klopotowska M, et al. The Tumor Microenvironment-A Metabolic Obstacle to NK Cells' Activity. Cancers (Basel) 2020;12(12).

72. Ljunggren HG, Malmberg KJ. Prospects for the use of NK cells in immunotherapy of human cancer. Nat Rev Immunol 2007;7(5):329–39.

73. Tonn T, Schwabe D, Klingemann HG, et al. Treatment of patients with advanced cancer with the natural killer cell line NK-92. Cytotherapy 2013;15(12):1563–70.

74. Seliktar-Ofir S, Merhavi-Shoham E, Itzhaki O, et al. Selection of Shared and Neoantigen-Reactive T Cells for Adoptive Cell Therapy Based on CD137 Separa-tion. Front Immunol 2017;8:1211.

75. Inozume T, Hanada K, Wang QJ, et al. Selection of CD8+PD-1+ lymphocytes in fresh human melanomas enriches for tumor-reactive T cells. J Immunother 2010; 33(9):956–64.

76. Riggan L, Shah S, O'Sullivan TE. Arrested development: suppression of NK cell function in the tumor microenvironment. Clin Transl Immunol 2021;10(1):e1238.

77. Crowe NY, Smyth MJ, Godfrey DI. A critical role for natural killer T cells in immunosurveillance of methylcholanthrene-induced sarcomas. J Exp Med 2002; 196(1):119–27.

78. Knochelmann HM, Smith AS, Dwyer CJ, et al. CAR T Cells in Solid Tumors: Blueprints for Building Effective Therapies. Front Immunol 2018;9:1740.

79. Kelly CM, Antonescu CR, Bowler T, et al. Objective Response Rate Among Patients With Locally Advanced or Metastatic Sarcoma Treated With Talimogene Laherparepvec in Combination With Pembrolizumab: A Phase 2 Clinical Trial. JAMA Oncol 2020;6(3):402–8.

80. Pollack SM. The potential of the CMB305 vaccine regimen to target NY-ESO-1 and improve outcomes for synovial sarcoma and myxoid/round cell liposarcoma patients. Expert Rev Vaccin 2018;17(2):107–14.

81. Somaiah N, Chawla SP, Block MS, et al. A Phase 1b Study Evaluating the Safety, Tolerability, and Immunogenicity of CMB305, a Lentiviral-Based Prime-Boost Vaccine Regimen, in Patients with Locally Advanced, Relapsed, or Metastatic Cancer Expressing NY-ESO-1. Oncoimmunology 2020;9(1):1847846.

82. Chawla SP, Van Tine BA, Pollack SM, et al. Phase II Randomized Study of CMB305 and Atezolizumab Compared With Atezolizumab Alone in Soft-Tissue Sarcomas Expressing NY-ESO-1. J Clin Oncol 2021;Jco2003452. https://doi. org/10.1200/JCO.20.03452.

83. Dancsok AR, Gao D, Lee AF, et al. Tumor-associated macrophages and macrophage-related immune checkpoint expression in sarcomas. Oncoimmunology 2020;9(1):1747340.

84. Chen L, Oke T, Siegel N, et al. The Immunosuppressive Niche of Soft-Tissue Sarcomas is Sustained by Tumor-Associated Macrophages and Characterized by Intratumoral Tertiary Lymphoid Structures. Clin Cancer Res 2020;26(15):4018–30.

85. Chawla, S.P., et al. RESULTS FROM THE CHONDROSARCOMA PHASE 1 STUDY EXPANSION COHORT OF THE TETRAVALENT DEATH RECEPTOR 5 AGONIST INBRX-109. in Connective Tissue Oncology Society Annual Meeting. November 19, 2020.

86. Coley WB. The treatment of malignant tumors by repeated inoculations of erysipelas. With a report of ten original cases. 1893. Clin Orthop Relat Res 1893; 1991(262):3–11.

87. Kawai, A., et al., Efficacy and safety of nivolumab monotherapy in patietns with unresectable clear cell sarcoma and alveolar soft part sarcoma (OSCAR trial, NCCH1510): A multicenter, Phase 2 clinical trial., in Connective Tissue Oncology Society Annual Meeting. November 19, 2020.

88. Hindi N, Rosenbaum E, Jonczak E, et al. Retrospective world-wide registry on the efficacy of immune checkpoint inhibitors in alveolar soft part sarcoma: Updated results from sixty patients. Jco 2021;39(15_suppl):11564.

89. Somaiah N, Conley AP, Lin HY, et al. A phase II multi-arm study of durvalumab and tremelimumab for advanced or metastatic sarcomas. Jco 2020; 38(15_suppl):11509.

90. Naqash AR, O'Sullivan Coyne GH, Moore N, et al. Phase II study of atezolizumab in advanced alveolar soft part sarcoma (ASPS). Jco 2021;39(15_suppl):11519.

91. Shi Y, Cai Q, Jiang Y, et al. Activity and Safety of Geptanolimab (GB226) for Patients with Unresectable, Recurrent, or Metastatic Alveolar Soft Part Sarcoma: A Phase II, Single-arm Study. Clin Cancer Res 2020;26(24):6445–52.

92. Yang J, Dong L, Yang S, et al. Safety and clinical efficacy of toripalimab, a PD-1 mAb, in patients with advanced or recurrent malignancies in a phase I study. Eur J Cancer 2020;130:182–92.

93. D'Angelo SP, Shoushtari AN, Keohan ML, et al. Combined KIT and CTLA-4 Blockade in Patients with Refractory GIST and Other Advanced Sarcomas: A Phase Ib Study of Dasatinib plus Ipilimumab. Clin Cancer Res 2017;23(12): 2972–80.

94. Gordon EM, Chua-Alcala VS, Kim K, et al. SAINT: Results of a phase 1/2 study of safety/efficacy using safe amounts of ipilimumab, nivolumab, and trabectedin as first-line treatment of advanced soft tissue sarcoma. Jco 2019;37(15_suppl): 11016.

95. Palmerini E, Lopez-Pousa A, Grignani G, et al. IMMUNOSARC: a collaborative Spanish (GEIS) and Italian (ISG) sarcoma groups phase I/II trial of sunitinib and nivolumab in advanced soft tissue and bone sarcoma: Results from the phase II part, bone sarcoma cohort. Jco 2020;38(15_suppl):11522.

Retroperitoneal and Mesenteric Liposarcomas

Caroline C.H. Siew, MBBS, MMed (Surgery), FRCS[a,b], Sameer S. Apte, MDCM, FRCSC[c],
Marco Baia, MD[d], David E. Gyorki, MBBS, MD, FRACS[c], Samuel Ford, MD, PhD, FRCS[d],
Winan J. van Houdt, MD, PhD, MS[a],*

KEYWORDS

- Liposarcoma • Retroperitoneal liposarcoma • Mesenteric liposarcoma
- Well-differentiated liposarcoma • Dedifferentiated liposarcoma

KEY POINTS

- Retroperitoneal liposarcomas are mainly well-differentiated or de-differentiated liposarcomas. Extended surgery with liberal organ resection is the cornerstone of treatment.
- Histologic subtype and grade determine oncological outcomes, with 8-year survival ranging between 30% and 80%.
- Local recurrence is a major issue, with rates around 40%.
- Neoadjuvant radiotherapy can be considered in well-differentiated liposarcomas or low-grade DDLPS.
- The role of neoadjuvant chemotherapy for high-grade DDLPS will be explored in the EORTC 1809 – STRASS2 trial.

INTRODUCTION

Retroperitoneal sarcomas (RPS) are a rare heterogeneous group of mesenchymal neoplasms, which represent around 15% of soft tissue sarcomas, with an estimated annual incidence of 5 per million.[1,2] The main histologic subtypes in the retroperitoneum are liposarcoma (LPS; 66%), leiomyosarcoma (LMS; 18%), solitary fibrous tumor (5%), malignant peripheral nerve sheath tumor (3%) and undifferentiated pleomorphic sarcoma (3%).[3,4] Each sarcoma histologic subtype demonstrates distinct clinical behavior, treatment response, and outcomes. Mesenteric sarcomas (MS)

[a] Department of Surgical Oncology, The Netherlands Cancer Institute – Antoni van Leeuwenhoek, Plesmanlaan 121, Amsterdam 1066 CX, the Netherlands; [b] Department of General Surgery, Tan Tock Seng Hospital, 11 Jalan Tan Tock Seng, 308433 Singapore; [c] Department of Surgical Oncology, Peter MacCallum Cancer Centre, 305 Grattan Street, Melbourne, Victoria, 3000 Australia; [d] The Sarcoma Unit, Queen Elizabeth Hospital Birmingham NHS Foundation Trust, Mindelsohn Way, Edgbaston, Birmingham B15 2GW, UK
* Corresponding author.
E-mail address: w.v.houdt@nki.nl

Surg Oncol Clin N Am 31 (2022) 399–417
https://doi.org/10.1016/j.soc.2022.03.005

are extremely rare, with dedifferentiated liposarcomas (DDLPS) being the predominant histologic subtype (48%), followed by leiomyosarcomas (23%) and well-differentiated liposarcomas (WDLPS; 14%).[5]

There are different biologic groups of liposarcomas: WDLPS, DDLPS, myxoid liposarcomas and pleomorphic liposarcomas. These various subtypes have different molecular backgrounds and genetic alterations, which presumably drive tumor initiation.[6] WDLPS and DDLPS are the most common and almost always associated with amplification of the chromosome segment 12q13-15, which harbors the oncogenes murine double minute 2 (*MDM2*), cyclin-dependent kinase (*CDK4*), and high mobility group A (*HMGA2*).[7,8] Myxoid liposarcomas are characterized by *FUS-DDIT3* translocations or *EWSR-DDIT3* fusions. They are primarily located in the extremity and rarely in the retroperitoneum as the primary location.[6] Pleomorphic liposarcomas are often high-grade lesions with the loss of p53 and retinoblastoma protein, and are associated with a poor prognosis.[9] They are usually aggressive with high risk of metastases but are rare in the retroperitoneum or mesentery.

Because retroperitoneal liposarcomas (RPLPS) and mesenteric liposarcomas (MLPS) mostly comprise of WDLPS and DDLPS, these entities will be the main focus of this review.

WORKUP
Presentation and Evaluation

RPLPS commonly present as a slowly enlarging, painless abdominal mass or an incidental finding on imaging.[10] Less commonly, patients present with clinically significant symptoms due to mass effect on surrounding structures (paraesthesia, lower extremity edema, deep vein thrombosis, back pain, early satiety, and bowel obstruction). Rarely, a rapidly expanding RPLPS presents with systemic manifestations such as night sweats, fevers, flu-like symptoms, or weight loss (<1% of patients).[11] Given the lack of symptoms, RPLPS tend to present late and are often large. Symptoms or signs suggesting compression of critical structures should be used to guide preoperative imaging assessment.

Given the heterogeneity and complexity of the disease, it is recommended that suspected RPLPS should be referred to high-volume sarcoma centers for evaluation and management. Assessment at a sarcoma center also facilitates inclusion in clinical trials or multiinstitutional prospective registries.

Imaging

International guidelines recommend computed tomography (CT) scan of the chest, abdomen, and pelvis with intravenous contrast as standard of care.[12-14] Cross-sectional imaging is essential for: (1) ruling out metastases (primarily liver and lung), (2) assessing the extent of the primary tumor and its anatomic relations, and (3) confirming resectability. Often, an arterial phase contrast CT is useful to aid in preoperative planning regarding proximity to major vascular structures. When resection of RPLPS requires a nephrectomy, assessment of the contralateral kidney function by differential renal scan or perfusion on arterial phase CT is advised. Extrapulmonary metastases to the bone and paraspinal soft tissue is common in myxoid liposarcomas (2% of RPLPS),[15] and these sites should be evaluated.[16] CT findings of WDLPS include abnormal retroperitoneal fat distribution, displacement of the intra-abdominal structures, fibrous septa (>2 mm), nodular soft tissue foci, and heterogenous fat density[17,18] (**Fig. 1**). DDLPS generally demonstrate a large proportion of solid soft tissue density on CT, with variable areas of heterogenous fat density[18] (**Fig. 2**).

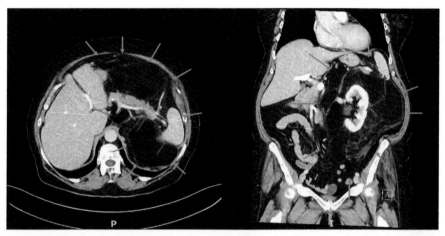

Fig. 1. Axial and coronal CT views of a well-differentiated retroperitoneal liposarcoma showing fat density, internal septa, and displaced abdominal viscera. Left Panel: Blue arrows – outline of tumor margin. Red arrows – pancreatic tail and spleen surrounded by tumor. Right panel: Blue arrows – outline of tumor margin. Red arrows – kidney and spleen surrounded by tumor.

Well-differentiated and de-differentiated LPS often coexist, necessitating careful evaluation by a sarcoma radiologist to delineate the extent of well-differentiated disease and proximity to critical structures. Importantly, preoperative planning does not reliably predict gross organ invasion in DDLPS, and the surgeon must consider this when interpreting imaging.[19]

Magnetic Resonance Imaging (MRI) is an alternative to CT when an iodinated contrast allergy is present.[17] Additionally, MRI is useful for determining anatomic

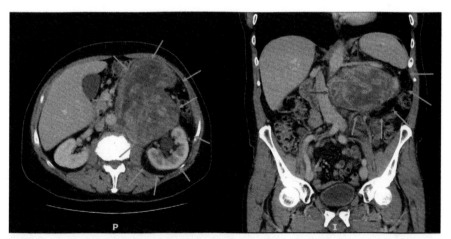

Fig. 2. Axial and coronal CT views of a grade III dedifferentiated retroperitoneal liposarcoma showing heterogenous soft-tissue density and sparse fat density. Left panel: Blue arrows – lateral tumor extent. Red arrow – tumor abutting left side of the aorta. Right panel: Blue arrows – lateral tumor extent. Red arrows – tumor displacing inferior vena cava, and left renal artery.

relationships of RPLPS to major nerves (sciatic or femoral), vessels, muscle, fascia, and the paraspinal nerve roots.[20] For RPLPS in the pelvis, MRI also helps to determine the proximity to rectum, sphincter muscles, bladder, ureters, gynecologic organs, and major neural foramina (sciatic, femoral, and obturator).[17,18]

The use of ^{18}F-fluorodeoxyglucose positron emission tomography (FDG-PET) may be complementary to CT and MRI in the work up of RPLPS. In 2 recent studies, FDG-avidity in RPS was highly associated with tumor grade, recurrence-free and overall survival.[21,22] FDG-PET also has an important role in increasing the diagnostic accuracy of tumor grading from percutaneous biopsies, by identifying the most metabolically active area to target[23,24] (**Fig. 3**). Additionally, in the context of equivocal or technically infeasible biopsy (eg, mesenteric LPS surrounded by bowel), high FDG-avidity can indicate a higher-grade tumor.[25] Accordingly, FDG-avidity can aid in the decision to manage the tumor as DDLPS or WDLPS and consideration for preoperative chemotherapy or radiotherapy. Finally, when CT findings are ambiguous in WDLPS, FDG-PET showing low FDG-avidity can corroborate low-tumor grade on biopsy.[26]

Biopsy

Mesenchymal tumors represent only a third of retroperitoneal lesions,[17] and other differentials such as lymphoma, germ cell tumor, or carcinomas will need to be considered in the evaluation of a retroperitoneal mass. Percutaneous core needle biopsy is, hence, recommended to confirm the diagnosis in suspected RPLPS.[27] Fine-needle aspiration (FNA) is low yield and should be avoided.[27] In a study of 503 retroperitoneal lesions, core biopsy differentiated malignant from benign tumors 98% of the time, and determined subtype with 88% to 90% accuracy.[28] Preoperative biopsy informs on tumor grade, which is a critical factor for surgical planning, selecting possible neoadjuvant therapies, and enrollment in clinical trials.[29] Core biopsy can also harvest sufficient tissue for molecular subtyping, genetic analysis, and tumor banking. A retroperitoneal approach with multiple, large (14G to 16G) coaxial cores is the preferred

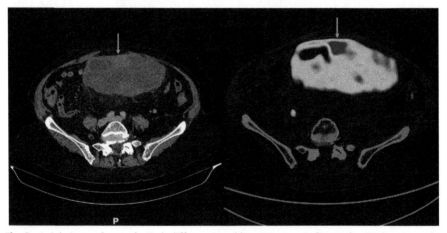

Fig. 3. Axial views of a grade III dedifferentiated liposarcoma. Left panel – CT showing relative homogeneity of tumor. Right panel – [18]FDG-PET avidity of superficial central part of lesion (*red area*) showing the highest-grade area of tumor to target during biopsy (*blue arrow*).

method of biopsy.[27,28,30] In a retrospective analysis of 498 patients who underwent core biopsy for RPS, needle-tract recurrences (2%) only occurred after a transabdominal, noncoaxial approach.[31]

Nearly all RPLPS display *MDM2* gene amplification by fluorescence in-situ hybridization (FISH) or by newer sequencing techniques.[32] *MDM2* FISH testing is particularly useful for differentiating low-grade RPLPS with scant mitoses from benign lipomas.[32] Similarly, the *DDIT3* gene rearrangements that characterize myxoid liposarcomas are detectable by FISH[33] or sequencing.

MANAGEMENT

All cases should be discussed in a multidisciplinary tumor board with sarcoma specialists from Radiology, Pathology, Surgical, Medical, and Radiation Oncology to determine the best treatment options.[12]

Surgery

Surgery is the cornerstone of treatment for RPLPS and a complete resection presents the only chance of cure. The goal of surgery is to perform a complete macroscopic resection, with a single specimen of the tumor and en bloc removal of involved organs[12] (**Fig. 4**). However, these are often large tumors in close proximity to organs and within the confines of the retroperitoneum, which makes resection with wide margins challenging. As a result, RPLPS are associated with a worse prognosis than extremity liposarcomas even for WDLPS, with locoregional recurrences accounting for most deaths.[34] Surgical planning should analyze anatomic relationships with other viscera, neurovascular structures, muscles, and bones. Imaging should be scrutinized for tumor extension out of the retroperitoneum, for example, through the inguinal canal, because this would require a different surgical approach. Features suggesting potential unresectability such as encasement of superior mesenteric vessels or celiac trunk, involvement of the suprahepatic veins or multifocal disease should also be assessed.[35]

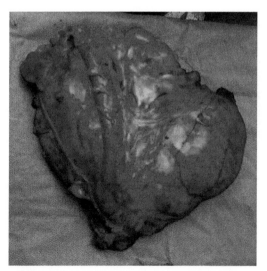

Fig. 4. Retroperitoneal liposarcoma resection specimen with en bloc removal of colon, kidney, distal pancreas, and spleen.

The surgical strategy for RPS resection has shifted during the years from mostly simple excisions of the tumor with resection of only contiguous involved organs to compartmental multivisceral resections en bloc with the tumor. It is impossible to distinguish normal fat from WDLPS; hence, all ipsilateral retroperitoneal fat should be resected (**Fig. 5**). There is no role for intraoperative frozen section because this is unreliable and difficult to interpret.[36]

Initial surgical series during 1982 to 2009 showed 5-year local recurrence-free survival rates of 50% to 60%.[35] In 2009, French and Italian sarcoma groups each published retrospective studies evaluating an aggressive surgical approach for primary RPS to improve surgical margins and hence local control.[37,38] A liberal approach to resection of organs close to the tumor regardless of invasion was described, and the technical details published in 2012.[35] The colon, kidney, and psoas were often resected with no increase in morbidity, whereas resections of the distal pancreas, spleen, and diaphragm had a slight increased risk of morbidity. Resection of major vessels was associated with the highest risk of complications; hence, subadventitial dissection of tumor is advised when the tumor is in close proximity to major vessels, whereas resection of major vessels with reconstruction is only performed for direct tumor invasion. The duodenum, head of pancreas, liver, and bone are also only resected if clearly infiltrated. The French series indicated a 3.29-fold lower rate of abdominal recurrence after complete compartmental resection.[37] The Italian series revealed significant improvement in 5-year overall survival from 48% to 66% and decrease in 5-year local recurrences from 49% to 28% with extended surgery.[39] However, this seems to mainly benefit low and intermediate grade tumors because high-grade tumors tend to develop distant metastases. Extended surgery in the French group led to 18% morbidity and 3% mortality, with a trend of increase in morbidity if more than 3 viscera were resected.[40] A Transatlantic Australasian Retroperitoneal Sarcoma Working Group (TARPSWG) report on postoperative morbidity after radical resection in specialist sarcoma centers showed 16.4% morbidity, 10.5% reoperation rate, and 1.8% 30-day mortality.[41] The most common adverse events were bleeding/hematoma (2.9%) and bowel anastomotic leakages (2.6%),

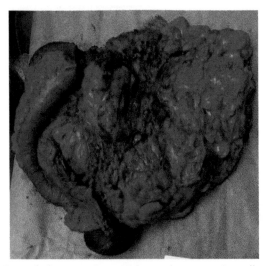

Fig. 5. Posterior view of the resection specimen demonstrating all retroperitoneal fat removed en bloc

but these had no impact on oncological outcome. Pancreaticoduodenectomy, vascular resection, and combined resections involving the colon, kidney, pancreas, and spleen were associated with higher risk of severe adverse events. The morbidity of this surgical approach within reasonable limits is comparable with other major abdominal surgeries.

Amid the shift in surgical approaches, there has been debate between various sarcoma centers regarding the optimal approach to RPS resection.[42] The rate of histologic organ invasion from retrospective reviews ranges from 26%[19] to 61%.[43] Some question the rationale for liberal removal of adjacent organs without evidence of tumor involvement.[44] Others view organ invasion as a marker of biologic aggressiveness and an extended surgical approach within acceptable limits offers the best chance of cure.[45] There is no standardized extent of surgical resection for RPLPS but the recently updated consensus approach from the TARPSWG for the management of primary RPS has acknowledged the more extended approach.[12] Nevertheless, treatment must be individualized with consideration of patient factors, tumor biology, and local tumor extent on preoperative imaging. The benefits of oncological resection need to be balanced with the operative morbidity and impact on quality of life for each patient.

The complex nature of the resection potentially requiring multiorgan resection may necessitate multidisciplinary expertise from vascular surgery, hepatobiliary surgery, urology, or orthopedic surgery. Complete resection significantly affects recurrence and survival, hence quality surgery is crucial. Surgical practice and therapeutic approaches for sarcoma vary across different institutes, and higher volume leads to higher quality care and better outcomes. A review of the National Cancer Data Base by Keung and colleagues found that surgery in high-volume hospitals was associated with fewer incomplete resections (1.6% vs 4.5%), lower 30-day mortality (1.9% vs 3.1%) and longer 5-year overall survival (57.7% vs 52%).[46] High-volume hospitals were defined as facilities averaging greater than 10 cases per year and additional analyses found progressive improvements in patient outcomes with increasing hospital case volume. Hence, the call for centralization of care for RPLPS to expert sarcoma centers, with a multicenter analysis identifying the threshold where hospital case volume impacts the overall survival as 13 procedures/year.[47]

Radiotherapy

Given the tendency for abdominal recurrence of RPLPS despite extended resection, preoperative, intraoperative, and postoperative radiotherapies have been used in the hope of improving local control. Several retrospective and some prospective studies have described increased local control but less impact on overall survival,[48–50] whereas other reports showed no benefit.[51]

With no definite evidence on its role and optimal timing, the use of radiotherapy has thus been variable with around 30% of RPS patients receiving radiotherapy and a recent trend toward preoperative therapy.[50,52] Preoperative radiotherapy is generally preferred to postoperative radiotherapy: adjacent viscera are displaced by tumor out of the treatment field, target volume definition is more accurate,[53] and an oxygenated tumor in situ is more radiosensitive with potential for downsizing, improved complete resection and lower risks of tumor seeding.[54] Intraoperative radiotherapy allows dose delivery directly to the tumor bed with promising results for local control but is not widely used due to significant toxicities such as bowel perforation, fistulas, strictures, and neuropathy.[55,56]

Following the attempted randomized trial by the American College of Surgeons Oncology Group to assess the role of preoperative radiotherapy for RPS, which closed due to poor accrual, the EORTC-62092 STRASS trial was conducted across 31 international centers to evaluate the impact of preoperative radiotherapy on abdominal recurrence in all histologic subtypes of RPS.[57] After a median follow-up of 43 months for 266 patients, the trial showed similar abdominal recurrence-free survival and overall survival at 3 years for surgery alone versus surgery with preoperative radiotherapy for localized primary RPS in general. However, liposarcomas compromised almost 75% of the cohort, and post hoc analysis demonstrated abdominal recurrence-free survival for RPLPS at 3 years was 65.2% in the surgery group compared with 75.7% in the radiotherapy plus surgery group (HR 0.6; 95% CI 0.38–1.02). The conclusion was that preoperative radiotherapy is currently not standard of care for RPS but could be beneficial for low-to-intermediate grade RPLPS.

Next, the STREXIT series was performed to explore the potential effect of radiotherapy on retroperitoneal liposarcoma recurrence that the subgroup analysis in the STRASS trial had suggested. Data were obtained from patients with primary RPS that were not enrolled in STRASS but were still treated at 10 STRASS trial centers during the trial period.[58] These patients in the STREXIT cohort underwent surgery with curative intent with or without preoperative radiotherapy. The cohort was evaluated after propensity score matching and subgroup analysis for RPLPS showed that radiotherapy correlated with better abdominal recurrence-free survival with an HR of 0.58. Further subgroup analyses on the pooled STRASS and STREXIT cohorts of 528 patients showed improved abdominal recurrence-free survival in WDLPS and grade I-II DDLPS with the addition of preoperative RT. The 5-year abdominal recurrence-free survival was 63.9% in the radiotherapy with surgery group compared with 51% in the group with surgery alone (HR 0.62; 95% CI 0.41–0.93). This benefit was not appreciated for grade III DDLPS. Overall survival for all RPS histologic subtypes and RPLPS were similar regardless of radiotherapy administration. The study suggests the use of preoperative radiotherapy in primary retroperitoneal WDLPS and grade I-II DDLPS can improve local control, but the effect on survival may require longer follow-up.

Chemotherapy

Systemic chemotherapy is used in neoadjuvant and adjuvant settings, advanced or metastatic disease. The role of chemotherapy is not clearly defined for RPLPS, and most data are obtained from trials on soft tissue sarcomas in general or extrapolated from studies on extremity sarcomas.[59] The chemosensitivity of liposarcomas is restricted to dedifferentiated liposarcomas with overall response rates of 21%[60] and higher response in the myxoid subtype.[61] Sarcoma subtypes have varying responses to different chemotherapy regimens. Common regimens for liposarcomas are doxorubicin alone or with ifosfamide and gemcitabine with docetaxel in a first-line setting, and trabectedin and erubulin in a second-line setting.[62]

Neoadjuvant chemotherapy has the potential advantage of evaluating tumor biology, addressing micrometastases to prevent the development of distant metastases and reducing tumor size, hence facilitating resection.[59] A retrospective multicenter study of 158 patients from 2008 to 2018 with primary RPS who received neoadjuvant chemotherapy followed by complete resection was performed to evaluate tumor responses and clinical outcomes.[63] Chemotherapy regimens were mostly anthracycline based but also included ifosfamide alone and gemcitabine plus docetaxel. The 71 DDLPS patients demonstrated partial response in 19.7%, stable disease in 52.1%, and progressive disease in 28.2%. WDLPS comprised 14 patients and demonstrated partial response in 21.4%, stable disease in 78.6%, and none progressed while on neoadjuvant systemic therapy. Tumor response to systemic therapy was predictive of clinical outcomes, with significantly worse overall survival for patients who had progressive disease. Following the findings of this pilot study, the EORTC-1809 STRASS2 trial will evaluate whether neoadjuvant chemotherapy will increase the disease-free survival in 2 types of high-risk RPS—grade III DDLPS and LMS.[64] A regimen of doxorubicin and ifosfamide will be administered for grade III DDLPS, whereas the combination of doxorubicin and dacarbazine has been selected for LMS. Patients will be randomized between 3 cycles of neoadjuvant chemotherapy followed by surgery or surgery alone. This multicenter phase III trial started recruiting in 2020 with estimated completion in 2028.

OUTCOMES, PROGNOSTIC FACTORS, AND NOMOGRAMS

The founders of TARPSWG published a retrospective series on 1007 primary RPS patients who underwent resection across 8 European and North American sarcoma reference centers between 2002 and 2011, evaluating treatment variations and patterns of recurrence.[50] Histologic subtype and grade had significant impact on oncological outcome and pattern of treatment failure. The 8-year overall survival exceeded 80% for WDLPS but was 43.9% for DDLPS (**Fig. 6** for the overall survival curve of WDLPS and DDLPS). Histologic grade is a major prognostic determinant and the French National Federation of Comprehensive Cancer (FNCLCC) grading system can be used to further prognosticate DDLPS.[65] The 8-year survival was 50% for grade II DDLPS and 30% for grade III DDLPS.[50] Deaths for WDLPS and grade II DDLPS were mostly related to local recurrence, given that WDLPS almost never metastasize and risk of distant metastases in DDLPS is less than 10%. However, grade III DDLPS have greater than 30% risk for distant metastases at 8 years.

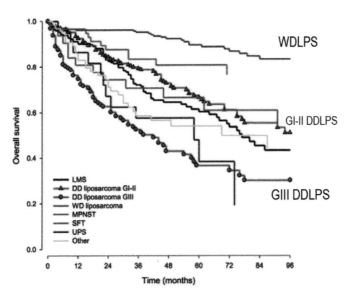

Fig. 6. Overall survival curve for retroperitoneal sarcomas according to histologic subtypes. (*From* Gronchi A et al. Variability in Patterns of Recurrence After Resection of Primary Retroperitoneal Sarcoma (RPS): A Report on 1007 Patients From the Multi-institutional Collaborative RPS Working Group. *Ann Surg.* May 2016;263(5):1002-9; with permission.)

RPLPS have a predilection for local recurrence. Local recurrence rates at 8 years in the TARPSWG series were more than 40% for DDLPS but ranged between 5% and 42.5% for WDLPS depending on treatment institution[50] (**Figs. 7** and **8** for crude cumulative incidences of local recurrence and distant metastases in WDLPS and DDLPS). The improved local control for WDLPS in some institutions highlighted the significance of extended surgical resections. An analysis by the Memorial Sloan Kettering Cancer Center of their cohort of 675 patients who had surgery for primary RPS from 1982 to 2010 demonstrated that DDLPS are more inclined to recur early, with 5-year local recurrence of 58%.[66] In comparison, WDLPS showed local recurrence rates of 39% at 5 years which gradually increased to 60% at 15 years.[66]

Known prognostic factors for survival include histologic subtype, grade, tumor size and multifocality, patient age, and treatment-related features including completeness of resection, tumor rupture, and center expertise.[37,38,50,67-71] Predictive nomograms have been described to integrate these variables and aid stratification of prognosis. The first nomogram for soft tissue sarcoma was designed at the Memorial Sloan Kettering Center (MSKCC) in 2002 and evaluated age, histology, tumor size, and depth to predict 12-year sarcoma-specific death.[72] RPS-specific nomograms were subsequently developed, with 4 currently available.

The MD Anderson Cancer Center described the first RPS-specific nomogram in 2010, which evaluated the following variables to predict median, 3-year and 5-year overall survival—age, presentation (primary or recurrent), tumor size, multifocality, histology, and completeness of resection.[73] The National Cancer Institute in Milan also developed a nomogram to predict 5-year and 10-year overall survival but focused on primary RPS.[74] Variables used were age, histology, grade, tumor size, and surgical margins. These nomograms did not address the risk of

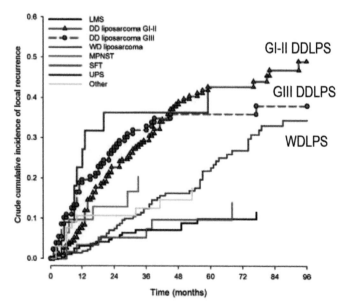

Fig. 7. Crude cumulative incidence of local recurrence for retroperitoneal sarcomas, according to histologic subtypes. (*From* Gronchi A et al. Variability in Patterns of Recurrence After Resection of Primary Retroperitoneal Sarcoma (RPS): A Report on 1007 Patients From the Multi-institutional Collaborative RPS Working Group. *Ann Surg.* May 2016;263(5):1002-9; with permission)

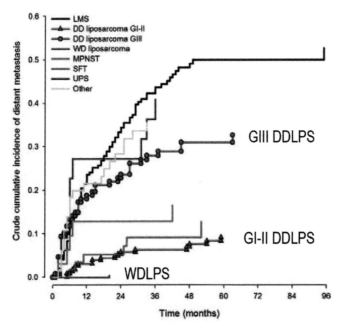

Fig. 8. Crude cumulative incidence of distant metastases for retroperitoneal sarcomas, according to histologic subtypes. (*From* Gronchi A et al. Variability in Patterns of Recurrence After Resection of Primary Retroperitoneal Sarcoma (RPS): A Report on 1007 Patients From the Multi-institutional Collaborative RPS Working Group. Ann Surg. May 2016;263(5):1002-9; with permission)

recurrence, until Gronchi and colleagues created 2 nomograms in 2013 for patients with primary resected RPS for the prediction of 7-year overall survival and disease-free survival.[75] Covariates include age, tumor size, histologic subtype, FNCLCC grade, multifocality and completeness of resection. These 2 nomograms have been endorsed by the eighth edition of the *American Joint Committee on Cancer (AJCC) Staging Manual* and are available as a smartphone application "Sarculator" for ease of daily use. The most recent nomograms for primary RPS from MSKCC are formulated to predict disease-specific death, local and distant recurrence at 3, 5, and 15 years, with each nomogram incorporating different variables.[66]

The use of nomograms to predict personalized prognosis will complement patient discussions and treatment planning, and is partially replacing the use of traditional classification systems. However, the allocation of patients into prognostic stage groups using the AJCC TNM staging system can still be used to compare patient groups.

RECURRENCE

Local recurrence is a significant issue in RPS and the predominant cause of mortality for RPLPS,[34] with 76% to 80% of liposarcomas recurring locally in the absence of distant metastases.[76–78] Surgical resection is usually the preferred option for treatment when feasible, but patient selection, the decision whether to use radiotherapy or chemotherapy and the choice of optimal timing for intervention is usually challenging. A period of observation to ascertain tumor biology can be useful for patient selection because locally recurrent liposarcomas with growth rates beyond 0.9 cm/

mo are associated with poor outcomes despite aggressive surgery.[79] Patients with multifocal intra-abdominal disease or concurrent distant metastases are generally not surgical candidates.[80,81]

The large retrospective series of resected primary RPS[50] was examined for recurrence and outcomes.[77] Among the 1007 patients, 219 experienced local recurrence, 146 had distant metastases, and 43 patients developed both local recurrence and distant metastases. RPLPS made up most of the patients with local recurrence only (80%) and 5-year overall survival was 29%.[77] Patients who underwent resection of the recurrence had improved 5-year overall survival of 43% versus 11% for those without surgery. However, 58% of the patients who had resection of their local recurrence had recurred locally again at 5 years. A recent multicenter study of patient outcomes following second recurrence of RPS after complete resection of a first local recurrence has shown a potential for achieving long-term survival with surgery.[78] Liposarcomas were the predominant histologic subtype among the 323 patients with local recurrence only, with 31% WDLPS and 46.1% DDLPS. Complete resection of this second recurrence was achieved in 61.9% of the patients with locally recurrence only, and yielded remarkable 5-year overall survival of 66.9% for WDLPS and 31.6% for DDLPS.[78] Complete resection of recurrent RPLPS is the only chance for prolonged survival albeit inferior to that of primary RPLPS and will unlikely achieve cure, which needs to be considered against the anticipated morbidity. There is no definite evidence for chemotherapy or radiotherapy in resectable recurrent RPLPS.[81] For unresectable patients, palliative chemotherapy may be considered in selected patients to improve their quality of life. Palliative radiotherapy and even surgery may be considered for symptom control.

SURVEILLANCE

There are few published protocols for the surveillance of resected soft tissue sarcomas, and none for retroperitoneal, abdominal, or pelvic disease.[82,83] Recommended surveillance protocols, published in international sarcoma management guidelines, extrapolate from evidence in lower limb sarcoma and expert opinion.[84,85] Wide differences between specialist centers are seen in the frequency and intensity of follow-up after RPS resection, ranging from no follow-up to regular cross-sectional imaging up to 10 years after surgery.[86,87] No prospective study has evaluated the impact of surveillance intensity on overall survival or considered a comparison with no surveillance. Retrospective data from single institutions have neither demonstrated a survival benefit with intensive surveillance nor any impact on the timing of intervention for WDLPS recurrence.[36,88] Nevertheless, postoperative imaging surveillance continues to be practiced in all major sarcoma centers. This requires significant resources, and the most intense protocol is associated with up to 20× increase in expenditure as compared with the least intense.[89]

QUALITY OF LIFE

Little is known regarding the impact of RPS management on health-related quality of life (HR-QoL). Patient reported outcomes are difficult to assess due to the heterogeneity of the disease and the varying magnitudes of intervention required. There is no sarcoma-specific HR-QoL instrument currently, and it is the subject of several ongoing initiatives. These include the intensive EORTC QOL group efforts, which will hopefully be ready for clinical implementation soon. A prospective series from a single institution, using generic HR-QoL tools, demonstrated that RPS patients were able to regain premorbid HR-QoL in 12 to 24 months following surgical resection. Despite this, chronic neuropathic pain frequently plagues patients who have extensive resection of the iliopsoas tract as part of surgical management.[90] The impact of surveillance imaging on HR-QoL has not been studied in patients with sarcoma but studies in other cancer types have demonstrated associations between increased health-care interaction and symptoms of anxiety and depression.[91,92]

MESENTERIC LIPOSARCOMA

MLPS is an extremely rare entity. In a recently described international retrospective series, WDLPS and DDLPS represented 14% and 48% of resected MS pathologic conditions respectively.[5] Forty-one percent of all MS are FNCLCC grade 3 compared with 27% for RPS with a corresponding reduction in 5-year overall survival at 50%. Wide surgical clearance of MS along with involved viscera is the management of choice, in a similar manner to RPS.[12] Preoperative biopsy is recommended if technically possible, including consideration of endoscopic ultrasound-guided FNA. The site of origin of MS makes these tumors more prone to peritoneal invasion and involvement of central structures such as the superior mesenteric artery, and increases the risk of unresectability.[93] MS exhibit marked variability in lesion size and surgical complexity to achieve a complete resection while maintaining enteric function. Multifocal primary MLPS is a particularly difficult entity to manage and disseminated disease may not be amenable to surgical clearance, with an extremely high recurrence risk due to potential field change. Neoadjuvant chemotherapy may have a role in down-staging DDLPS to facilitate resection against critical structures but is generally a feature of institution-specific protocols.[63,94] The proximity of small bowel limits the utility of neoadjuvant radiotherapy. Active management of local recurrence is encouraged and management strategies include surgical resection, ablative therapy, or systemic therapy.[78] Systemic metastases tend to be hepatic rather than pulmonary, and this reflects the portal venous drainage of MS.

COLLABORATION

There are still many areas where improvements can be made, such as exploring the role of new systemic agents for LPS or fine-tuning personalized approaches for locally recurrent disease. However, given the rarity of both RPLPS and MLPS, collaboration is critical to garner greater knowledge and understanding of the disease. Close collaboration between many centers around the globe has been achieved by the TARPSWG. The TARPSWG was established in 2013 as an international network of sarcoma referral centers with interest in this rare disease.[95] The alliance has enabled multi-center studies with large patient numbers for better understanding of the biology and behavior of RPS. The group has published consensus statements for the management of RPS, and their cooperation was an important motor behind the success of the EORTC-STRASS trials. The prospective Retroperitoneal Sarcoma Registry was established in 2017 by the TARPSWG to collect standardized clinical data of primary RPS patients, and the analysis will allow for greater insights into this entity or research opportunities.[29]

SUMMARY

Surgery remains the mainstay of treatment of RPLPS and MLPS, and an aggressive surgical approach with relatively liberal organ resections is currently considered the standard of care. Patient outcomes are improved with treatment at high-volume sarcoma centers. Local recurrence is the most common cause of death in WDLPS and low-grade DDLPS, whereas mortality in high-grade DDLPS is due to both local recurrences and distant metastases. Neoadjuvant radiotherapy may be beneficial in WDLPS and low-grade DDLPS but not in high grade DDLPS. Neoadjuvant chemotherapy for high-grade DDLPS is currently being evaluated in a multicenter phase III trial (STRASS 2). Treatment of recurrence is a crucial issue and resection can provide the possibility for prolonged survival but this needs to be determined on an individual basis.

CLINICS CARE POINTS

- Extended surgery with liberal organ resection is the cornerstone of treatment of retroperitoneal liposarcoma.
- Complete initial resection offers the best chance of cure, and treatment should be done in high-volume (threshold of 13 procedures/y) expert sarcoma centers.
- Histologic subtype and grade determine oncological outcomes—local recurrences are the major cause of death in well-differentiated liposarcomas (WDLPS) and low-grade dedifferentiated liposarcomas (DDLPS), whereas high-grade DDLPS develop both local recurrences and distant metastases.
- Individualized treatment strategies should be discussed with each patient, balancing the oncological benefit with potential morbidity.
- Neoadjuvant radiotherapy can be considered in WDLPS or low-grade DDLPS.
- The role of neoadjuvant chemotherapy for high-grade DDLPS will be explored in the EORTC 1809 – STRASS2 trial.
- Mesenteric liposarcomas have a larger proportion of high-grade lesions than retroperitoneal liposarcomas and poorer prognosis.

DISCLOSURE

No conflicts of interest, No sources of funding

REFERENCES

1. Porter GA, Baxter NN, Pisters PW. Retroperitoneal sarcoma: a population-based analysis of epidemiology, surgery, and radiotherapy. Cancer Apr 1 2006;106(7): 1610–6.
2. Gatta G, Capocaccia R, Botta L, et al. Burden and centralised treatment in Europe of rare tumours: results of RARECAREnet—a population-based study. Lancet Oncol 2017;18(8):1022–39.
3. Soft tissue and bone tumours. WHO classification of tumours series; 5th edition, Vol. 3. International Agency for Research on Cancer (IARC); 2020.
4. Callegaro D, Raut CP, Ng D, et al. Has the Outcome for Patients Who Undergo Resection of Primary Retroperitoneal Sarcoma Changed Over Time? A Study of Time Trends During the Past 15 years. Ann Surg Oncol 2021; 28(3):1700–9.
5. Tattersall HL, Hodson J, Cardona K, et al. Primary mesenteric sarcomas: Collaborative experience from the Trans-Atlantic Australasian Retroperitoneal Sarcoma Working Group (TARPSWG). J Surg Oncol 2021;123(4):1057–66.
6. Crago AM, Dickson MA. Liposarcoma: Multimodality Management and Future Targeted Therapies. Surg Oncol Clin N Am 2016;25(4):761–73.

7. Mandahl N, Akerman M, Aman P, et al. Duplication of chromosome segment 12q15-24 is associated with atypical lipomatous tumors: a report of the CHAMP collaborative study group. CHromosomes And MorPhology. Int J Cancer 1996; 67(5):632–5.

8. Barretina J, Taylor BS, Banerji S, et al. Subtype-specific genomic alterations define new targets for soft-tissue sarcoma therapy. Nat Genet 2010;42(8):715–21.

9. Dalal KM, Kattan MW, Antonescu CR, et al. Subtype specific prognostic nomogram for patients with primary liposarcoma of the retroperitoneum, extremity, or trunk. Ann Surg 2006;244(3):381–91.

10. Taguchi S, Kume H, Fukuhara H, et al. Symptoms at diagnosis as independent prognostic factors in retroperitoneal liposarcoma. Mol Clin Oncol 2016;4(2): 255–60.

11. Storm FK, Mahvi DM. Diagnosis and management of retroperitoneal soft-tissue sarcoma. Ann Surg 1991;214(1):2–10.

12. Swallow CJ, Strauss DC, Bonvalot S, et al. Management of Primary Retroperitoneal Sarcoma (RPS) in the Adult: An Updated Consensus Approach from the Transatlantic Australasian RPS Working Group. Ann Surg Oncol 2021;28:7873–88.

13. Mv Mehren, Kane JM, Bui MM, et al. NCCN Guidelines Insights: Soft Tissue Sarcoma, Version 1.2021: Featured Updates to the NCCN Guidelines. J Natl Compr Cancer Netw 2020;18(12):1604–12.

14. Gronchi A, Miah AB, Dei Tos AP, et al, GENTURIS. Soft tissue and visceral sarcomas: ESMO-EURACAN-GENTURIS Clinical Practice Guidelines for diagnosis, treatment and follow-up. Ann Oncol 2021;32(11):1348–65.

15. Setsu N, Miyake M, Wakai S, et al. Primary Retroperitoneal Myxoid Liposarcomas. Am J Surg Pathol 2016;40(9):1286–90.

16. Moreau L-C, Turcotte R, Ferguson P, et al. Myxoid \ round cell liposarcoma (MRCLS) revisited: an analysis of 418 primarily managed cases. Ann Surg Oncol 2012;19(4):1081–8.

17. Messiou C, Morosi C. Imaging in retroperitoneal soft tissue sarcoma. J Surg Oncol 2018;117(1):25–32.

18. Messiou C, Moskovic E, Vanel D, et al. Primary retroperitoneal soft tissue sarcoma: Imaging appearances, pitfalls and diagnostic algorithm. Eur J Surg Oncol Jul 2017;43(7):1191–8.

19. Fairweather M, Wang J, Jo VY, et al. Surgical Management of Primary Retroperitoneal Sarcomas: Rationale for Selective Organ Resection. Ann Surg Oncol 2018;25(1):98–106.

20. Craig WD, Fanburg-Smith JC, Henry LR, et al. Fat-containing lesions of the retroperitoneum: radiologic-pathologic correlation. Radiographics 2009;29(1):261–90.

21. Subramaniam S, Callahan J, Bressel M, et al. The role of 18F-FDG PET/CT in retroperitoneal sarcomas—A multicenter retrospective study. J Surg Oncol 2021;123(4):1081–7.

22. Rhu J, Hyun SH, Lee K-H, et al. Maximum standardized uptake value on 18F-fluorodeoxyglucose positron emission tomography/computed tomography improves outcome prediction in retroperitoneal liposarcoma. Scientific Rep 2019; 9(1):6605.

23. Hain SF, O'Doherty MJ, Bingham J, et al. Can FDG PET be used to successfully direct preoperative biopsy of soft tissue tumours? Nucl Med Commun 2003; 24(11):1139–43.

24. Young R, Snow H, Hendry S, et al. Correlation between percutaneous biopsy and final histopathology for retroperitoneal sarcoma: a single-centre study. ANZ J Surg 2020;90(4):497–502.

25. Rakheja R, Makis W, Skamene S, et al. Correlating Metabolic Activity on ^{18}F-FDG PET/CT With Histopathologic Characteristics of Osseous and Soft-Tissue Sarcomas: A Retrospective Review of 136 Patients. Am J Roentgenol 2012;198(6):1409–16.

26. Parkes A, Urquiola E, Bhosale P, et al. PET/CT Imaging as a Diagnostic Tool in Distinguishing Well-Differentiated versus Dedifferentiated Liposarcoma. Sarcoma 2020;2020:8363986.

27. Fairweather M, Raut CP. To Biopsy, or Not to Biopsy: Is There Really a Question? Ann Surg Oncol 2019;26(13):4182–4.

28. Strauss DC, Qureshi YA, Hayes AJ, et al. The role of core needle biopsy in the diagnosis of suspected soft tissue tumours. J Surg Oncol 2010;102(5):523–9.

29. van Houdt WJ, Raut CP, Bonvalot S, et al. New research strategies in retroperitoneal sarcoma. The case of TARPSWG, STRASS and RESAR: making progress through collaboration. Curr Opin Oncol 2019;31(4):310–6.

30. Berger-Richardson D, Burtenshaw SM, Ibrahim AM, et al. Early and Late Complications of Percutaneous Core Needle Biopsy of Retroperitoneal Tumors at Two Tertiary Sarcoma Centers. Ann Surg Oncol 2019;26(13):4692–8.

31. Van Houdt WJ, Schrijver AM, Cohen-Hallaleh RB, et al. Needle tract seeding following core biopsies in retroperitoneal sarcoma. Eur J Surg Oncol 2017; 43(9):1740–5.

32. Weaver J, Downs-Kelly E, Goldblum JR, et al. Fluorescence in situ hybridization for MDM2 gene amplification as a diagnostic tool in lipomatous neoplasms. Mod Pathol 2008;21(8):943–9.

33. Baranov E, Black MA, Fletcher CDM, et al. Nuclear expression of DDIT3 distinguishes high-grade myxoid liposarcoma from other round cell sarcomas. Mod Pathol 2021;34(7):1367–72.

34. Brennan MF, Antonescu CR, Moraco N, et al. Lessons learned from the study of 10,000 patients with soft tissue sarcoma. Ann Surg 2014;260(3):416–21.

35. Bonvalot S, Raut CP, Pollock RE, et al. Technical considerations in surgery for retroperitoneal sarcomas: position paper from E-Surge, a master class in sarcoma surgery, and EORTC-STBSG. Ann Surg Oncol 2012;19(9):2981–91.

36. Singer S, Antonescu CR, Riedel E, et al. Histologic subtype and margin of resection predict pattern of recurrence and survival for retroperitoneal liposarcoma. Ann Surg 2003;238(3):358–70.

37. Bonvalot S, Rivoire M, Castaing M, et al. Primary retroperitoneal sarcomas: a multivariate analysis of surgical factors associated with local control. J Clin Oncol 2009;27(1):31–7.

38. Gronchi A, Lo Vullo S, Fiore M, et al. Aggressive surgical policies in a retrospectively reviewed single-institution case series of retroperitoneal soft tissue sarcoma patients. J Clin Oncol 2009;27(1):24–30.

39. Gronchi A, Miceli R, Colombo C, et al. Frontline extended surgery is associated with improved survival in retroperitoneal low- to intermediate-grade soft tissue sarcomas. Ann Oncol 2012;23(4):1067–73.

40. Bonvalot S, Miceli R, Berselli M, et al. Aggressive surgery in retroperitoneal soft tissue sarcoma carried out at high-volume centers is safe and is associated with improved local control. Ann Surg Oncol 2010;17(6):1507–14.

41. MacNeill AJ, Gronchi A, Miceli R, et al. Postoperative Morbidity After Radical Resection of Primary Retroperitoneal Sarcoma: A Report From the Transatlantic RPS Working Group. Ann Surg 2018;267(5):959–64.

42. Gronchi A, Pollock R. Surgery in retroperitoneal soft tissue sarcoma: a call for a consensus between Europe and North America. Ann Surg Oncol 2011;18(8): 2107–10.

43. Mussi C, Colombo P, Bertuzzi A, et al. Retroperitoneal sarcoma: is it time to change the surgical policy? Ann Surg Oncol 2011;18(8):2136–42.

44. Ikoma N, Roland CL, Torres KE, et al. Concomitant organ resection does not improve outcomes in primary retroperitoneal well-differentiated liposarcoma: A retrospective cohort study at a major sarcoma center. J Surg Oncol 2018; 117(6):1188–94.

45. Strauss DC, Renne SL, Gronchi A. Adjacent, Adherent, Invaded: A Spectrum of Biologic Aggressiveness Rather Than a Rationale for Selecting Organ Resection in Surgery of Primary Retroperitoneal Sarcomas. Ann Surg Oncol 2018; 25(1):13–6.

46. Keung EZ, Chiang YJ, Cormier JN, et al. Treatment at low-volume hospitals is associated with reduced short-term and long-term outcomes for patients with retroperitoneal sarcoma. Cancer 2018;124(23):4495–503.

47. Villano AM, Zeymo A, Chan KS, et al. Identifying the Minimum Volume Threshold for Retroperitoneal Soft Tissue Sarcoma Resection: Merging National Data with Consensus Expert Opinion. J Am Coll Surg 2020;230(1):151–160 e2.

48. Albertsmeier M, Rauch A, Roeder F, et al. External Beam Radiation Therapy for Resectable Soft Tissue Sarcoma: A Systematic Review and Meta-Analysis. Ann Surg Oncol 2018;25(3):754–67.

49. Diamantis A, Baloyiannis I, Magouliotis DE, et al. Perioperative radiotherapy versus surgery alone for retroperitoneal sarcomas: a systematic review and meta-analysis. Radiol Oncol 2020;54(1):14–21.

50. Gronchi A, Strauss DC, Miceli R, et al. Variability in Patterns of Recurrence After Resection of Primary Retroperitoneal Sarcoma (RPS): A Report on 1007 Patients From the Multi-institutional Collaborative RPS Working Group. Ann Surg 2016; 263(5):1002–9.

51. Haas RLM, Bonvalot S, Miceli R, et al. Radiotherapy for retroperitoneal liposarcoma: A report from the Transatlantic Retroperitoneal Sarcoma Working Group. Cancer 2019;125(8):1290–300.

52. Bates JE, Dhakal S, Mazloom A, et al. The Benefit of Adjuvant Radiotherapy in High-grade Nonmetastatic Retroperitoneal Soft Tissue Sarcoma: A SEER Analysis. Am J Clin Oncol 2018;41(3):274–9.

53. Baldini EH, Wang D, Haas RL, et al. Treatment Guidelines for Preoperative Radiation Therapy for Retroperitoneal Sarcoma: Preliminary Consensus of an International Expert Panel. Int J Radiat Oncol Biol Phys 2015;92(3):602–12.

54. Pawlik TM, Ahuja N, Herman JM. The role of radiation in retroperitoneal sarcomas: a surgical perspective. Curr Opin Oncol 2007;19(4):359–66.

55. Jones JJ, Catton CN, O'Sullivan B, et al. Initial results of a trial of preoperative external-beam radiation therapy and postoperative brachytherapy for retroperitoneal sarcoma. Ann Surg Oncol 2002;9(4):346–54.

56. Krempien R, Roeder F, Oertel S, et al. Intraoperative electron-beam therapy for primary and recurrent retroperitoneal soft-tissue sarcoma. Int J Radiat Oncol Biol Phys 2006;65(3):773–9.

57. Bonvalot S, Gronchi A, Le Péchoux C, et al. Preoperative radiotherapy plus surgery versus surgery alone for patients with primary retroperitoneal sarcoma (EORTC-62092: STRASS): a multicentre, open-label, randomised, phase 3 trial. Lancet Oncol 2020;21(10):1366–77.

58. Callegaro D, Gronchi A, et al. Preoperative radiotherapy in patients with primary retroperitoneal sarcoma: EORTC-62092 trial (STRASS) vs off-trial (STREXIT) results. Annals of Surgery 2022;in press.

59. Almond LM, Gronchi A, Strauss D, et al. Neoadjuvant and adjuvant strategies in retroperitoneal sarcoma. Eur J Surg Oncol 2018;44(5):571–9.

60. Livingston JA, Bugano D, Barbo A, et al. Role of chemotherapy in dedifferentiated liposarcoma of the retroperitoneum: defining the benefit and challenges of the standard. Scientific Rep 2017;7(1).

61. Jones RL, Fisher C, Al-Muderis O, et al. Differential sensitivity of liposarcoma subtypes to chemotherapy. Eur J Cancer 2005;41(18):2853–60.

62. Constantinidou A, Jones RL. Systemic therapy in retroperitoneal sarcoma management. J Surg Oncol 2018;117(1):87–92.

63. Tseng WW, Barretta F, Conti L, et al. Defining the role of neoadjuvant systemic therapy in high-risk retroperitoneal sarcoma: A multi-institutional study from the Transatlantic Australasian Retroperitoneal Sarcoma Working Group. Cancer 2021;127(5):729–38.

64. Surgery With Our Without Neoadjuvant Chemotherapy in High Risk RetroPeritoneal Sarcoma. https://ClinicalTrials.gov/show/NCT04031677.

65. Gronchi A, Collini P, Miceli R, et al. Myogenic differentiation and histologic grading are major prognostic determinants in retroperitoneal liposarcoma. Am J Surg Pathol 2015;39(3):383–93.

66. Tan MC, Brennan MF, Kuk D, et al. Histology-based Classification Predicts Pattern of Recurrence and Improves Risk Stratification in Primary Retroperitoneal Sarcoma. Ann Surg 2016;263(3):593–600.

67. Toulmonde M, Bonvalot S, Meeus P, et al. Retroperitoneal sarcomas: patterns of care at diagnosis, prognostic factors and focus on main histological subtypes: a multicenter analysis of the French Sarcoma Group. Ann Oncol 2014;25(3):735–42.

68. Stoeckle E, Coindre JM, Bonvalot S, et al. Prognostic factors in retroperitoneal sarcoma: a multivariate analysis of a series of 165 patients of the French Cancer Center Federation Sarcoma Group. Cancer 2001;92(2):359–68.

69. Anaya DA, Lahat G, Liu J, et al. Multifocality in retroperitoneal sarcoma: a prognostic factor critical to surgical decision-making. Ann Surg 2009;249(1):137–42.

70. Anaya DA, Lev DC, Pollock RE. The role of surgical margin status in retroperitoneal sarcoma. J Surg Oncol 2008;98(8):607–10.

71. Keung EZ, Hornick JL, Bertagnolli MM, et al. Predictors of outcomes in patients with primary retroperitoneal dedifferentiated liposarcoma undergoing surgery. J Am Coll Surg 2014;218(2):206–17.

72. Kattan MW, Leung DH, Brennan MF. Postoperative nomogram for 12-year sarcoma-specific death. J Clin Oncol 2002;20(3):791–6.

73. Anaya DA, Lahat G, Wang X, et al. Postoperative nomogram for survival of patients with retroperitoneal sarcoma treated with curative intent. Ann Oncol 2010;21(2):397–402.

74. Ardoino I, Miceli R, Berselli M, et al. Histology-specific nomogram for primary retroperitoneal soft tissue sarcoma. Cancer 2010;116(10):2429–36.

75. Gronchi A, Miceli R, Shurell E, et al. Outcome prediction in primary resected retroperitoneal soft tissue sarcoma: histology-specific overall survival and disease-free survival nomograms built on major sarcoma center data sets. J Clin Oncol 2013;31(13):1649–55.

76. Stojadinovic A, Yeh A, Brennan MF. Completely resected recurrent soft tissue sarcoma: primary anatomic site governs outcomes. J Am Coll Surg 2002;194(4):436–47.

77. MacNeill AJ, Miceli R, Strauss DC, et al. Post-relapse outcomes after primary extended resection of retroperitoneal sarcoma: A report from the Trans-Atlantic RPS Working Group. Cancer 2017;123(11):1971–8.

78. van Houdt WJ, Fiore M, Barretta F, et al. Patterns of recurrence and survival probability after second recurrence of retroperitoneal sarcoma: A study from TARPSWG. Cancer 2020;126(22):4917–25.
79. Park JO, Qin LX, Prete FP, et al. Predicting outcome by growth rate of locally recurrent retroperitoneal liposarcoma: the one centimeter per month rule. Ann Surg 2009;250(6):977–82.
80. Hamilton TD, Cannell AJ, Kim M, et al. Results of Resection for Recurrent or Residual Retroperitoneal Sarcoma After Failed Primary Treatment. Ann Surg Oncol 2017;24(1):211–8.
81. Trans-Atlantic RPSWG. Management of Recurrent Retroperitoneal Sarcoma (RPS) in the Adult: A Consensus Approach from the Trans-Atlantic RPS Working Group. Ann Surg Oncol 2016;23(11):3531–40.
82. Glasbey JC, Bundred J, Tyler R, et al. The impact of postoperative radiological surveillance intensity on disease free and overall survival from primary retroperitoneal, abdominal and pelvic soft-tissue sarcoma. Eur J Surg Oncol 2021;47(7):1771–7.
83. Raut CP, Callegaro D, Miceli R, et al. Predicting Survival in Patients Undergoing Resection for Locally Recurrent Retroperitoneal Sarcoma: A Study and Novel Nomogram from TARPSWG. Clin Cancer Res 2019;25(8):2664–71.
84. Casali PG, Abecassis N, Aro HT, et al. Soft tissue and visceral sarcomas: ESMO-EURACAN Clinical Practice Guidelines for diagnosis, treatment and follow-up. Ann Oncol 2018;29(Suppl 4):iv51–67.
85. Yahya Zaidi M, Cardona K. Post-operative surveillance in soft tissue sarcoma: using tumor-specific recurrence patterns to direct approach. Chin Clin Oncol 2018;7(4):45.
86. Cipriano CA, Jang E, Tyler W. Sarcoma Surveillance: A Review of Current Evidence and Guidelines. J Am Acad Orthop Surg 2020;28(4):145–56.
87. Gerrand CH, Billingham LJ, Woll PJ, et al. Follow up after Primary Treatment of Soft Tissue Sarcoma: A Survey of Current Practice in the United Kingdom. Sarcoma 2007;34128.
88. Richardson K, Potter M, Damron TA. Image intensive soft tissue sarcoma surveillance uncovers pathology earlier than patient complaints but with frequent initially indeterminate lesions. J Surg Oncol 2016;113(7):818–22.
89. Goel A, Christy ME, Virgo KS, et al. Costs of follow-up after potentially curative treatment for extremity soft-tissue sarcoma. Int J Oncol 2004;25(2):429–35.
90. Fiore M, Brunelli C, Miceli R, et al. A Prospective Observational Study of Multivisceral Resection for Retroperitoneal Sarcoma: Clinical and Patient-Reported Outcomes 1 Year After Surgery. Ann Surg Oncol 2021;28(7):3904–16.
91. Bauml JM, Troxel A, Epperson CN, et al. Scan-associated distress in lung cancer: Quantifying the impact of "scanxiety. Lung Cancer 2016;100:110–3.
92. Tyldesley-Marshall N, Greenfield S, Neilson SJ, et al. The role of Magnetic Resonance Images (MRIs) in coping for patients with brain tumours and their parents: a qualitative study. BMC cancer 2021;21(1):1013.
93. Perhavec A, Provenzano S, Baia M, et al. Inoperable Primary Retroperitoneal Sarcomas: Clinical Characteristics and Reasons Against Resection at a Single Referral Institution. Ann Surg Oncol 2021;28(2):1151–7.
94. Pasquali S, Palassini E, Stacchiotti S, et al. Neoadjuvant treatment: a novel standard? Curr Opin Oncol 2017;29(4):253–9.
95. Callegaro D, Raut CP, Swallow CJ, et al. Retroperitoneal sarcoma: the Transatlantic Australasian Retroperitoneal Sarcoma Working Group Program. Curr Opin Oncol 2021;33(4):301–8.

Management of Myxofibrosarcoma and Undifferentiated Pleomorphic Sarcoma

Aimee M. Crago, MD, PhD, FSSO[a],*, Kenneth Cardona, MD, FSSO[b],
Hanna Koseła-Paterczyk, MD, PhD[c], Piotr Rutkowski, MD, PhD[d]

KEYWORDS

- Undifferentiated pleomorphic sarcoma • Myxofibrosarcoma
- Malignant fibrous histiocytoma • Soft tissue sarcoma • Limb-sparing surgery
- systemic therapy

KEY POINTS

- Undifferentiated pleomorphic sarcoma (UPS) and myxofibrosarcoma (MFS) are genomically complex tumors commonly diagnosed in the extremity and trunk of older patients.
- Although genomically similar, the presence of myxoid stroma is associated with the diagnosis of MFS as opposed to UPS; tumors with highest proportion of myxoid stroma are associated with the lowest rates of metastasis in MFS/UPS.
- MFS has a locally aggressive phenotype. Preoperative assessment with MRI allows for the identification of infiltrative tumor "tails" that are resected en bloc with dominant tumor nodules to minimize local recurrence.
- Adjuvant radiation mitigates risks of local recurrence in UPS/MFS, and there is growing evidence of survival benefit associated with the use of perioperative chemotherapy in patients with high-risk of metastatic disease including those with larger UPS/MFS.
- Treatments for advanced disease include anthracycline-based therapies in the first-line treatment and gemcitabine–docetaxel combination; recent research demonstrates the efficacy of immunotherapy in a proportion of patients.

[a] Department of Surgery, Gastric and Mixed Tumor Service, Memorial Sloan Kettering Cancer Center, 1275 York Avenue, H1220, New York, NY, USA; [b] Division of Surgical Oncology, Department of Surgery, Sarcoma Disease Team, Winship Cancer Institute, Emory University Hospital Midtown, Emory University School of Medicine, 550 Peachtree St, NEMOT, 9th floor, Atlanta, GA 30322, USA; [c] Maria Sklodowska-Curie National Research Institute of Oncology, Deputy for Clinical Oncology Unit in Department of Soft Tissue/Bone, Sarcoma and Melanoma, Warsaw, Poland; [d] Maria Sklodowska-Curie National Research Institute of Oncology, Sarcoma and Melanoma, Roentgena 5, 02-781 Warszawa, Poland
* Corresponding author.
E-mail address: cragoa@mskcc.org
Twitter: @AimeeCragoMD (A.M.C.); @kencardonaMD (K.C.); @rutkowskip1972 (P.R.)

Surg Oncol Clin N Am 31 (2022) 419–430
https://doi.org/10.1016/j.soc.2022.03.006
1055-3207/22/© 2022 Elsevier Inc. All rights reserved.

surgonc.theclinics.com

INTRODUCTION

Undifferentiated pleomorphic sarcoma (UPS) and myxofibrosarcoma (MFS) are the most common histologic subtypes of soft tissue sarcoma (STS) found in the trunk and extremities, together representing approximately 25% of STS diagnosed in these locations. The lesions are rarely identified in the retroperitoneum (**Fig. 1**). They are generally diagnosed during the sixth and seventh decades and present as a painless mass. Preoperative evaluation includes cross-sectional imaging of the tumor, tissue sampling to establish diagnosis and staging to rule out metastases, particularly pulmonary disease. Surgery forms the backbone of therapeutic algorithms for localized disease, although adjuvant radiation plays a role in preventing local recurrence in many patients and neoadjuvant chemotherapy can be considered in a subset of high-risk cases. Systemic therapies for advanced disease include cytotoxic regimens based on, among others, doxorubicin and novel therapeutics such as PD-L1 inhibitors.

PATIENT EVALUATION OVERVIEW
Histologic Diagnosis

Core biopsy and histologic evaluation by an expert STS pathologist establishes the diagnosis of UPS/MFS. UPS, which represents a diagnosis of exclusion, was previously termed malignant fibrous histiocytoma (MFH). The term historically encompassed a *catch-all* for many of the high-grade, poorly differentiated STS with large and irregular nuclei. Although UPS may still represent a heterogeneous group of lesions with variable outcomes, differing progenitor cells and complex karyotypes, modern genomic analysis and immunohistochemical staining techniques have allowed for the term to be more narrowly defined. Many MFH described in historic series were likely dedifferentiated liposarcomas, malignant peripheral nerve sheath tumors, poorly differentiated leiomyosarcomas, or malignant solitary fibrous tumors, each of which can seem similar to UPS microscopically. Clinical findings as well as directed staining for markers such as MDM2 and CDK4, loss of H2k27me3, smooth muscle markers such as SMA, desmin, and caldesmin, and nuclear STAT6 can rule out these respective histologies.[1–4]

Genomic analysis shows significant similarity between UPS and MFS, previously termed myxoid MFH. Both histologies are commonly characterized by complex genomic karyotypes. Loss of *TP53*, *RB*, and *PTEN* are consistently reported copy number alterations observed in at least 10% to 20% of UPS and MFS; mutations in

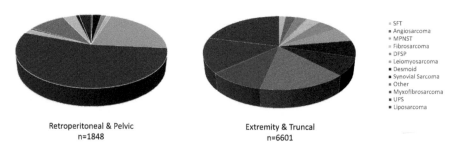

Fig. 1. Histologic classification of STS tumors diagnosed in patients admitted to MSKCC between 1982 and 2021. Liposarcoma, leiomyosarcoma, solitary fibrous tumor, and malignant peripheral nerve sheath tumor represent common histologies in the retroperitoneum and pelvis. UPS/MFH, myxofibrosarcoma, synovial sarcoma, and dermatofibrosarcoma protuberans represent a greater proportion of those tumors diagnosed in the extremity and trunk.

these genes are also identified in both tumor types.[5–8] Copy number alterations affect additional cell cycle regulators such as *CCNE1* and mutations have been observed in *ATRX*, which control telomere length and cellular senescence.[5] Despite these genetic similarities, on histologic evaluation, MFS differs from UPS in that it is associated with an infiltrative and multinodular growth pattern, myxoid stroma in portions of the tumor, spindled and vacuolated cells, and distinctive curvilinear vessels (**Fig. 2**). The tumors can be high grade or low grade, defined in large part by tumor cellularity, whereas UPS is almost uniformly high grade.[9,10]

Outcome is Determined by Histology

Early analysis of MFH outcomes showed poor prognosis with high rates of distal metastases. In a study of 100 patient diagnosed with MFH before 2001, 5-year distant recurrence free survival (DRFS) was only 64%.[11] A similar study analyzing 239 patients undergoing complete surgical resection of MFH between 1982 and 1996 had a 5-year disease-specific survival (DSS) of 65%.[12] Commonly described risk factors, such as tumor size more than 10 cm, were associated with poor outcomes in this study. Because more precise subclassification of pleomorphic sarcomas was described, risk was also shown to be closely associated with presumed histologic origin. For example, in a study by Fletcher and colleagues, 30 of the MFH were reclassified as having myogenic origin (eg, pleomorphic rhabdomyosarcoma, leiomyosarcoma), a finding associated with significantly worse outcomes as compared with the group as a whole.[11]

There is some debate in the literature regarding the percent of the tumor that is required to be myxoid to define a tumor as being an MFS as opposed to UPS and how this in turn may associate with prognosis. A modern series of UPS and MFS was examined in attempt to define the histologic characteristics of each tumor and

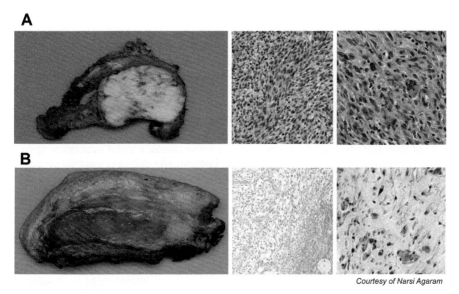

Courtesy of Narsi Agaram

Fig. 2. Gross and microscopic images depicting a representative (*A*) UPS and (*B*) MFS. The latter has a myxoid appearance on gross specimens, and thin, pale, myxoid stroma with curvilinear vessels. UPS is characterized by densely packed cells with large, pleomorphic nuclei, and numerous mitotic bodies.

describe outcomes more precisely after classification using updated ancillary pathology techniques. Tumors were resected between 1992 and 2013 and meticulous rereview of slides was performed to exclude subtypes of pleomorphic sarcoma other than UPS and MFS.[10] The percent of each UPS or MFS that was composed of myxoid stroma was characterized and cut point analysis was used to determine thresholds defining subgroups of the cancers with significant differences in outcome. Tumors with less than 5% myxoid stromal were associated with a DSS of only 36% (vs 60% for those with ≥5% myxoid component). The authors suggested that such a cut point would be appropriate to differentiate UPS and MFS for clinical decision-making. A second subgroup of MFS, defined by those tumors with greater than 70% myxoid content, was associated with particularly good prognosis and a DSS of 66% 5 years after resection (compared with 52% for tumors with 5%–69% myxoid component).

This analysis did not show a significant difference in local recurrence free survival (LRFS) between UPS and MFS but, historically, MFS has been thought to be associated with high rates of recurrent disease (greater than 25% local recurrence risk 5 years after surgery). This finding is thought to be related to its infiltrative nature and has been correlated in multiple studies with close or microscopically positive margins.[13–15] Up to half of these recurrences can be observed outside the direct surgical or radiation field given the multinodular growth pattern of MFS.[16] Second local recurrences can occur in more than half of those patients after the initial recurrence with multiple recurrences historically requiring amputation even at specialty centers.[17] Of note, local recurrence is more commonly observed in high-grade tumors as opposed to low-grade tumors, although this may be a function of a more rapid rate of recurrence in high-grade tumors. Low-grade tumors often recur as high-grade disease associated with an increased risk of distal metastases.[9]

Imaging Work-Up

Distant metastases in high-grade UPS/MFS are most commonly identified in the lung; therefore, staging with chest X-ray or CT is generally sufficient before the treatment of localized disease. Cross-sectional MRI is ideal for defining the extent of local disease before planned resection (**Fig. 3**). UPS often presents as a heterogeneously enhancing mass in the soft tissues. Signals on T1 sequences are similar to those observed for muscle. Central regions of hyperintensity on T2 sequences can represent necrosis or hemorrhage. This can sometimes lead to misdiagnosis of benign hematoma. Although this may be a reasonable consideration in patients prescribed anticoagulants or with history of acute injury, even in these cases, careful evaluation to rule out peripheral nodularity (ie, with subtraction imaging and diffusion weighted imaging on MRI) and consideration of biopsy to rule out occult malignancy should be considered before any attempt at draining the lesion is performed.

Appearance of MFS on MRI imaging is similar to UPS on T1 sequences but on T2 sequences, the lesions are hyperintense, reflecting the myxoid component in the tumors. It is common, particularly in tumors located in the superficial tissues and along fascial planes between muscle compartments to observe multifocality of gross tumor nodules and infiltrative "tails," which can represent microscopic extension of the tumor from areas of gross disease. These "tails" can be differentiated from edema, also hyperintense on T2 sequences, on postcontrast images. MFS-associated "tails" enhance but tumor-associated edema does not. Identification of these curvilinear enhancing "tails" can also be helpful in differentiating MFS from other subtypes of myxoid neoplasm (eg, intramuscular myxoma; see **Fig. 3**).[18,19]

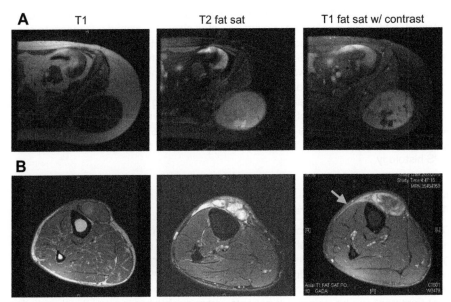

Fig. 3. Although both (*A*) UPS and (*B*) MFS seem similar on T1 sequences, MFS is hyperintense on T2 sequences and can have infiltrative, enhancing tails that extend outward from gross disease (*arrow*).

SURGICAL TREATMENT OPTIONS

Retrospective clinical trials have shown a clear association between complete R0 resection and decreased rates of local recurrence in UPS and MFS. For example, in 425 patients treated by the French National Group, the 5-year local recurrence free rate after R1 resection was 51.6% versus 75.6% after R0 resection.[13] Given such findings, the goal of surgery in UPS/MFS should generally be complete microscopic resection.

As for most high-grade sarcomas, R0 resection of UPS is generally attained by resecting a 1 cm margin of normal tissue around the lesion or removing adjacent fascial margins. In the extremity and trunk, obtaining adequate margins may be difficult due to proximity to neurovascular bundles. When major nerves or vessels are encased by high-grade tumors, these require en bloc resection with the tumor. Arteries can be reconstructed when distal ischemia is a concern. Morbidity related to resection of major nerves can be mitigated by bracing or, in the upper extremity, tendon transfer. Encasement of major neurovascular bundles is rare, however. In most cases, tumors instead displace the structures, and resection is performed by removing the perineurium and vascular sheath. Risk of local recurrence resulting from microscopically positive margins is accepted because local recurrences do not seem to negatively affect the survival and can be mitigated with adjuvant or neoadjuvant radiation.

The infiltrative nature of MFS requires modification of surgery with 2 cm margins resected en bloc with the tumor where feasible. The planned resection bed should include enhancing tails that are visualized during imaging work-up. As previously noted, these tails represent microscopic tumor extension and if not removed increase risk of microscopically positive margins and local recurrence. Such surgery may require the removal of significant portions of skin or create large areas of "dead space" that affect healing; hence, complex reconstruction with rotational or free flaps may be required to reconstruct the operative defect. This reconstruction may be performed in a delayed fashion to confirm by formal pathologic review that microscopically negative margins have been obtained. After initial resection, a vacuum-assisted closure is placed and reconstruction performed as a second procedure after permanent histologic sections have been reviewed. In a series of 53 MFS patients, delayed closured after resection and VAC placement was associated with a lower rate of local recurrence when compared with outcomes in patients treated with immediate reconstruction.[20]

Careful surgical planning and improved understanding of the biology of MFS has resulted in improved rates of local recurrence. In modern series of patients treated at major sarcoma centers are reported to range from 18% to 25%.[10,13,15] These rates are not significantly different than those seen in modern series of the less infiltrative UPS histology.

ADJUVANT THERAPIES
Adjuvant and Neoadjuvant radiation

Decisions regarding the role of adjuvant radiation in treatment of UPS/MFS are generally based on the outcomes of a randomized phase III trial examining limb-sparing surgery after radiation. In the classic study, Yang and colleagues estimated risks of local recurrence after adjuvant radiation were reduced from 22% to 0% 10 years after STS resection. The study did not show that radiation affects overall survival (OS), so adjuvant treatment can be deferred in patients where morbidity associated with radiation may be high or in instances where risk of local recurrence may be low at baseline. For example, prospective data obtained after observation of small, high-grade tumors (T1, <5 cm) showed baseline rates of local recurrence were 7.6% 5 years after R0 resection, a rate that may not justify risk of radiation if recurrence could be managed with salvage surgery.[21] Similarly, a range of retrospective studies has associated low-grade lesions with reduced risk of local recurrence, so observation may be appropriate after resection of these tumors. Baseline risk of local recurrence in STSs can be calculated using a nomogram recently published by Cahlon and colleagues.[22]

Detailed analysis of radiation use in MFS has been performed given its infiltrative nature and associated risk of local recurrence and close or microscopically positive margins after resection. A subset of these studies have shown radiation to be associated with improved rates of local recurrence in a subset (though not all) retrospective analyses.[13] Selection bias may be the cause of variable results. Radiation would, therefore, generally be applied to patients with larger, high-grade tumors with microscopically positive margins as opposed to those with low-grade lesions resected with wide margins where salvage of local recurrence would not be morbid. Such an argument is strengthened by results presented in Mutter and colleagues. Although rates of microscopically positive margins were higher after resections for MFS than a control group of leiomyosarcomas, use of adjuvant radiation was more common in patients with MFS and 5-year LRFS rates were similar in both cohorts (14.6 vs 13.2%, respectively), suggesting the use of adjuvant radiation can optimize local control and compensate for the locally aggressive behavior of MFS.[16]

Adjuvant Chemotherapy

There is growing evidence of the efficacy of adjuvant, doxorubicin-based chemotherapy in a patient with high-risk STS including a subset of UPS/MFS. Retrospective analyses have shown associations between improved outcomes and the use of adjuvant anthracyclines and ifosfamide in large, high-grade sarcomas and in an older meta-analysis of 14 studies using perioperative chemotherapy, a modest benefit was observed in patients receiving adjuvant therapy (4% improvement in OS after 10 years). An update of this meta-analysis included 4 additional trials in which doxorubicin dosing was intensified and combinations with ifosfamide were used. This report showed an absolute risk reduction of death of 11% associated with adjuvant doxorubicin and ifosfamide (AI; 41% versus 30% in patients who did not receive adjuvant therapy.[23]

Recently, the results of the negative EORTC-STBSG 62931 trial (assessing the use of 5 cycles of AI vs no preoperative chemotherapy) were also reanalyzed to examine this question. Specifically, the subset of patients with predicted OS less than 60% 10 years after treatment (as calculated using the Sarculator nomogram that integrates risk based on characteristics such as age, histology, tumor size, and grade) were studied. The revision showed that in these patients, the use of preoperative chemotherapy was associated with significant increase in disease-free survival (DFS; HR = 0.49) and OS (HR = 0.50)[24,25] In EORTC-STBSG 62931, patients with MFH/UPS accounted for 22% of the chemotherapy cohort and 33% of the control population. No benefit has been seen in the prescription of histology-specific regimens (eg, gemcitabine and docetaxel for UPS) as opposed to standard AI in a prospective trial (ISG-STS 1001) of neoadjuvant therapy and AI chemotherapy was related to improved OS and DFS.[26] However, the use of preoperative AI in high-risk STS patients in ISG-STS 1001 was again associated with a better survival than predicted by Sarculator nomogram, which adds the additional evidence for the efficacy of neoadjuvant AI in this patient population.[27]

UPS/MFS greater than 10 cm have generally been associated with metastatic risk significant enough to consider systemic therapy, although risk stratification may be improved using nomograms that integrate multiple tumor and patient characteristics. The results presented in Lee and colleagues, also suggest that in UPS/MFS, patient selection may be further tailored by considering the percent myxoid component of the tumor specifically when considering UPS/MFS as UPS defined by a percent tumor myxoid component of less than 5%, risks of death from disease have been reported to be as high as 64%, so that adjuvant chemotherapy may be of benefit in select patients even with tumors 5 to 10 cm in diameter. For tumors with significant myxoid components (>70%), 5-year DRFS is 65% (vs 24% for tumors with <5% myxoid stroma), so that the treatment may not be associated with as significant a benefit and should be reserved for patients with larger tumors per standard protocols.

MEDICAL TREATMENT OPTIONS FOR ADVANCED DISEASE

Doxorubicin used alone or in combination with ifosfamide remains the standard first-line systemic treatment in patients with metastatic, locally advanced unresectable STS including UPS/MFS.[28] In a randomized study by Judson and colleagues, doxorubicin in monotherapy was compared with a combination of AI in the first-line palliative treatment of patients with high-grade STS. There was no significant difference in OS between both groups (median OS 12.8 for doxorubicin vs 14.3 months in AI) but median progression-free survival (PFS) was significantly higher for the AI group than for the doxorubicin group (7.4 vs 4.6 months) and more patients in the combination arm had an overall response (26% vs 14%). Combination chemotherapy was associated with a significantly higher risk of grade 3/4 side effects of the treatment, however. Based on the results of this study, intensive combination chemotherapy ought to be prescribed when the aim for treatment is tumor shrinkage to provide relief from symptoms or before possible surgical excision of the metastases whereas single agent doxorubicin may be more appropriate for palliating asymptomatic patents.[29]

Alternative regimens include gemcitabine used alone or in combination, especially with docetaxel. In a study by Maki and colleagues of 19 patients diagnosed with

UPS, 32% had documented responses and median PFS was 6.2 months in patients treated with gemcitabine–docetaxel.[30] The GeDDis trial compared gemcitabine plus docetaxel with doxorubicin alone in the first-line treatment of palliative therapy in 257 patients diagnosed with STS, 12% to 13% of whom were diagnosed with UPS. PFS after 24 weeks (the primary endpoint) was 46% in both arms though OS was slightly better for doxorubicin. Gemcitabine plus docetaxel was more toxic and harder to administer than doxorubicin, so the combined regimen remains second line therapy in patients with metastatic UPS.[31] Gemcitabine can also be combined with dacarbazine; in a Spanish study comparing gemcitabine plus dacarbazine versus dacarbazine alone, UPS patients were 19 of the 113 included patients. Median PFS was 4.2 months for combination versus 2 months for dacarbazine monotherapy (hazard ratio 0.58) and median OS was 16.8 months versus 8.2 months.[30] Targeted therapy was considered in the PALETTE trial, a randomized, placebo-controlled trial assessing the efficacy of pazopanib, a multikinase inhibitor, in patients with previously treated advanced STS including UPS/MFS. The drug prolonged PFS by 3 months when compared with placebo, and thus it can be considered for patients with metastatic UPS/MFS.[32]

A promising treatment option for advanced UPS/MFS is immunotherapy; it is one of the few STS subtypes with noted responses to treatment and prolonged survival. A large study of immunotherapy in sarcomas was published in 2017 (SARC028 Trial). This two-cohort, single-arm, open-label, phase 2 study enrolled 86 patients with STS or bone sarcoma. Ten patients with UPS were included. Seven (18%) of 40 patients with STS had an objective response, including 4 (40%) of 10 patients with UPS. Responses were reasonably durable, with a median duration of response being 33 weeks (median PFS for UPS cohort 30 weeks). The median OS for patients with STS was 49 weeks (95% CI 34–73). The median OS for patients with UPS had not been reached at the time of analysis.[33] An expansion cohort increasing the number of UPS patients examined to 40 was reported at the American Society of Clinical Oncology conference in 2019. Overall response rate (by RECIST v1.1) in the UPS cohort was 23% (9/40), median PFS was 3 months, 12-week PFS rate was 50%, and median OS of 12 months.[34]

Combination of nivolumab and ipilimumab was also studied sarcoma patients. An open-label, unblinded, noncomparative, multicenter randomized phase II study enrolled 96 patients, who received either nivolumab or nivolumab and ipilimumab. Patients were heavily pretreated, with 61% having received at least 3 prior chemotherapy lines. Median overall response rates were 5% in the nivolumab monotherapy group and 16% in the combination arm with responses observed in UPS/MFS patients treated with a combination of nivolumab and ipilimumab.[35]

FUTURE DIRECTIONS

Recent trials have established a role for immunotherapy in the third-line setting for patients with advanced disease and ongoing studies are examining potential predictive markers and neoadjuvant approaches such as prescription in combination with radiation. For example, results of immunotherapy in a preoperative setting were presented on ASCO 2020. A randomized, phase II noncomparative trial was presented evaluating the efficacy of 3 to 4 cycles of neoadjuvant nivolumab or a combination of ipilimumab/nivolumab in patients with resectable retroperitoneal dedifferentiated liposarcoma or extremity/truncal UPS. Median pathologic response in 9 UPS patients (all of whom received concurrent neoadjuvant radiation) was 95%. Given association of pathologic response and ultimate outcome in STS, this is a promising finding.[36]

It is clear that rates and durability of response to immunotherapy may be less impressive than in other cancer types, so parallel genomic and translational studies continue to examine the role of targeted therapy in these diseases. The TCGA analysis confirmed not only mutations and copy number alterations in *TP53*, *RB1*, and *PTEN* affecting UPS and MFS but noted common copy number alterations affecting Hippo pathways components *VGLL3* and *YAP1*.[5] A second study examining MFS independently identified a high-risk subset of lesions characterized by increased expression of *ITGA10*. The gene product integrin α-10 was shown to interact with Rictor and TRIO, both encoded on a chromosome 5 amplicon to activate the oncogenic RAC/PAK and AKT/mTOR pathways.[37] This suggests a basis for clinical trials to examine inhibitors of these pathways in patients with advanced disease.

CLINICS CARE POINTS

- Core biopsy should be performed to establish the diagnosis of undifferentiated pleomorphic sarcoma (UPS)/myxofibrosarcoma (MFS).

- Myxoid stroma, fibrous septa, and curvilinear vessels suggest a diagnosis of MFS; low-grade and high-grade forms are observed. UPS is an intermediate-grade or high-grade lesions composed of irregular, pleomorphic cells seen in several sarcomas, so ancillary techniques should be used to rule out histologies such as liposarcoma, leiomyosarcoma, malignant peripheral nerve sheath tumor, and solitary fibrous tumor.

- Cross-sectional MRI of the primary lesion is performed in parallel with pulmonary staging and can be useful particularly in MFS to delineating nonpalpable tumor "tails" that extend outward from the gross nodules.

- Surgical resection of UPS should be performed with 1 cm margins or with resection of adjacent fascia. Adjacent, but not encased, neurovascular bundles can be preserved by resection of the perineurium and vascular sheath.

- The locally aggressive nature of MFS means that 2 cm margins should be planned when morbidity is not prohibitive and tumor "tails" identified on MRI should be resected en bloc with the primary lesion.

- If R1 resection of high-grade tumors is planned to reduce minimize surgical morbidity, adjuvant or neoadjuvant radiation can be used to mitigate risk of local recurrence.

- Neo-/adjuvant chemotherapy should be considered in patients with tumors at high-risk for metastasizing (high-grade MFS more than 10 cm in size and UPS at least 5 cm in greatest diameter).

- Advanced disease is generally treated with anthracycline-based regimens (the first-line therapy) or gemcitabine/docetaxel combinations. Pazopanib can be considered in progressive cases, anti-PD1 demonstrates promising activity in proportion of patients.

DISCLOSURE

A.M. Crago: Advisory Board, Springworks Therapeutics. K. Cardona: none to report. H. Kosela-Paterczyk: none to report. P. Rutkowski: honoraria for lectures and Advisory Boards from BMS < MSD, Novartis, Pierre Fabre, Sanofi, Merck, and Blueprint Medicines outside of the scope of this study. A.Crago - NIH/NCI P50-CA217694, P30-CA008748.

REFERENCES

1. Prieto-Granada CN, Wiesner T, Messina JL, Jungbluth AA, Chi P, Antonescu CR. Loss of H3K27me3 Expression Is a Highly Sensitive Marker for Sporadic and Radiation-induced MPNST. Am J Surg Pathol 2016;40(4):479–89.
2. Cheah AL, Billings SD, Goldblum JR, Carver P, Tanas MZ, Rubin BP. STAT6 rabbit monoclonal antibody is a robust diagnostic tool for the distinction of solitary fibrous tumour from its mimics. Pathology 2014;46(5):389–95.
3. Doyle LA, Vivero M, Fletcher CD, Mertens F, Hornick JL. Nuclear expression of STAT6 distinguishes solitary fibrous tumor from histologic mimics. Mod Pathol 2014;27(3):390–5.
4. Dry SMaF, Leiomyosarcoma S. WHO classification of Tumours of soft tissue and bone. 5th edition. IARC; 2020. p. 195–7.
5. Cancer Genome Atlas Research Network. Electronic address edsc, Cancer Genome Atlas Research N. Comprehensive and Integrated Genomic Characterization of Adult Soft Tissue Sarcomas. Cell 2017;171(4):950–965 e28.
6. Barretina J, Taylor BS, Banerji S, et al. Subtype-specific genomic alterations define new targets for soft-tissue sarcoma therapy. Nat Genet 2010;42(8):715–21.
7. Chibon F, Mairal A, Freneaux P, et al. The RB1 gene is the target of chromosome 13 deletions in malignant fibrous histiocytoma. Cancer Res 2000;60(22):6339–45.
8. Perot G, Chibon F, Montero A, et al. Constant p53 pathway inactivation in a large series of soft tissue sarcomas with complex genetics. Am J Pathol 2010;177(4): 2080–90.
9. Mentzel T, Calonje E, Wadden C, et al. Myxofibrosarcoma. Clinicopathologic analysis of 75 cases with emphasis on the low-grade variant. Am J Surg Pathol 1996;20(4):391–405.
10. Lee AY, Agaram NP, Qin LX, et al. Optimal Percent Myxoid Component to Predict Outcome in High-Grade Myxofibrosarcoma and Undifferentiated Pleomorphic Sarcoma. Ann Surg Oncol 2016;23(3):818–25.
11. Fletcher CD, Gustafson P, Rydholm A, Willen H, Akerman M. Clinicopathologic re-evaluation of 100 malignant fibrous histiocytomas: prognostic relevance of subclassification. J Clin Oncol 2001;19(12):3045–50.
12. Salo JC, Lewis JJ, Woodruff JM, Leung DH, Brennan MF. Malignant fibrous histiocytoma of the extremity. Cancer 1999;85(8):1765–72.
13. Boughzala-Bennadji R, Stoeckle E, Le Pechoux C, et al. Localized Myxofibrosarcomas: Roles of Surgical Margins and Adjuvant Radiation Therapy. Int J Radiat Oncol Biol Phys 2018;102(2):399–406.
14. Look Hong NJ, Hornicek FJ, Raskin KA, et al. Prognostic factors and outcomes of patients with myxofibrosarcoma. Ann Surg Oncol 2013;20(1):80–6.
15. Sanfilippo R, Miceli R, Grosso F, et al. Myxofibrosarcoma: prognostic factors and survival in a series of patients treated at a single institution. Ann Surg Oncol 2011; 18(3):720–5.
16. Mutter RW, Singer S, Zhang Z, Brennan MF, Alektiar KM. The enigma of myxofibrosarcoma of the extremity. Cancer 2012;118(2):518–27.
17. Haglund KE, Raut CP, Nascimento AF, Wang Q, George S, Baldini EH. Recurrence patterns and survival for patients with intermediate- and high-grade myxofibrosarcoma. Int J Radiat Oncol Biol Phys 2012;82(1):361–7.
18. Lefkowitz RA, Landa J, Hwang S, et al. Myxofibrosarcoma: prevalence and diagnostic value of the "tail sign" on magnetic resonance imaging. Skeletal Radiol 2013;42(6):809–18.

19. Waters B, Panicek DM, Lefkowitz RA, et al. Low-grade myxofibrosarcoma: CT and MRI patterns in recurrent disease. AJR Am J roentgenology 2007;188(2):W193–8.
20. Fourman MS, Ramsey DC, Kleiner J, et al. Temporizing Wound VAC Dressing Until Final Negative Margins are Achieved Reduces Myxofibrosarcoma Local Recurrence. Ann Surg Oncol 2021. https://doi.org/10.1245/s10434-021-10242-4.
21. Pisters PW, Pollock RE, Lewis VO, et al. Long-term results of prospective trial of surgery alone with selective use of radiation for patients with T1 extremity and trunk soft tissue sarcomas. Ann Surg 2007;246(4):675–81.
22. Cahlon O, Brennan MF, Jia X, Qin LX, Singer S, Alektiar KM. A postoperative nomogram for local recurrence risk in extremity soft tissue sarcomas after limb-sparing surgery without adjuvant radiation. Ann Surg 2012;255(2):343–7.
23. Pervaiz N, Colterjohn N, Farrokhyar F, Tozer R, Figueredo A, Ghert M. A systematic meta-analysis of randomized controlled trials of adjuvant chemotherapy for localized resectable soft-tissue sarcoma. Cancer 2008;113(3): 573–81.
24. Pasquali S, Pizzamiglio S, Touati N, et al. The impact of chemotherapy on survival of patients with extremity and trunk wall soft tissue sarcoma: revisiting the results of the EORTC-STBSG 62931 randomised trial. Eur J Cancer 2019;109:51–60.
25. Callegaro D, Miceli R, Bonvalot S, et al. Development and external validation of two nomograms to predict overall survival and occurrence of distant metastases in adults after surgical resection of localised soft-tissue sarcomas of the extremities: a retrospective analysis. Lancet Oncol 2016;17(5):671–80.
26. Gronchi A, Ferrari S, Quagliuolo V, et al. Histotype-tailored neoadjuvant chemotherapy versus standard chemotherapy in patients with high-risk soft-tissue sarcomas (ISG-STS 1001): an international, open-label, randomised, controlled, phase 3, multicentre trial. Lancet Oncol 2017;18(6):812–22.
27. Pasquali S, Palmerini E, Quagliuolo V, et al. Neoadjuvant chemotherapy in high-risk soft tissue sarcomas: A Sarculator-based risk stratification analysis of the ISG-STS 1001 randomized trial. Cancer 2022;128(1):85–93.
28. Casali PG, Abecassis N, Aro HT, et al. Soft tissue and visceral sarcomas: ESMO-EURACAN Clinical Practice Guidelines for diagnosis, treatment and follow-up. Ann Oncol 2018;29(Suppl 4):iv51–67.
29. Judson I, Verweij J, Gelderblom H, et al. Doxorubicin alone versus intensified doxorubicin plus ifosfamide for first-line treatment of advanced or metastatic soft-tissue sarcoma: a randomised controlled phase 3 trial. Lancet Oncol 2014; 15(4):415–23.
30. Maki RG, Wathen JK, Patel SR, et al. Randomized Phase II Study of Gemcitabine and Docetaxel Compared With Gemcitabine Alone in Patients With Metastatic Soft Tissue Sarcomas: Results of Sarcoma Alliance for Research Through Collaboration Study 002. J Clin Oncol 2007;25(19):2755–63.
31. Seddon B, Strauss SJ, Whelan J, et al. Gemcitabine and docetaxel versus doxorubicin as first-line treatment in previously untreated advanced unresectable or metastatic soft-tissue sarcomas (GeDDiS): a randomised controlled phase 3 trial. Lancet Oncol 2017;18(10):1397–410.
32. van der Graaf WT, Blay JY, Chawla SP, et al. Pazopanib for metastatic soft-tissue sarcoma (PALETTE): a randomised, double-blind, placebo-controlled phase 3 trial. Lancet 2012;379(9829):1879–86.
33. Tawbi HA, Burgess M, Bolejack V, et al. Pembrolizumab in advanced soft-tissue sarcoma and bone sarcoma (SARC028): a multicentre, two-cohort, single-arm, open-label, phase 2 trial. Lancet Oncol 2017;18(11):1493–501.

34. Burgess MA, Bolejack V, Schuetze S, et al. Clinical activity of pembrolizumab (P) in undifferentiated pleomorphic sarcoma (UPS) and dedifferentiated/pleomorphic liposarcoma (LPS): Final results of SARC028 expansion cohorts. J Clin Oncol 2019;37(15_suppl):11015.

35. D'Angelo SP, Mahoney MR, Van Tine BA, et al. Nivolumab with or without ipilimumab treatment for metastatic sarcoma (Alliance A091401): two open-label, non-comparative, randomised, phase 2 trials. Lancet Oncol 2018;19(3):416–26.

36. Roland CL, Keung EZ-Y, Lazar AJ, et al. Preliminary results of a phase II study of neoadjuvant checkpoint blockade for surgically resectable undifferentiated pleomorphic sarcoma (UPS) and dedifferentiated liposarcoma (DDLPS). J Clin Oncol 2020;38(15_suppl):11505.

37. Okada T, Lee AY, Qin LX, et al. Integrin-alpha10 Dependency Identifies RAC and RICTOR as Therapeutic Targets in High-Grade Myxofibrosarcoma. Cancer Discov 2016;6(10):1148–65.

Gastrointestinal Stromal Tumor

New Insights for a Multimodal Approach

Ashwyn K. Sharma, MD[a,b], Teresa S. Kim, MD[c],
Sebastian Bauer, MD[d,e], Jason K. Sicklick, MD[a,b,*]

KEYWORDS

- Gastrointestinal Stromal Tumor • Next Generation Sequencing
- Tyrosine Kinase Inhibitors • Immunotherapy

KEY POINTS

- GIST has been shown to have numerous genetic alterations that dictate its response to chemotherapy, and therefore genetic testing should always be performed when possible.
- Most localized GIST can be treated with surgery alone. Adjuvant and neoadjuvant therapy are reserved for those with high risk of recurrence and with tumors that would result in difficult/extensive surgery, respectively.
- There are multiple chemotherapy options available other than imatinib that can be used for treatment of GIST. Immunotherapy options have been explored but are still an active area of research.
- Surgery may play a role in metastatic GIST, and debulking operations may prove beneficial in very select patients, though more research is needed.

INTRODUCTION

Gastrointestinal stromal tumor (GIST), although rare, with an incidence of approximately 7 to 19 cases per million annually around the world, is the most common sarcoma of the gastrointestinal (GI) tract.[1,2] These tumors are hypothesized to arise from the interstitial cells of Cajal (ICCs), or the pacemaker cells of the GI tract. Although

a Department of Surgery, Division of Surgical Oncology, University of California San Diego, San Diego, CA, USA; b Moores Cancer Center, University of California San Diego School of Medicine, 3855 Health Sciences Drive, Box 0987, La Jolla, CA 92093, USA; c Department of Surgery, University of Washington, 1959 NE Pacific Street, Box 356410, Seattle, WA 98195, USA; d Department of Medical Oncology, Sarcoma Center, West German Cancer Center, University Hospital Essen Hufelandstr. 55, Essen 45122, Germany; e DKTK Partner Site Essen, German Cancer Consortium (DKTK), Heidelberg, Germany
* Corresponding author. Moores Cancer Center, University of California San Diego School of Medicine, 3855 Health Sciences Drive, Box 0987, La Jolla, CA 92093.
E-mail address: jsicklick@health.ucsd.edu

Surg Oncol Clin N Am 31 (2022) 431–446
https://doi.org/10.1016/j.soc.2022.03.007
1055-3207/22/© 2022 Elsevier Inc. All rights reserved.

these tumors can occur anywhere throughout the gut, they are most often found in the stomach (55%) and small intestine (30%). A minority of these tumors are found in the colon, rectum, and esophagus, as well as even outside the GI tract (ie, extraintestinal). The clinical presentation is often nonspecific, and symptoms can include abdominal pain, nausea, vomiting, increasing abdominal girth, loss of appetite, early satiety, acute bleeding, or chronic anemia.

GIST is characteristically known for oncogenic gain-of-function mutations in the *KIT* or *PDGFRA* genes, as well as other drivers, including alterations in *SDHx* subunits, *NF1*, *BRAF*, *FGFR1*, and *ETV6-NTRK3* fusions. As a result of the identification of genomic alterations in *KIT* in the late 1990s, GIST has become the paradigm for precision oncology and multimodal therapies. Thus, genomic testing, targeted neoadjuvant and adjuvant therapy, as well as surgical resection are all key components for treating this disease. In this article, the authors highlight the importance of genomic testing of GIST, the use of neoadjuvant and adjuvant therapy for localized disease, surgical principles for GIST, as well as current and new approaches for addressing metastatic disease.

DIAGNOSTICS AND GENOMIC TESTING
Mutation Profiling

Historically, GIST was considered a morbid disease associated with a high mortality. In addition, GIST were often misclassified as other tumors, including leiomyoma, leiomyosarcoma, and histiocytomas.[3] However, in 1998, Hirota and colleagues[4] demonstrated that GIST characteristically express KIT (c-KIT or CD117) like ICCs, the putative cells of origin for these tumors. At the same time, research in chronic myelogenous leukemia and the discovery of the Philadelphia chromosome (*BCR-ABL*) led to the development of a tyrosine kinase inhibitor (TKI) called STI-571, later named imatinib (Gleevac or Gleevec). It was soon discovered that imatinib not only was effective against chronic myelogenous leukemias harboring *BCR-ABL,* but also effective against the KIT receptor as well. Within a few years, the first patients with advanced GIST were treated with imatinib and demonstrated tremendous objective radiologic responses and improvements in survival compared with historical controls. After imatinib rapidly moved through phase 2 and 3 trials, the Food and Drug Administration (FDA) granted approval for imatinib in the treatment of GIST in February 2002. This was followed shortly thereafter by the European Medicine Agency approval.

Despite the significant improvement in prognosis for patients with GIST, the past 20 years have led to multiple discoveries that have added more complexity and nuance to the treatment of GIST. One year after the FDA approval of imatinib, Heinrich and colleagues[5] discovered that 35% of patients with non-*KIT* mutant GIST harbored activating mutations in the *PDGFRA* gene. Shortly after this, reports were published highlighting patients with neurofibromatosis type 1 caused by germline *NF1* mutations having a higher predilection for developing GIST.[6] In 2007, McWhinney and colleagues[7] demonstrated that multiple families with mutations within the succinate dehydrogenase gene (*SDH A/B/C/D*) developed GIST. One year later, it was discovered that 7% of patients with non-*KIT* and non-*PDGFRA* mutant GIST had activating mutations in *BRAF V600E*, like melanoma.[8] Finally, over the last 10 years, discovery of GIST arising owing to hypermethylation of the *SDHC* promoter ("epimutation") and gene fusions in *ETV6-NTRK3* and *FGFR1* have also been described.[9–12] Thus, over the past 20 years, the genomic landscape of GIST has dramatically expanded.

Today, approximately 60% to 70% of patients with GIST harbor somatic tumor mutations in *KIT*.[11] Even within *KIT* mutant tumors, there remains substantial genomic diversity. Of all *KIT* mutant GIST, 67% will have mutations affecting *KIT* exon 11, 10% to 15% affecting *KIT* exon 9, and 1% each affecting exons 13, 17, and 18. After this, approximately 10% of GIST have *PDGFRA* mutations and 7% have germline mutations in 1 of 4 *SDH* genes (ie, *SDHA*, *SDHB*, *SDHC*, and *SDHD*). The remainder of tumors most often have mutations in *NF1*, *BRAF*, *KRAS*, *ETV6-NTRK3*, *FGFR1* gene fusions, or unknown mutations in descending order. Furthermore, these differing mutation profiles confer different tumor biologies, responses to imatinib therapy, and responses to other therapies. As a result, tumor mutational profiling has become more pertinent for identifying which patients will respond to therapies and for subsequently guiding individualized treatment.

Next-Generation Sequencing

Next-generation sequencing (NGS) is a method of simultaneously sequencing millions of fragments of DNA and has been quickly adopted for clinical purposes.[13] It is an established test for determining both germline and somatic mutations in patients based on tissue and/or blood samples. With the ever-growing genetic diversity of GIST, NGS has become a powerful tool in tailoring management for GIST patients.

As we have learned about each GIST subtype, it has become evident that each mutated gene confers differences in tumor biology, primary tumor location, clinical phenotype, metastasis patterns, outcomes, and importantly, imatinib responsiveness. Ultimately, the driving mutation in GIST determines the likelihood of treatment success or even failure. For example, the MetaGIST trial, a meta-analysis of 2 clinical trials that studied outcomes of low- and high-dose (400 mg vs 800 mg) imatinib in patients with advanced GIST, determined that high-dose imatinib (800 mg) confers an advantage in progression-free survival (PFS) in patients who possessed a *KIT* exon 9 mutation.[14] As a result, both the National Comprehensive Cancer Network and the European Society for Medical Oncology have deemed mutational analyses and genetic testing standard practice for GIST and strongly encourage including these tests in the diagnostic workup for GIST, particularly in those patients for whom systemic therapy is being considered.[15,16]

However, despite these recommendations, the reality is that most patients do not undergo genetic testing. In a study by Florindez and Trent,[17] *KIT* mutation testing was assessed on 3866 patients using the using the Surveillance, Epidemiology, and End Results (SEER) database in the United States from 2010 to 2015. They found that only 26.7% of patients underwent genetic testing. Similar studies in the Netherlands have noted that only a third of patients with GIST undergo mutational testing.[18] Many barriers for genetic testing have been proposed, including inadequate tissue availability and high testing costs. High costs have traditionally been a major barrier to testing in single-payer health care systems of developed countries, such as the United Kingdom, Israel, and Japan, as well as in developing countries. However, a study by Banerjee and colleagues[19] used a Markov model to assess the economic cost-effectiveness of genetic testing versus empiric first-line imatinib therapy in patients with metastatic GIST. Tailoring therapy (ie, imatinib 400 mg vs imatinib 800 mg vs other agents) based on NGS data ultimately remained cost-effective for genetic testing costs up to $3730 (USD). Thus, genetic testing is recommended to be performed on all patients with metastatic GIST in whom systemic therapy is being considered and should be strongly considered in any nonmetastatic patient in whom systemic therapy is being considered.

MANAGEMENT OF LOCALIZED DISEASE

Surgery remains the mainstay treatment for localized GIST. The surgical procedure to be performed should aim to resect the tumor with histologically negative margins (ie,

R0). Every effort should be made to avoid rupturing the tumor capsule during resection. Because most GIST tends to not metastasize to lymph nodes (except SDH-deficient GIST and some fusion-driven GIST), lymphadenectomy is generally not indicated.

Small Gastrointestinal Stromal Tumor

Small GIST are defined as GIST that are less than 2 cm in size.[20] Moreover, there are subsets of small GIST. GIST that are less than 1 cm in size are termed micro-GIST, whereas those between 1 and 2 cm are designated as mini-GIST.[21] Previous studies have demonstrated that these tumors generally have lower proliferative capacity, and lower mitotic rates.[22] Based on autopsy studies of patients over 50 years old, it is estimated that up to 23% of people will have a small, incidental GIST.[23] Most of these tumors tend to be asymptomatic and have benign behavior in that they rarely tend to undergo disease progression or metastasis. However, for unknown reasons, a very small subset of small GIST may have more aggressive biology. In one SEER study of 378 patients with GIST less than 2 cm, 11.4% had regional/distant metastatic disease.[24] The annual incidence rate was 4.2 per 10,000,000 (10M), and the 5-year GIST-specific mortality was 34%. This suggested that although quite rare, a subset of these small GIST has an underappreciated disease-specific mortality, which should be kept in mind when evaluating patients with small GIST.

Most small GIST are located within the stomach and diagnosed incidentally during endoscopy or during pathologic analysis of tissue obtained from other operations, such as gastric sleeve resections for morbid obesity or during other cancer operations. However, a small proportion of these small GIST are also found in the small intestine, colon, and rectum. These tumors tend to have higher mitotic rates and worse prognoses than small gastric GIST. Therefore, despite low mitotic rates, less than 2 cm small bowel GIST may exhibit significant growth and progression.[25]

Pathologic examination of tissue samples is required for the diagnosis of small GIST. Given that these tumors are less than 2 cm, endoscopic ultrasound-guided with fine needle aspiration (EUS-FNA) is an ideal approach to diagnose these tumors. Once the diagnosis is established, the treatment for these tumors depends on several factors. First, any small GIST within the small intestine, colon, or rectum should ultimately be resected in good surgical candidates. Second, for small gastric GIST, treatment depends on the presence of high-risk features on EUS-FNA or pathology. Features such as irregular borders, cystic spaces, ulceration, echogenic foci, heterogeneity, and high mitotic rate indicate potentially more aggressive disease and merit surgical resection. Small GIST without these features can potentially be surveilled endoscopically or radiographically, although some centers suggest no follow-up may be necessary for these tumors. Moreover, for those being followed, the frequency and length of time for follow-up are not well established.

Gastrointestinal Stromal Tumor in Adolescents and Young Adults

Classically, GIST is a disease of older adults. The median age of diagnosis for patients with GIST is 64 years of age, with most tumors having mutations in *KIT* or *PDGFRA*. Studies have demonstrated that approximately 5% to 6.8% of GIST are in adolescent and young adult (AYA) patients. Fero and colleagues[26] performed a US population-based analysis of patients diagnosed with GIST in the SEER database. These AYA patients were more likely to have small intestine GIST and were more often managed operatively. Nonoperative management in this population was associated with a 2-fold increased risk of death from GIST. In addition, IJzerman and colleagues[27] performed an analysis of the Dutch GIST Registry and found that AYA patients similarly had a high percentage of small intestine GIST and a high percentage of non-*KIT/PDGFRA* mutations. Finally, a related study was reported by the Weldon and colleagues[28] from the National Institutes of Health (NIH) Pediatric and Wildtype GIST Clinic. They sought to determine the effect of surgical resection on event-free survival (EFS, defined as freedom from disease progression or recurrence). Among 76 participants in this retrospective study, repeated resection after the initial resection was significantly associated with decreasing postoperative EFS ($P<.01$). They found no improvement in EFS with more extensive or serial resections, although this may have been affected more by disease biology and patient selection than from surgical management. Thus, cytoreductive surgical management should be individualized for each patient, but is certainly warranted in cases of tumor bleeding or obstruction.

Indications for Adjuvant Therapy

Adjuvant therapy for localized GIST may be necessary in certain circumstances. The modified NIH criteria were proposed to identify patients with high-risk GIST and those with a high likelihood of recurrence.[29] It uses 4 variables: tumor size, mitotic rate (per 5 mm^2), tumor location, and tumor rupture. Patients with a high risk of recurrence based on these criteria, which include the presence of tumor rupture, tumor size greater than 10 cm, mitotic index greater than 10/5 mm^2, or tumor size greater than 5 cm with mitotic index greater than 5/5 mm^2, may be considered high risk and therefore benefit from adjuvant therapy following resection.

The ACOSOG Z9001 Trial studied whether adjuvant imatinib therapy following resection could lead to increased overall survival (OS) and recurrence-free survival (RFS) in patient with resected GIST greater than 3 cm.[30] This study did show an improvement in RFS but no improvement in OS. The SSG XVIII/AIO trial demonstrated that 3 years of adjuvant imatinib following complete tumor resection prolongs RFS in patients with high risk of recurrence, and longer treatments of imatinib increases the time to GIST recurrence.[31,32] The most recent long-term follow-up of these patients showed that 3 years of adjuvant imatinib provides a 13% survival benefit after 10 years over 1 year of treatment. Longer treatment durations have also been studied, including the PERSIST-5 trial, a phase 2 trial that followed patients who underwent 5 years of adjuvant imatinib therapy.[33] This study demonstrated an estimated 5-year RFS of 90% and OS of 95%. However, without randomization or a matched control to patients receiving 3 years of imatinib, it cannot be concluded that 5 years of adjuvant therapy is superior to 3 years. The SSG XII Trial (NCT02413736) is currently underway to study this question in more detail. Based on the results of these trials, 3 years of adjuvant therapy is currently the standard of care. However, although adjuvant therapy reduces the risk of relapse and the risk of death in high-risk patients, the overall risk remains substantial in these patients.

Neoadjuvant Therapy for Locally Advanced Gastrointestinal Stromal Tumor

For certain patients with locally advanced GIST, neoadjuvant therapy may be indicated. In some cases, GIST may be in particularly difficult anatomic locations (including the rectum, esophagus, esophagogastric junction, and duodenum), or may be advanced to the point where surgical intervention would confer extreme morbidity to the patient and/or require a multivisceral resection to remove all gross tumor. In these circumstances, neoadjuvant therapy for GIST should be considered.

When considering neoadjuvant therapy, factors to consider include the mutational profile of the tumor, duration of therapy, and the extent of response. Before any initiation of medical therapy including imatinib, mutational profiling of the tumor should be performed. This is to ensure that the tumor is responsive to medical therapy and does not possess a resistant mutation (for instance, a GIST with a *PDGFRA* D842V mutation has primary resistance to imatinib, and an alternative agent, such as avapritinib, would be indicated). As mentioned above, genetic testing is recommended to be performed on all GIST patients in whom systemic therapy is being considered.

Several studies have explored the duration of neoadjuvant therapy and extent of response before surgery. Rutkowski and colleagues[34] performed a pooled analysis of 161 patients who underwent neoadjuvant imatinib therapy for nonmetastatic, locally advanced GIST. The median duration of therapy was 9.2 months, with R0 resection achieved in 83% of patients. In a more recent retrospective study by Cavnar and colleagues,[35] 150 patients with locally advanced GIST underwent neoadjuvant imatinib therapy for a median of 7.1 months, with partial response (PR) or stable disease (SD) seen in 40% and 51% of patients, respectively, by RECIST criteria. Posttreatment high mitotic rates were noted to be predictive of lower OS. Moreover, R2 resection and utilization of adjuvant imatinib therapy were also factors that affected rates of relapse or recurrence.

Ultimately, if neoadjuvant therapy is to be considered, mutational testing should be performed. Neoadjuvant therapy is often administered for 6 to 9 months before surgery, based on achieving maximal response to therapy. Finally, adjuvant therapy should be administered to reduce risk of recurrence and improve disease-free survival in the appropriately selected patients.

Surgical Approaches for Rectal Gastrointestinal Stromal Tumor

Rectal GIST is a rare entity, comprising approximately 5% of all GIST. Like other rectal tumors, symptoms are nonspecific and can include pain, bleeding, changes in bowel habits, and occasionally urinary symptoms. These tumors tend to occur in the lower segment of the rectum, with some studies indicating up to 85% of rectal GIST presents within 5 cm of the anal verge.[36] Although for any localized GIST, surgery is first line, rectal GIST is unique in that their anatomic location makes surgical resection more difficult. Moreover, rectal GIST is associated with higher rates of recurrence, and the rate of tumor rupture in these tumors is more than 4 times higher than the rate in nonrectal GIST.[37] Moreover, these tumors have a higher risk of lung metastasis than other GIST subtypes. Therefore, computed tomographic (CT) chest scan should be included in the staging workup.

Given the limited operative space and possible sphincter involvement, the surgical procedure of choice varies and is not standardized. Historically, a wide variety of procedures, including local excision, low anterior resection, abdominoperineal resection, and total pelvic exenterations, were performed for these tumors, to achieve oncologic resection with negative margins. However, with the advent of imatinib, treatment paradigms have changed substantially, and combined multimodal therapy with neoadjuvant imatinib followed by surgical resection has become the standard of care with the goal of performing less morbid operations.

Perioperative imatinib has been shown to improve outcomes, improving OS, disease-free survival, and RFS.[38] As discussed previously, given the difficult anatomic location of these tumors, neoadjuvant imatinib can potentially result in tumor shrinkage and subsequently lead to greater preservation of the rectum and anal sphincter, as well as allow for more minimally invasive approaches. In one series, 92% of patients receiving preoperative imatinib treatment underwent resection (via low anterior resection or local excision), compared with only 48% of patients who did not receive neoadjuvant therapy.[39] In addition, neoadjuvant imatinib has been shown to be associated with improved R0 surgical margins during resection. Interestingly, one study demonstrated that even with positive margins after resection, patients who received adjuvant imatinib therapy resulted in no recurrences over the study period (1982–2016) at a single high-volume center.[39] However, another study of 48 patients from an international patient registry with localized rectal GIST found that disease recurrence remains prevalent in one-third of patients treated during the imatinib era. Thus, treating physicians should remain vigilant in their follow-up of these patients.[40]

METASTATIC AND UNRESECTABLE GASTROINTESTINAL STROMAL TUMOR

For metastatic and unresectable GIST, the mainstay of treatment involves systemic therapy. This section reviews current standards of care for metastatic GIST, new approaches and targeted therapies, and the role of surgery in these patients.

Currently Food and Drug Administration–Approved Systemic Therapy

Imatinib

Traditional cytotoxic chemotherapy was ineffective for GIST and did not substantially affect the natural history of the disease, as response rates were often less than 5%. Thus, a prognosis of advanced GIST was dismal before the early 2000s.

In 2002, imatinib was approved by the FDA for the treatment of advanced GIST. It is a selective TKI, targeting the KIT and platelet-derived growth factor receptor-alpha (PDGFRA) receptor tyrosine kinases. This approval came after a multicenter, randomized trial that evaluated the efficacy of imatinib in 147 patients with advanced GIST.[41] In this trial, 53.7% of patients were found to have a PR to imatinib based on RECIST criteria, although no patients had a complete response (CR). Overall, the clinical benefit rate (CBR) of imatinib was 81%. As a result, imatinib soon became FDA approved as first-line therapy for patients with advanced and metastatic GIST.

In patients with metastatic disease, imatinib should be continued until progression is documented. In some studies, approximately 10% of patients will achieve long-term disease control with imatinib alone.[42] Discontinuation of imatinib is associated with a risk of progression, regardless of the pattern of response achieved with imatinib before interruption of therapy.[43] Despite the promise of imatinib, most patients will eventually develop resistance to the drug. Some studies indicate that up to 40% of primary localized GIST will develop recurrence within 5 years, and moreover, discontinuation of adjuvant imatinib after years of treatment results in progression of disease in high-risk patients.[44]

Sunitinib

Sunitinib (Sutent) is another TKI that is now the approved second-line therapy for GIST. It has both antitumor and antiangiogenic activity, by targeting multiple receptors, including VEGFR1, VEGFR2, PDGFRA, PDGFRB, KIT, FLT3, RET, and CSF1R.[45] In a randomized, double-blind, placebo-controlled multicenter international trial for patients with imatinib-resistant GIST, sunitinib demonstrated significantly longer PFS compared with placebo (median 27.3 weeks vs 6.4 weeks for placebo),[46] despite only a 7% PR rate. Thus, sunitinib was FDA approved for the management of advanced imatinib-resistant GIST in 2006.

Like imatinib, mutation status correlates with the efficacy of sunitinib. For example, primary *KIT* exon 9 mutants have higher response rates compared with *KIT* exon 11 mutations.[47] In addition, patients with *KIT* exon 13 or 14 secondary mutations had longer PFS and OS when treated with sunitinib as compared with those with *KIT* exon 17 or 18 secondary mutations.

Regorafenib

Regorafenib (Stivarga) is another TKI with similar activity against multiple targets, including angiogenic (VEGFR1-3, TIE2), stromal (PDGFR-β, FGFR), and oncogenic receptor tyrosine kinases (KIT, RET, and RAF).[48] The GRID trial, an international, multicenter, randomized, placebo-controlled phase 3 trial, randomized 240 GIST patients with advanced GIST with failure of previous imatinib or sunitinib to regorafenib or placebo.[49] Overall, patients receiving regorafenib had longer median PFS (4.8 months vs 0.9 months for placebo). In addition, 75.9% of patients receiving regorafenib had either PR or SD, compared with 38.4% in the placebo arm. As a result, the FDA approved regorafenib in the third-line setting for use in patients with advanced GIST refractory to imatinib and sunitinib.

Ripretinib

Ripretinib is the latest novel TKI for *KIT* mutant GIST with a dual switch pocket inhibitory mechanism of action that blocks the kinase from achieving an active state, and thereby results in inhibition of downstream signal transduction. A phase 1, two-part dose-escalation/expansion trial was performed for 184 patients with advanced GIST that had at least one prior line of therapy.[50] Ripretinib was generally well tolerated and was found to have an objective response rate (ORR) of 11.3%, with median PFS ranging from 5.5 months (if on fourth-line treatment or greater) to 10.7 months (second line). The subsequent INVICTUS study further evaluated the efficacy of ripretinib. This study was a double-blind, randomized, placebo-controlled phase 3 trial of 129 patients with GIST who had progressed on at least imatinib, sunitinib, or regorafenib.[51] Patients who received ripretinib had increased median PFS compared with those in the placebo group (median 6.3 months vs 1.0 months), as well as increased OS (median 15.1 months vs 6.6 months). In addition, patients receiving ripretinib showed a higher ORR compared with those receiving the placebo (9% vs 0%). Ripretinib received FDA approval for treatment of adult patients with advanced GIST who have previously received 3 or more TKIs.

Most recently, the randomized, open-label, phase 3 INTRIGUE trial (NCT03673501) was performed. This trial aimed to compare the efficacy of ripretinib with sunitinib in patients with advanced GIST who have progressed on imatinib. However, on interim analysis, the study failed to meet its efficacy endpoint and was halted early. Thus, sunitinib remains the second-line therapy for advanced GIST. At the time of drafting this article, the detailed trial results have not been published.

Avapritinib

Patients with *PDGFRA* mutant GIST account for about 10% of all GIST. The most common mutant, *PDGFRA* exon 18, D842V, is known for primary imatinib and sunitinib resistance. As a result, survival rates for these patients were historically poor in patients with advanced disease. Avapritinib (Ayvakit) was developed as a selective TKI that was recently developed to target KIT and PDGFRA. The NAVIGATOR trial, a two-part, open-label, dose escalation/dose expansion phase 1 study, studied 237 patients with advanced GIST, including 56 patients with *PDGFRA* D842V mutant tumors.[52] In the *PDGFRA* D842V population, avapritinib elicited an ORR of 89%, which included an 8% CR rate and an 82% PR rate. The median duration of response was not reached (range, 1.9+ months to 20.3+ months). The 98% CBR of avapritinib led the FDA to approve avapritinib in January 2020 in the first-line setting for adults with advanced *PDGFRA* exon 18 mutant GIST.

Based on these promising results, the VOYAGER trial was conducted, randomizing 476 patients to avapritinib versus regorafenib, with PFS being the primary endpoint.[53] In this population, only 3.8% of patients had a *PDGFRA* exon 18 mutation, and only 2.3% had a *PDGFRA* D842V mutation, whereas 28.6% of patients had unknown mutation status. Ultimately, although the ORR in the avapritinib arm was higher than that in the regorafenib arm (17.1 vs 7.2%), there was no difference in median PFS. Like the

NAVIGATOR trial, the patients with *PDGFRA* D842V mutations demonstrated significantly higher PFS in the avapritinib arm (median not reached) compared with the regorafenib arm (median 4.5 months). One potential limitation of this study was that the patient population included those with various *KIT* and *PDGFRA* mutant GIST. As such, the investigators postulated that the relative efficacy of avapritinib and regorafenib might be influenced by the underlying mutational landscape. Knowledge of this landscape was limited given that more than a quarter of patients did not have baseline tumor mutation status.

Larotrectinib and entrectinib

Gene fusions involving 1 of the 3 tropomyosin receptor kinases (TRK) NTRK1, NTRK2, and NTRK3 have been found in multiple diverse cancers in both children and adults. Recently, gene fusions have been reported in GIST, with Shi and colleagues[11] identifying *FGFR1* gene fusions as well at *ETV-NTRK3* fusions, suggesting that these are additional actionable targets for treating GIST.

Two additional inhibitors, larotrectinib and entrectinib, are highly specific small molecule inhibitors of TRK family of proteins. Drilon and colleagues[54] enrolled 55 patients with solid organ tumors with identified *NTRK* gene fusions by molecular profiling and performed a combined phase 1 to 2 study using larotrectinib in a histology-agnostic fashion. The ORR by RECIST criteria was 75%. In this study, 2 of 3 patients with GIST had PRs. Thus, larotrectinib was approved by the FDA in 2018 for any solid tumor bearing an *NTRK* fusion and was the first drug to be approved for cancers with a specific genomic alteration rather than tissue type. In addition, 3 clinical studies of entrectinib (ALKA-372-001, STARTRK-1, and STARTRK-2) enrolled patients aged 18 years or older with metastatic or locally advanced *NTRK* fusion-positive solid tumors. Subjects received entrectinib orally at a dose of at least 600 mg once per day. An integrated efficacy and safety analysis of these trials demonstrated that at a median follow-up of 12.9 months, 57% of patients had an objective response, with 7% achieving a CR and 50% achieving a PR[55] with a median duration of response of 10 months. Based on these results, the FDA approved entrectinib for adults and pediatric patients 12 years of age and older with solid tumors that have an *NTRK* gene fusion without a known acquired resistance mutation. Ultimately, these recent approvals of tissue agnostic therapies underscore the importance of categorizing GIST by their specific genomic alterations, rather than treating this disease as a one-size-fits-all entity.

New Approaches: Immunotherapy for Gastrointestinal Stromal Tumor

Therapeutic enhancement of the antitumor immune response via immune checkpoint blockade (ICB) has revolutionized treatment of a minority of solid cancers, such as melanoma and non–small cell lung cancer. However, the role of immunotherapy in GIST remains to be defined. Recent studies have investigated the role of ICB for GIST given that these tumors have immune infiltrates within the tumor microenvironment.

It has been found that GIST tends to have a high proportion of tumor-associated macrophages and T cells in both treated and untreated tumors.[56,57] In addition, natural killer (NK) and B cells have also been found within the GIST microenvironment. Interestingly, these populations have been found to correlate with clinical outcomes. For instance, Rusakiewicz and colleagues[58] demonstrated that high densities of CD3+ tumor-infiltrating lymphocytes, as well as the density of NK infiltrate predicted PFS. In addition, *in silico* immune signature gene expression analysis of 31 GIST demonstrated that the immune microenvironment of GIST is remarkably like that of melanoma, suggesting that GIST may benefit from immunotherapy.[56] Reiterating the importance of tumor mutation profiling, a recent study of RNA sequencing of 75 human GISTs demonstrated that *PDGFRA*-mutated tumors were more heavily infiltrated with activated immune cells than tumors with *KIT* mutations, suggesting a link between oncogene signaling and tumor immunogenicity.[59]

Not only do these tumors have immune infiltrates, but also imatinib has been shown to have both stimulatory and suppressive immunologic effects in GIST. In a mouse model of *KIT* exon 11–mutated GIST, imatinib therapy activated CD8$^+$ T cells and induced regulatory T-cell apoptosis within GIST by reducing tumor cell expression of the immunosuppressive enzyme IDO.[60] Imatinib has also been shown to activate NK cells by inhibiting KIT, which results in the release of cancer neoantigens from tumor lysis and decreases in the expression of PD-L1 to thereby decrease immune escape.[61] These findings suggest that immunotherapy in combination with imatinib may also be effective. However, in both a mouse model of GIST and human GIST specimens, chronic imatinib therapy caused reversible M2/immunosuppressive polarization of macrophages[57] and dampened innate immune responses by decreasing type I interferon signaling.[62] These studies highlight the complexity of the GIST immune microenvironment pre–imatinib and post–imatinib therapy.

Preclinical studies in murine GIST have also demonstrated synergy between targeted therapy, for example, imatinib, and clinically available immune checkpoint blocking agents, such as anti-CTLA-4 (ipilimumab).[60] Given these findings, 2 clinical trials have explored immunotherapy in GIST, with mixed to disappointing results. A phase Ib study of dasatinib plus ipilimumab was conducted based on preclinical evidence that demonstrated that combined KIT and CTLA-4 blockade was synergistic.[63] Twenty-eight patients were included in this study, of which 20 patients were diagnosed with GIST. However, no patient experienced a PR or CR by RECIST criteria, and the median PFS was only 2.8 months. The study was in part limited by the use of a less-effective TKI, dasatinib, rather than first-line imatinib. Nevertheless, similar results were reported from a phase I trial of imatinib and ipilimumab in 35 advanced solid tumor patients, including 12 with GIST: only 2 patients experienced a PR, 1 with wild-type GIST, and 1 with KIT-mutated melanoma.[64]

Dual ICB targeting both CTLA-4 and PD-1 has demonstrated improved efficacy in other cancer types, such as melanoma.[65] In GIST, a randomized, unblinded phase 2 trial was performed on 36 patients with advanced GIST refractory to at least imatinib. They compared nivolumab alone versus nivolumab plus ipilimumab.[66] Patients in the nivolumab had a CBR of 52.6% (no PR, all SD) with a median PFS of 11.7 weeks, whereas those in the combination nivolumab plus ipilimumab arm had a CBR of 31.3% (1 PR, remainder SD) with a median PFS of 8.3 weeks. The trial did not meet its primary endpoint of response rate greater than 15%, highlighting the ongoing need for better predictors of immunotherapy response (ie, patient selection), and more precise targeting of immunosuppressive mechanisms in TKI-treated GIST.

Additional preclinical studies suggest new approaches to translate to clinical trials. For example, in a mouse model of GIST, imatinib was found to be more effective when combined with ICB targeting the PD-1/PD-L1 axis.[67] Current trials investigating this therapeutic combination are ongoing. Approaches targeting the innate immune response have also demonstrated preclinical efficacy in GIST, including the combination of imatinib with an agonist antibody targeting the macrophage costimulatory receptor CD40.[68] Improving the understanding of the immune system and GIST, particularly in the context of targeted therapy, will be critical to incorporating immunotherapy into future GIST management. At this time, given the overall disappointing clinical trial results to date, immunotherapy is not currently a part of the standard of care for GIST.

The Role of Surgery in Metastatic Gastrointestinal Stromal Tumor

Treatment with imatinib and latter-line options, such as sunitinib and regorafenib, remains the standard of care for patients with metastatic GIST. However, these treatments are not curative, and many tumors have primary resistance or develop secondary resistance (eg, *KIT* exon 13/144 or 17/18 mutations) to these TKIs. Debulking or cytoreductive surgery has been considered a treatment option for metastatic GIST that may improve outcomes. The rationale for this is based on observations that increased baseline tumor burden and tumor size can be determinants for subsequent imatinib resistance. By performing debulking surgery, the risk of secondary mutations may be decreased and thus improve outcomes.

Debulking surgery seems to be most effective for patients who have demonstrated response to TKI therapy. Fairweather and colleagues[69] sought to determine treatment recommendations for patients with metastatic GIST. They reported on 400 operations on 323 patients with metastatic GIST treated with TKIs from 2001 to 2014. Based on imaging, patients were characterized as having responsive disease (RD), SD, unifocal progressive disease (UPD), or multifocal progressive disease (MPD). Those patients that demonstrated better radiographic response from imatinib were found to have longer median PFS (RD, 36 months; SD, 30 months; UPD, 11 months; MPD, 6 months) from the time of surgery, as well as improved median OS (RD, not reached; SD, 110 months; UPD, 59 months; MPD, 24 months).

A large European retrospective study showed long-term disease control in patients with metastatic GIST that responded to imatinib and in whom complete macroscopic resection (R0/R1) was achieved.[70] Patients with R0/R1 surgery had a median OS of 8.7 compared with 5.3 years in those with incomplete resection, suggesting a survival advantage of more than 3 years. However, neither radical nor debulking surgery was associated with longer disease control when surgery was performed in patients progressing on or after imatinib. This suggests that complete resection of residual metastatic disease before disease progression on imatinib is associated with a longer median OS.

Despite these encouraging retrospective studies, randomized clinical trials examining the benefit of debulking surgery for metastatic GIST have failed because of poor accrual rates. However, one clinical trial, despite closing early, enrolled 41 patients and studied the possible benefit of debulking surgery versus imatinib therapy alone.[71] For the 41 patients in this cohort, 2-year PFS was 88% in the surgery arm versus 57.7% in the imatinib arm. The median OS was not reached in the surgery arm, whereas median OS was 49 months in the imatinib arm, suggesting a possible benefit for debulking surgery in GIST. However, it is unlikely that further studies will be conducted to ask this question, and we will need to rely on retrospective data. In those patients who are considered for resection following sunitinib and regorafenib treatment, surgeons must bear in mind that these drugs can impact wound healing, although there is less for debulking surgery following later lines of therapy.

Ultimately, surgery in patients with metastatic GIST on imatinib may be considered in select patients, particularly those with RD to TKI and ideally earlier in their disease course, particularly before progression on systemic therapy begins. Surgery should be performed on carefully selected patients, and if feasible for the patient, should be discussed 6 to 12 months after initiation of treatment of metastatic disease.

SUMMARY

Over the past 20 years, GIST has evolved into an increasingly complex clinical entity with ever more challenges as patients live longer with their disease. Surgical resection is the gold standard and mainstay of treatment for GIST. It should always be considered with a new diagnosis of GIST, as well as in properly selected patients with metastatic disease. The wide variety of genetic alterations in these tumors and corresponding differences in tumor biologies from these alterations mandate that genetic testing be performed whenever possible. Based on these results, imatinib or other TKIs may be necessary and can be tailored to properly treat advanced tumors in a mutation-specific fashion. As more research on GIST is conducted, and new treatment strategies become available, a thorough understanding of the multidisciplinary and multimodal approach for treating GIST will become ever more paramount to effectively treat patients with this disease.

REFERENCES

1. Ma GL, Murphy JD, Martinez ME, et al. Epidemiology of gastrointestinal stromal tumors in the era of histology codes: results of a population-based study. Cancer Epidemiol Biomarkers Prev 2015;24(1):298–302.
2. Coe TM, Sicklick JK. Epidemiology of GIST. In: Scoggins CR, Raut CP, Mullen JT, editors. Gastrointestinal stromal tumors: bench to bedside. Cham: Springer International Publishing; 2017. p. 7–15.
3. Roland CL, Feig BW. History of GIST. In: Scoggins CR, Raut CP, Mullen JT, editors. Gastrointestinal stromal tumors: bench to bedside. Cham: Springer International Publishing; 2017. p. 1–5.
4. Hirota S, Isozaki K, Moriyama Y, et al. Gain-of-function mutations of c-kit in human gastrointestinal stromal tumors. Science 1998;279(5350):577–80.
5. Heinrich MC, Corless CL, Duensing A, et al. PDGFRA activating mutations in gastrointestinal stromal tumors. Science 2003;299(5607):708–10.
6. Miettinen M, Fetsch JF, Sobin LH, et al. Gastrointestinal stromal tumors in patients with neurofibromatosis 1: a clinicopathologic and molecular genetic study of 45 cases. Am J Surg Pathol 2006;30(1):90–6.
7. McWhinney SR, Pasini B, Stratakis CA, et al. Familial gastrointestinal stromal tumors and germ-line mutations. N Engl J Med 2007;357(10):1054–6.
8. Agaram NP, Wong GC, Guo T, et al. Novel V600E BRAF mutations in imatinib-naive and imatinib-resistant gastrointestinal stromal tumors. Genes Chromosomes Cancer 2008;47(10):853–9.
9. Killian JK, Miettinen M, Walker RL, et al. Recurrent epimutation of SDHC in gastrointestinal stromal tumors. Sci Transl Med 2014;6(268):268ra177.
10. Brenca M, Rossi S, Polano M, et al. Transcriptome sequencing identifies ETV6-NTRK3 as a gene fusion involved in GIST. J Pathol 2016;238(4):543–9.
11. Shi E, Chmielecki J, Tang CM, et al. FGFR1 and NTRK3 actionable alterations in "wild-type" gastrointestinal stromal tumors. J Transl Med 2016;14(1):339.
12. Haller F, Moskalev EA, Faucz FR, et al. Aberrant DNA hypermethylation of SDHC: a novel mechanism of tumor development in Carney triad. Endocr Relat Cancer 2014;21(4):567–77.
13. Yohe S, Thyagarajan B. Review of clinical next-generation sequencing. Arch Pathol Lab Med 2017;141(11):1544–57.
14. Gastrointestinal Stromal Tumor Meta-Analysis G. Comparison of two doses of imatinib for the treatment of unresectable or metastatic gastrointestinal stromal tumors: a meta-analysis of 1,640 patients. J Clin Oncol 2010;28(7):1247–53.
15. Casali PG, Blay JY, Abecassis N, et al. Gastrointestinal stromal tumours: ESMO-EURACAN-GENTURIS Clinical Practice Guidelines for diagnosis, treatment and follow-up. Ann Oncol 2022;33(1):20–33.
16. Network NCC. Gastrointestinal stromal tumors (version 1.2022). 2022. Available at: https://www.nccn.org/professionals/physician_gls/pdf/gist.pdf.

17. Florindez J, Trent J. Low frequency of mutation testing in the United States: an analysis of 3866 GIST patients. Am J Clin Oncol 2020;43(4):270–8.
18. Verschoor AJ, Bovee J, Overbeek LIH, et al. The incidence, mutational status, risk classification and referral pattern of gastro-intestinal stromal tumours in the Netherlands: a nationwide pathology registry (PALGA) study. Virchows Arch 2018;472(2):221–9.
19. Banerjee S, Kumar A, Lopez N, et al. Cost-effectiveness analysis of genetic testing and tailored first-line therapy for patients with metastatic gastrointestinal stromal tumors. JAMA Netw Open 2020;3(9):e2013565.
20. Fernandez JA, Gomez-Ruiz AJ, Olivares V, et al. Clinical and pathological features of "small" GIST (</=2 cm). What is their prognostic value? Eur J Surg Oncol 2018;44(5):580–6.
21. Nishida T, Goto O, Raut CP, et al. Diagnostic and treatment strategy for small gastrointestinal stromal tumors. Cancer 2016;122(20):3110–8.
22. Rossi S, Gasparotto D, Toffolatti L, et al. Molecular and clinicopathologic characterization of gastrointestinal stromal tumors (GISTs) of small size. Am J Surg Pathol 2010;34(10):1480–91.
23. Agaimy A, Wunsch PH, Hofstaedter F, et al. Minute gastric sclerosing stromal tumors (GIST tumorlets) are common in adults and frequently show c-KIT mutations. Am J Surg Pathol 2007;31(1):113–20.
24. Coe TM, Fero KE, Fanta PT, et al. Population-based epidemiology and mortality of small malignant gastrointestinal stromal tumors in the USA. J Gastrointest Surg 2016;20(6):1132–40.
25. Agaimy A, Wunsch PH, Dirnhofer S, et al. Microscopic gastrointestinal stromal tumors in esophageal and intestinal surgical resection specimens: a clinicopathologic, immunohistochemical, and molecular study of 19 lesions. Am J Surg Pathol 2008;32(6):867–73.
26. Fero KE, Coe TM, Fanta PT, et al. Surgical management of adolescents and young adults with gastrointestinal stromal tumors: a US population-based analysis. JAMA Surg 2017;152(5):443–51.
27. NS IJ, Drabbe C, den Hollander D, et al. Gastrointestinal stromal tumours (GIST) in young adult (18-40 years) patients: a report from the Dutch GIST Registry. Cancers (Basel) 2020;12(3). https://doi.org/10.3390/cancers12030730.
28. Weldon CB, Madenci AL, Boikos SA, et al. Surgical management of wild-type gastrointestinal stromal tumors: a report from the National Institutes of Health Pediatric and Wildtype GIST Clinic. J Clin Oncol 2017;35(5):523–8.
29. Joensuu H. Risk stratification of patients diagnosed with gastrointestinal stromal tumor. Hum Pathol 2008;39(10):1411–9.
30. Dematteo RP, Ballman KV, Antonescu CR, et al. Adjuvant imatinib mesylate after resection of localised, primary gastrointestinal stromal tumour: a randomised, double-blind, placebo-controlled trial. Lancet 2009;373(9669):1097–104.
31. Joensuu H, Eriksson M, Sundby Hall K, et al. One vs three years of adjuvant imatinib for operable gastrointestinal stromal tumor: a randomized trial. JAMA 2012; 307(12):1265–72.
32. Joensuu H, Eriksson M, Sundby Hall K, et al. Survival outcomes associated with 3 years vs 1 year of adjuvant imatinib for patients with high-risk gastrointestinal stromal tumors: an analysis of a randomized clinical trial after 10-year follow-up. JAMA Oncol 2020;6(8):1241–6.
33. Raut CP, Espat NJ, Maki RG, et al. Efficacy and tolerability of 5-year adjuvant imatinib treatment for patients with resected intermediate- or high-risk primary

gastrointestinal stromal tumor: the PERSIST-5 Clinical Trial. JAMA Oncol 2018; 4(12):e184060.

34. Rutkowski P, Gronchi A, Hohenberger P, et al. Neoadjuvant imatinib in locally advanced gastrointestinal stromal tumors (GIST): the EORTC STBSG experience. Ann Surg Oncol 2013;20(9):2937–43.

35. Cavnar MJ, Seier K, Gonen M, et al. Prognostic factors after neoadjuvant imatinib for newly diagnosed primary gastrointestinal stromal tumor. J Gastrointest Surg 2021;25(7):1828–36.

36. Shu P, Sun XF, Fang Y, et al. Clinical outcomes of different therapeutic modalities for rectal gastrointestinal stromal tumor: summary of 14-year clinical experience in a single center. Int J Surg 2020;77:1–7.

37. Farid M, Lee MJ, Chew MH, et al. Localized gastrointestinal stromal tumor of the rectum: an uncommon primary site with prominent disease and treatment-related morbidities. Mol Clin Oncol 2013;1(1):190–4.

38. Jakob J, Mussi C, Ronellenfitsch U, et al. Gastrointestinal stromal tumor of the rectum: results of surgical and multimodality therapy in the era of imatinib. Ann Surg Oncol 2013;20(2):586–92.

39. Cavnar MJ, Wang L, Balachandran VP, et al. Rectal gastrointestinal stromal tumor (GIST) in the era of imatinib: organ preservation and improved oncologic outcome. Ann Surg Oncol 2017;24(13):3972–80.

40. Stuart E, Banerjee S, de la Torre J, et al. Frequent rectal gastrointestinal stromal tumor recurrences in the imatinib era: retrospective analysis of an International Patient Registry. J Surg Oncol 2019;120(4):715–21.

41. Demetri GD, von Mehren M, Blanke CD, et al. Efficacy and safety of imatinib mesylate in advanced gastrointestinal stromal tumors. N Engl J Med 2002;347(7):472–80.

42. Heinrich MC, Rankin C, Blanke CD, et al. Correlation of long-term results of imatinib in advanced gastrointestinal stromal tumors with next-generation sequencing results: analysis of phase 3 SWOG Intergroup Trial S0033. JAMA Oncol 2017;3(7):944–52.

43. Patrikidou A, Chabaud S, Ray-Coquard I, et al. Influence of imatinib interruption and rechallenge on the residual disease in patients with advanced GIST: results of the BFR14 prospective French Sarcoma Group randomised, phase III trial. Ann Oncol 2013;24(4):1087–93.

44. Le Cesne A, Ray-Coquard I, Bui BN, et al. Discontinuation of imatinib in patients with advanced gastrointestinal stromal tumours after 3 years of treatment: an open-label multicentre randomised phase 3 trial. Lancet Oncol 2010;11(10):942–9.

45. Papaetis GS, Syrigos KN. Sunitinib: a multitargeted receptor tyrosine kinase inhibitor in the era of molecular cancer therapies. BioDrugs 2009;23(6):377–89.

46. Demetri GD, van Oosterom AT, Garrett CR, et al. Efficacy and safety of sunitinib in patients with advanced gastrointestinal stromal tumour after failure of imatinib: a randomised controlled trial. Lancet 2006;368(9544):1329–38.

47. Heinrich MC, Maki RG, Corless CL, et al. Primary and secondary kinase genotypes correlate with the biological and clinical activity of sunitinib in imatinib-resistant gastrointestinal stromal tumor. J Clin Oncol 2008;26(33):5352–9.

48. Wilhelm SM, Dumas J, Adnane L, et al. Regorafenib (BAY 73-4506): a new oral multikinase inhibitor of angiogenic, stromal and oncogenic receptor tyrosine kinases with potent preclinical antitumor activity. Int J Cancer 2011;129(1):245–55.

49. Demetri GD, Reichardt P, Kang YK, et al. Efficacy and safety of regorafenib for advanced gastrointestinal stromal tumours after failure of imatinib and sunitinib (GRID): an international, multicentre, randomised, placebo-controlled, phase 3 trial. Lancet 2013;381(9863):295–302.

50. Janku F, Abdul Razak AR, Chi P, et al. Switch control inhibition of KIT and PDGFRA in patients with advanced gastrointestinal stromal tumor: a phase I study of ripretinib. J Clin Oncol 2020;38(28):3294–303.
51. Blay JY, Serrano C, Heinrich MC, et al. Ripretinib in patients with advanced gastrointestinal stromal tumours (INVICTUS): a double-blind, randomised, placebo-controlled, phase 3 trial. Lancet Oncol 2020;21(7):923–34.
52. Heinrich MC, Jones RL, von Mehren M, et al. Avapritinib in advanced PDGFRA D842V-mutant gastrointestinal stromal tumour (NAVIGATOR): a multicentre, open-label, phase 1 trial. Lancet Oncol 2020;21(7):935–46.
53. Kang YK, George S, Jones RL, et al. Avapritinib versus regorafenib in locally advanced unresectable or metastatic gi stromal tumor: a randomized, open-label phase III study. J Clin Oncol 2021;39(28):3128–39.
54. Drilon A, Laetsch TW, Kummar S, et al. Efficacy of larotrectinib in TRK fusion-positive cancers in adults and children. N Engl J Med 2018;378(8):731–9.
55. Doebele RC, Drilon A, Paz-Ares L, et al. Entrectinib in patients with advanced or metastatic NTRK fusion-positive solid tumours: integrated analysis of three phase 1-2 trials. Lancet Oncol 2020;21(2):271–82.
56. Pantaleo MA, Tarantino G, Agostinelli C, et al. Immune microenvironment profiling of gastrointestinal stromal tumors (GIST) shows gene expression patterns associated to immune checkpoint inhibitors response. Oncoimmunology 2019;8(9): e1617588.
57. Cavnar MJ, Zeng S, Kim TS, et al. KIT oncogene inhibition drives intratumoral macrophage M2 polarization. J Exp Med 2013;210(13):2873–86.
58. Rusakiewicz S, Semeraro M, Sarabi M, et al. Immune infiltrates are prognostic factors in localized gastrointestinal stromal tumors. Cancer Res 2013;73(12): 3499–510.
59. Vitiello GA, Bowler TG, Liu M, et al. Differential immune profiles distinguish the mutational subtypes of gastrointestinal stromal tumor. J Clin Invest 2019;129(5): 1863–77.
60. Balachandran VP, Cavnar MJ, Zeng S, et al. Imatinib potentiates antitumor T cell responses in gastrointestinal stromal tumor through the inhibition of Ido. Nat Med 2011;17(9):1094–100.
61. Borg C, Terme M, Taieb J, et al. Novel mode of action of c-kit tyrosine kinase inhibitors leading to NK cell-dependent antitumor effects. J Clin Invest 2004;114(3): 379–88.
62. Liu M, Etherington MS, Hanna A, et al. Oncogenic KIT modulates type I IFN-mediated antitumor immunity in GIST. Cancer Immunol Res 2021;9(5):542–53.
63. D'Angelo SP, Shoushtari AN, Keohan ML, et al. Combined KIT and CTLA-4 blockade in patients with refractory GIST and other advanced sarcomas: a phase Ib study of dasatinib plus ipilimumab. Clin Cancer Res 2017;23(12):2972–80.
64. Reilley MJ, Bailey A, Subbiah V, et al. Phase I clinical trial of combination imatinib and ipilimumab in patients with advanced malignancies. J Immunother Cancer 2017;5:35.
65. Wolchok JD, Chiarion-Sileni V, Gonzalez R, et al. Overall survival with combined nivolumab and ipilimumab in advanced melanoma. N Engl J Med 2017;377(14): 1345–56.
66. Singh AS, Hecht JR, Rosen L, et al. A randomized phase II study of nivolumab monotherapy or nivolumab combined with ipilimumab in patients with advanced gastrointestinal stromal tumors. Clin Cancer Res 2021. https://doi.org/10.1158/1078-0432.CCR-21-0878.

67. Seifert AM, Zeng S, Zhang JQ, et al. PD-1/PD-L1 blockade enhances T-cell activity and antitumor efficacy of imatinib in gastrointestinal stromal tumors. Clin Cancer Res 2017;23(2):454–65.

68. Zhang JQ, Zeng S, Vitiello GA, et al. Macrophages and CD8(+) T cells mediate the antitumor efficacy of combined CD40 ligation and imatinib therapy in gastrointestinal stromal tumors. Cancer Immunol Res 2018;6(4):434–47.

69. Fairweather M, Balachandran VP, Li GZ, et al. Cytoreductive surgery for metastatic gastrointestinal stromal tumors treated with tyrosine kinase inhibitors: a 2-institutional analysis. Ann Surg 2018;268(2):296–302.

70. Bauer S, Rutkowski P, Hohenberger P, et al. Long-term follow-up of patients with GIST undergoing metastasectomy in the era of imatinib – analysis of prognostic factors (EORTC-STBSG Collaborative Study). Eur J Surg Oncol 2014;40(4):412–9.

71. Du CY, Zhou Y, Song C, et al. Is there a role of surgery in patients with recurrent or metastatic gastrointestinal stromal tumours responding to imatinib: a prospective randomised trial in China. Eur J Cancer 2014;50(10):1772–8.

Management of Desmoid Tumors

Gaya Spolverato, MD[a],*, Giulia Capelli, MD[a], Bernd Kasper, MD, PhD[b],
Mrinal Gounder, MD[c]

KEYWORDS

- Desmoid tumors • Desmoid-type fibromatosis • Aggressive fibromatosis
- Active surveillance • Outcomes

KEY POINTS

- Active surveillance, defined as serial MRI (ie, at 1–2 months after diagnosis and then every 3–6 months), is considered the first line of treatment for most patients with desmoid tumors (DT), according to international guidelines.
- Switching from active surveillance to treatment is considered in case of progressive symptoms and/or persistent interval growth.
- The choice of the first-line systemic therapy and the management of recurrence still represent a therapeutic challenge, for which well-defined and shared guidelines are lacking.
- Currently available treatments include tyrosine kinase inhibitors, liposomal doxorubicin, low-dose chemotherapy with IV methotrexate + vinblastine/vinorelbine, or oral vinorelbine alone. Some evidence exists concerning the efficacy and safety of pegylated liposomal doxorubicin, whereas studies are ongoing to test nirogacestat and tegavivint as new therapeutic agents.
- Function and structure preservation and attention to patients' quality of life are currently considered necessary in the management of patients with DT.

INTRODUCTION

Desmoid tumors (DT), also known as desmoid fibromatosis, are rare fibroblastic neoplasms that arise from the deep soft tissues and show a locally aggressive behavior in the absence of metastatic potential.[1] The incidence is 5 to 6 cases per million a year, with a peak in the third and fourth decades of life and a 2:1 female:male predominance.[2,3] Approximately 5% to 10% of cases are associated with familial adenomatous polyposis (FAP).[2]

[a] Department of Surgical, Oncological and Gastroenterological Sciences, University of Padova, Via Giustiniani 2, Padua 35121, Italy; [b] Sarcoma Unit, Mannheim University Medical Center, University of Heidelberg, Theodor-Kutzer-Ufer 1-3, Mannheim 68167, Germany; [c] Sarcoma Medical Oncology, Memorial Sloan Kettering Cancer Center and Weill Cornell Medical College, 300 East 66th Street, BAIC 1075, New York, NY 10065, USA
* Corresponding author.
E-mail address: gaya.spolverato@unipd.it

Surg Oncol Clin N Am 31 (2022) 447–458
https://doi.org/10.1016/j.soc.2022.03.008
surgonc.theclinics.com
1055-3207/22/© 2022 Elsevier Inc. All rights reserved.

DT can arise from multiple abdominal and extra-abdominal locations, including the extremities, limb, girdles, thoracic wall, breast, and head and neck.[4] The occurrence of DT in the abdominal wall is more common in women, particularly during or after pregnancy,[5] whereas localizations in the abdominal wall and in the mesentery are more common in patients with FAP.[6]

DT require a multidisciplinary management in order to address symptoms while offering the best chances of care.[7]

A paradigm shift has occurred when upfront surgery has been replaced by active surveillance in most patients.[8] When active treatment is required, several systemic and local treatments are considered, including tyrosine kinase inhibitors (TKIs), conventional chemotherapy, and radiotherapy (RT).[9] Acknowledging the possible involvement of aberrancies in the Notch pathway in the development of DT, γ-secretase inhibitors have also been considered more recently as possible therapeutic agents for patients with nonresectable disease.[10]

In order to address the scarcity of prospective studies and meta-analyses, and in the effort of harmonizing treatment strategies worldwide, global consensus meetings were held in the recent years, leading to the release of evidence-based guidelines.[8,9]

The aim of the current article is to conduct a systematic review to summarize the recent literature on the management of DT, with a particular focus on the role of active surveillance and the most recent advances in systemic and local therapies.

MOLECULAR ASPECTS

The current guidelines recommend mutational analysis for the diagnosis of DT.[8,9] Approximately 90% of DT are characterized by point mutations on exon 3 of the *CTNNB1* gene, determining a disruption of the Wnt/Beta-catenin signaling.[11] Three specific amino-acid changes, T41A, S45F, and S45P, are responsible for the constitutive activation of the Wnt/Beta-catenin signaling cascade in most patients with DT. In a minority of patients, DT are associated with a mutation in the *APC* gene on chromosome 5, a negative regulator of beta-catenin stability, which is responsible for FAP.[2] Particularly, mutations happening between codons 543 to 713 and 1310 to 2011 of *APC* were associated with an increased risk to develop DT in FAP patients.[12] Because *CTNNB1* mutations and *APC* mutations are mutually exclusive, current guidelines strongly recommend that patients with DT with a *CTNNB1* wild-type status are investigated for FAP with a colonoscopy and/or a germline testing.[9]

The presence of different *CTNNB1* mutations has been found to affect the risk of recurrence of DT following active treatment. A recent meta-analysis showed that patients with DT with a *CTNNB1* S45F mutation had a higher risk of recurrence following surgery compared with T41A, S45P, and *CTNNB1* wild-type patients, even though this association appeared to be mediated by tumor size.[13] Patients with an S45F mutation were also found to have a poor response to meloxicam and imatinib.[14,15]

Timbergen and colleagues[16] stated the hypothesis that prognostic differences in *CTNNB1*-mutated patients could be determined by the presence of different methylation patterns. Nevertheless, a genome-wide analysis of 29 DT cases failed to demonstrate differences in DNA methylation patterns of patients harboring either an S45F or a T41A mutation. On the other hand, DNA methylation patterns seemed to correlate with tumor size, thus suggesting that methylation alterations in DT may develop with a stepwise modality.

Finally, Bräutigam and colleagues[17] aimed to evaluate the role of hormonal receptors and PARP-1 expression as risk factors for DT recurrence. Although the expression of hormonal receptors did not seem to affect recurrence risk, the expression of

PARP-1 in all 69 cases included in the analysis led to the hypothesis that there is a possible role of this gene in the pathogenesis of DT. Nevertheless, PARP-1 expression resulted in being extremely heterogeneous depending on the cutoff used, so caution is needed in interpreting these findings.

ACTIVE SURVEILLANCE

Active surveillance, defined as serial MRI (ie, at 1–2 months after diagnosis and then every 3–6 months), is considered the first approach to most patients with DT, according to international guidelines.[2,8,9] Treatment is currently reserved to patients presenting with complications or with large tumors located in potentially life-threatening sites. Special consideration concerning active surveillance as a first-line treatment should be given to specific conditions. Front-line therapies should be considered in particular situations, including patients with chronic pain, pregnancy, and FAP-associated DT. This indication is supported by the evidence that up to 60% of patients with DT do not progress, and up to 30% experience spontaneous tumor regression. Regression can also occur after initial progressions, as reported in some prospective observational studies.[18]

Although the behavior of DT is difficult to predict, tumor location seems to play a major role in the definition of prognosis, with abdominal wall tumors being more indolent than extra-abdominal ones. In a study by Bonvalot and colleagues[19] on 147 patients with abdominal wall DT, about one-third of patients managed with active surveillance did not show disease progression at 36 months, whereas another third experienced spontaneous regression.

Several studies supported the noninferiority of active surveillance compared with surgery in terms of disease-free survival (DFS) also in extra-abdominal DT. In 2009, Fiore and colleagues[20] analyzed the long-term outcomes of 142 patients treated at 2 major centers in France and Italy and found a 5-year progression-free survival (PFS) of approximately 50% in patients managed conservatively; the rate of progression was similar to those who received medical treatment as first line. Similar results were achieved by Penel and colleagues[21] on a series of 771 patients: slightly more than 50% of patients did not experience progression at 2 years, and long-term outcomes were comparable between patients treated conservatively and those who received upfront surgery. Interestingly, patients with tumors located in unfavorable sites seemed to benefit most from an initial management with active surveillance. Favorable long-term outcomes of active surveillance compared with upfront surgery were also confirmed by a recent study by Ruspi and colleagues[22] on 87 consecutive patients treated at Humanitas Clinical and Research Center in Milan. It should be noted that, although PFS represents an adequate end point to evaluate the efficacy of treatments, studies investigating the optimal management of DT should also take into account quality of life (QoL), functional impairment, use of narcotics, and impact on activities of daily living. A Dutch prospective trial is currently recruiting, evaluating these critical endpoints in adult patients with DT.[23]

According to a recent meta-analysis, including 25 studies and 3527 patients, most patients who are initially managed with active surveillance never progress, whereas only one-third needs to switch to another treatment, such as systemic treatment and surgery, after a period of time ranging from 6.5 to 19.7 months.[24] Of note, an initial conservative approach does not jeopardize the efficacy of following treatments, either surgical or medical, in the event of progression or recurrence,[8] as confirmed by several studies.[20,25] In an analysis of 216 patients managed with active surveillance, Colombo and colleagues[25] found a 5-year crude cumulative incidence of 5% (95%

confidence interval [CI]: 1.7%, 14%) of conversion to surgery and of 51% (95% CI: 41%, 65%) of conversion to other treatments. Moreover, no differences were found on overall survival at 5 and 10 years compared with patients who underwent front-line surgery.

These results, along with the consideration of surgery-related morbidity, including postoperative pain and loss of function, further confirm active surveillance as a good initial choice for the management of most patients with DT.

Patients who experience acute and/or chronic pain and functional impairment are frequently candidates to more aggressive first-line therapies. Nevertheless, the pathogenesis of pain could be multifactorial, and surgical resection could fail to achieve pain control. Thus, the indication to active surveillance as a first-line treatment should be maintained in this subset of patients, whenever possible.[8,26]

Similarly, although DT can appear or progress during pregnancy,[17] they usually tend to regress after delivery; thus, pregnancy per se does not constitute an indication for first-line aggressive treatment.[5,26]

In FAP-associated DT, resection of the primary tumor or early start of a pharmacologic treatment needs to be considered earlier, owing to a higher risk of complications, including intestinal obstruction, perforation, and mesenteric ischemia. Nevertheless, treatment should aim to preserve an adequate digestive function, so as to minimize the impact on patient's QoL. Thus, it is acceptable to treat complications without proceeding to resection of the primary tumor, in case this should result in an excessive sacrifice in terms of function.[26] On the other hand, upfront pharmacologic treatment with low-dose methotrexate and vinca alkaloids or TKIs can be considered in order to reduce morbidity and loss of function connected to surgical treatment.[27]

A recent study by Duhil de Bénazé and colleagues[28] analyzed the outcomes of 81 pediatric patients treated for DT in France. Overall, 52/80 participants (65%) answered the QoL questionnaires, of whom only 30 underwent active surveillance as a first-line treatment. Moreover, the study did not use a validated desmoid patient-reported outcomes (PRO) tool. Thus, despite that the study showed good results in terms of functional impairment, pain management, and social behavior in this population, the results should be interpreted with caution and need further confirmation from specifically designed studies.

Active surveillance should also be considered in patients undergoing incomplete surgery (ie, positive surgical margins). In 2003, Gronchi and colleagues[29] analyzed a series of 203 patients undergoing surgery for primary or recurrent extra-abdominal DT and found that microscopically positive margins did not affect DFS. Similarly, Crago and colleagues,[30] analyzing a cohort of 495 patients with DT who underwent surgery at Memorial Sloan Kettering Cancer Center between 1982 and 2011, did not find any significant association between the status of surgical margins (R0 vs R1) and the risk of recurrence. Based on these findings, active surveillance is currently recommended by international guidelines for the management of patients following R1 surgical resection.[9] At the 2021 ASCO Annual Meeting, Braggio and colleagues[31] presented the initial results of the natural history study from The Desmoid Tumor Research Foundation (DTRF), showing that approximately half of included patients had been managed with active surveillance at diagnosis. Active surveillance was also used as a first-line option in nearly 40% of 487 patients from the NetSARC and CONTICABASE French databases, with good results in terms of PFS, as reported by Bouttefroy and colleagues[32] at ESMO Virtual Congress 2020. A prospective trial is currently active in France, with the primary aim to assess the incidence of DT from 2016 on, and that will furnish data concerning the management of these patients and tumor response to treatments in terms of PFS. The initial results of the National

Clinical-biological Prospective Cohort of Incident Cases of Aggressive Fibromatosis trial are expected to be presented during ESMO 2021.[33]

INDICATIONS FOR TREATMENTS

According to a recent consensus statement,[26] active treatment of DT should be offered in case of intra-abdominal complications, particularly in patients with FAP-associated DT, and in patients with large tumors located in sites where progression could become life-threatening (ie, neck, mediastinum, and mesentery).

Switching from active surveillance to treatment is considered in the case of progressive symptoms and/or persistent interval growth.[2] The decision to undertake an active treatment should be shared with the patient, considering clinical and radiological findings, symptoms, and functional limitations. Recent guidelines suggest to consider switching from active surveillance to treatment after at least 3 consecutive reevaluations, and possibly after at least 1 year from the diagnosis.

In the case of disease progression, the first-line treatment is represented by either surgery or systemic therapies, based on tumor location. Surgery can be considered, taking into account some expected morbidities, for abdominal wall DT, whereas for all other locations, surgery represents a second-line therapy after failure of systemic treatments, such as chemotherapy and molecular targeted therapies.

SYSTEMIC TREATMENTS

Systemic treatments may represent the first line of treatment of intra-abdominal, retroperitoneal, and pelvic DT, along with tumors involving the extremities, girdles, thoracic wall, thoracic cavity, and head and neck region.[9] Systemic therapy should also be considered in patients who are at high risk of recurrence, such as young patients, those with an extremity location, and those with large tumors.[34]

Antihormonal therapies and nonsteroidal anti-inflammatory drugs showed limited efficacy in patients with DT and are not generally recommended.[35–38] Currently available treatments include TKI, liposomal doxorubicin, low-dose chemotherapy with IV methotrexate + vinblastine/vinorelbine, or oral vinorelbine alone.[8,9,21,39–45] TKI, such as sorafenib and pazopanib, were found to be safe and effective, with manageable side effects owing to their low dosage.[42,44–48] Recently, promising results in terms of disease control were achieved with apatinib and anlotinib in patients with DT located to the extremities, with an acceptable safety profile.[49,50]

Low-dose chemotherapy with methotrexate and vinblastine/vinorelbine also showed favorable results: in a randomized trial on 72 patients treated at 12 centers from the French Sarcoma Group, the investigators reported a PFS of 79% at 1 and 2 years.[45] Recently, a phase II trial showed that biweekly administration of methotrexate and vinblastine was well tolerated and more effective compared with weekly administration.[51] Weekly methotrexate + vinca alkaloids were also found to be active and tolerated in patients with FAP-associated DT allowing for disease control in 95% of patients.[52] Finally, oral vinorelbine was found to be effective, safe, and well tolerated in patients with progressive DT following active surveillance.[53] Nevertheless, chemotherapy regimens with methotrexate and vinca alkaloids are known to be associated with some relevant side effects, including myelosuppression with grade 3 or 4 neutropenia, which occurs in a significant rate of patients.[45]

Some studies also reported promising results using pegylated liposomal doxorubicin, which has been shown to be associated with a lower risk of neutropenia and cardiac toxic effects compared with parenteral doxorubicin.[54,55] Recently, a systematic review and meta-analysis conducted by the guideline committee for clinical care of extra-abdominal desmoid-type fibromatosis in Japan reported a good efficacy of doxorubicin-based and liposomal doxorubicin chemotherapy, with a lower rate of G3 or G4 complications for liposomal doxorubicin chemotherapy regimens. These findings led to the committee formulating a weak recommendation favoring the use of doxorubicin-based chemotherapy regimens in patients with DT, despite a low evidence level.[56]

Recently, nirogacestat (PF-03084014), an orally available drug with effect on the Notch signaling, was also proved to be effective and safe in patients with DT.[10,57,58] The DeFi study, a randomized double-blind international clinical trial, is ongoing, comparing the efficacy of nirogacestat versus placebo in adult patients with progressing DT,[59] whereas the RINGSIDE trial, designed to evaluate the efficacy and safety of another inhibitor of the Notch pathway, AL102, is currently recruiting.[60]

Finally, tegavivint, an inhibitor of the Wnt and beta-catenin pathway, is currently being tested as a new therapeutic agent.

Because of the absence of comparative studies, the treatment plan should take into account the anticipated toxicity, switching from less toxic to more toxic agents in a stepwise fashion. In order to guide the treatment choice, The Desmoid Tumor Working Group, an international group of multidisciplinary clinicians and patient advocates, developed a model including the following variables: level of evidence, overall response rate, PFS rate, ease of administration, and expected toxicity.[9]

LOCAL TREATMENTS

RT is currently considered a treatment following surgery or systemic therapies, particularly when surgery carries a high risk of morbidity.[2] Definitive RT at moderate doses (ie, 50 Gy) can achieve local control in approximately 70% of patients, even though long-term side effects should be taken into account, particularly in young patients.[61] One issue with RT is the risk of radiation-associated sarcomas[62]; therefore, RT is not generally recommended, unless in refractory disease where other options have been exhausted.

Recently, cryotherapy, defined as the administration of repeated cycles of freezing or passive thawing of the tumor, has been proposed as an alternative to RT.[63,64] The phase II trial (CRYODESMO-O1) conducted on 50 patients with extra-abdominal progressive disease following at least 2 lines of systemic treatments, with functional symptoms or pain, and with inoperable tumors, showed favorable results in terms of efficacy, with an observed nonprogression rate at 12 months of 85.8%. The investigators also reported promising results in terms of safety, pain management, and QoL.[65]

ASSESSMENT OF TUMOR GROWTH DURING OBSERVATION AND RESPONSE TO TREATMENT

DT have an unpredictable behavior: some of them progress locally, whereas others remain stable or even spontaneously regress during time.[20,66,67]

Several studies were conducted in order to identify radiological signs of progression during active surveillance and to assess risk factors of a more aggressive behavior. Recently, Cassidy and colleagues[68] analyzed 37 patients managed with active surveillance at Memorial Sloan Kettering Cancer Center, finding that the presence of hyperintense T2 signal in ≥90% of baseline tumor volume was related to disease progression. Moreover, Murahashi and colleagues[69] found that the so-called black fiber sign (ie, the presence of low-signal-intensity bands) on T1- or T2-weighted images was a predictor of an indolent behavior. In a retrospective case series of 59 patients, the absence of the black fiber sign was related to a higher risk of progression and need to switch to an active treatment.

Some investigators also proposed patient-tailored follow-up strategies depending on the predicted risk of progression, based on the presence of radiologic risk factors. Gondim Teixeira and colleagues[70] conducted a retrospective analysis of 48 patients with DT, finding that muscle/tumor T2 signal ratio was related with tumor growth. Based on the observation that tumors with T2 signal ratios lower than 1 tended to have an indolent behavior, the investigators proposed a 12-month interval for active surveillance of these patients.

Radiologic findings are also used to predict response to treatment in patients undergoing systemic therapies and recurrence following radical surgery. According to international guidelines, response evaluation should be defined according to Response Evaluation Criteria in Solid Tumors version 1.1 (RECIST 1.1).[9] Nevertheless, RECIST criteria can be difficult to apply in a clinical setting, partly because of the difficulties in assessing tissue cellularity.

During the last few years, radiomics has been used to identify prognostic factors of response to treatment. A multicentric study conducted by the French Sarcoma Group led to the development of a radiomics score that showed better performances in predicting PFS (CI 0.84; 95% CI, 0.71–0.96) compared with conventional radiologic criteria.[71] Radiomics was also proposed for the differential diagnosis of DT from soft tissue sarcomas. A radiomics model proposed by Timbergen and colleagues[72] showed good accuracy; nevertheless, radiomics is currently unable to predict the mutational status and cannot be considered an alternative to histology.

QUALITY OF LIFE

Because DT are locally aggressive tumors often arising in young patients, maintaining a good QoL is pivotal. Since the late 1990s, when Brennan and colleagues first compared the results of major amputation to observation in patients with recurrent desmoids of the extremity,[66] function and structure preservation have been considered necessary in the management of patients with DT.

In a recent work, Newman and colleagues[73] examined the associations between treatment modalities and Patient-reported Outcomes Measurement Information System function scores. Function scores were found to be lower in patients who underwent multiple surgical resections or RT. The investigators also reported that patients managed with local treatments had similar event-free survival rates compared with those receiving systemic treatment, thus further confirming the primary role of systemic therapies in the management of these patients.

Acknowledging the need for specific tools to assess QoL of patients with rare neoplastic conditions, Gounder and colleagues[74] also used PROs in order to develop a model to rate QoL of patients with DT. Their work resulted in an 11-item symptom scale and a 17-item impact scale, named the GODDESS (Gounder/DTRF Desmoid Symptom/Impact Scale), which is currently available in multiple languages and is being validated in the ongoing phase 3 trials.[74–77]

SUMMARY AND OPEN QUESTIONS

The management of DT is shifting more and more toward conservative and patient-tailored strategies, also thanks to the employment of radiologic and radiomics criteria, which are able to predict the risk of progression and the response to treatment. In order to offer better chances at PFS and an acceptable QoL, case discussion in the context of a multidisciplinary tumor board at a center of excellence is highly recommended.

The assessment of tumor mutational status and the discovery of new mutations could provide enhanced prognostic tools to guide the choice of primary treatment, in the case of failure of active surveillance.

Surgery is still considered a first-line active treatment in only few selected cases and for the management of selected intra-abdominal complications.

The choice of the first-line systemic treatment continues to be a matter of debate; according to current guidelines, no specific criteria exist to select the appropriate treatment based on tumor location.

Finally, recurrence still represents a therapeutic challenge, for which well-defined and shared guidelines are still lacking, the next project for The Desmoid Tumor Working Group.

DISCLOSURE

The authors have no commercial or financial conflicts of interest to declare. No funding was received for this article.

REFERENCES

1. Fiore M, Crago A, Gladdy R, et al. The landmark series: desmoid. Ann Surg Oncol 2021;28(3):1682–9.
2. Kasper B, Baumgarten C, Garcia J, et al. An update on the management of sporadic desmoid-type fibromatosis: a European Consensus Initiative between Sarcoma PAtients EuroNet (SPAEN) and European Organization for Research and Treatment of Cancer (EORTC)/Soft Tissue and Bone Sarcoma Group (STBSG). Ann Oncol 2017;28(10):2399–408.
3. Cuomo P, Scoccianti G, Schiavo A, et al. Extra-abdominal desmoid tumor fibromatosis: a multicenter EMSOS study. BMC Cancer 2021;21(1):437.
4. Board. WCoTE. Soft tissue and bone tumours. 5th edition ed. Lyon2020.
5. Fiore M, Coppola S, Cannell AJ, et al. Desmoid-type fibromatosis and pregnancy: a multi-institutional analysis of recurrence and obstetric risk. Ann Surg 2014; 259(5):973–8.
6. Cojocaru E, Gennatas S, Thway K, et al. Approach to screening for familial adenomatous polyposis (FAP) in a cohort of 226 patients with desmoid-type fibromatosis (DF): experience of a specialist center in the UK. Fam Cancer 2021;1: 69–74.
7. Gronchi A, Jones RL. Treatment of desmoid tumors in 2019. JAMA Oncol 2019; 5(4):567–8.
8. Kasper B, Raut CP, Gronchi A. Desmoid tumors: to treat or not to treat, that is the question. Cancer 2020;126(24):5213–21.
9. The management of desmoid tumours: a joint global consensus-based guideline approach for adult and paediatric patients. Eur J Cancer 2020;127:96–107.
10. Kummar S, O'Sullivan Coyne G, Do KT, et al. Clinical activity of the γ-secretase inhibitor PF-03084014 in adults with desmoid tumors (aggressive fibromatosis). J Clin Oncol 2017;35(14):1561–9.
11. Crago AM, Chmielecki J, Rosenberg M, et al. Near universal detection of alterations in CTNNB1 and Wnt pathway regulators in desmoid-type fibromatosis by whole-exome sequencing and genomic analysis. Genes Chromosomes Cancer 2015;54(10):606–15.

12. Slowik V, Attard T, Dai H, et al. Desmoid tumors complicating familial adenomatous polyposis: a meta-analysis mutation spectrum of affected individuals. BMC Gastroenterol 2015;15:84.

13. Timbergen MJM, Colombo C, Renckens M, et al. The prognostic role of β-catenin mutations in desmoid-type fibromatosis undergoing resection only: a meta-analysis of individual patient data. Ann Surg 2021;273(6):1094–101.

14. Hamada S, Futamura N, Ikuta K, et al. CTNNB1 S45F mutation predicts poor efficacy of meloxicam treatment for desmoid tumors: a pilot study. PLoS One 2014; 9(5):e96391.

15. Kasper B, Gruenwald V, Reichardt P, et al. Correlation of CTNNB1 mutation status with progression arrest rate in RECIST progressive desmoid-type fibromatosis treated with imatinib: translational research results from a phase 2 study of the German Interdisciplinary Sarcoma Group (GISG-01). Ann Surg Oncol 2016; 23(6):1924–7.

16. Timbergen MJM, Boers R, Vriends ALM, et al. Differentially methylated regions in desmoid-type fibromatosis: a comparison between CTNNB1 S45F and T41A tumors. Front Oncol 2020;10:565031.

17. Bräutigam K, Lindner J, Budczies J, et al. PARP-1 expression as a prognostic factor in desmoid-type fibromatosis. Ann Diagn Pathol 2020;44:151442.

18. Colombo C, Fiore M, Grignani G, et al. A prospective observational study of active surveillance in primary desmoid fibromatosis. Clin Cancer Res 2022. https://doi.org/10.1158/1078-0432.CCR-21-4205. clincanres.4205.

19. Bonvalot S, Ternès N, Fiore M, et al. Spontaneous regression of primary abdominal wall desmoid tumors: more common than previously thought. Ann Surg Oncol 2013;20(13):4096–102.

20. Fiore M, Rimareix F, Mariani L, et al. Desmoid-type fibromatosis: a front-line conservative approach to select patients for surgical treatment. Ann Surg Oncol 2009;16(9):2587–93.

21. Penel N, Le Cesne A, Bonvalot S, et al. Surgical versus non-surgical approach in primary desmoid-type fibromatosis patients: a nationwide prospective cohort from the French Sarcoma Group. Eur J Cancer 2017;83:125–31.

22. Ruspi L, Cananzi FCM, Sicoli F, et al. Event-free survival in desmoid-type fibromatosis (DTF): a pre-post comparison of upfront surgery versus wait-and-see approach. Eur J Surg Oncol 2021;47(5):1196–200.

23. Quality of life of patients with desmoid-type fibromatosis (QUALIFIED) [updated April 2, 2021 August 31, 2021]. ClinicalTrials.gov Identifier: NCT04289077]. Available at: https://clinicaltrials.gov/ct2/show/NCT04289077.

24. Timbergen MJM, Schut AW, Grünhagen DJ, et al. Active surveillance in desmoid-type fibromatosis: a systematic literature review. Eur J Cancer 2020;137:18–29.

25. Colombo C, Miceli R, Le Péchoux C, et al. Sporadic extra abdominal wall desmoid-type fibromatosis: surgical resection can be safely limited to a minority of patients. Eur J Cancer 2015;51(2):186–92.

26. Improta L, Tzanis D, Bouhadiba T, et al. Desmoid tumours in the surveillance era: what are the remaining indications for surgery? Eur J Surg Oncol 2020;46(7): 1310–4.

27. Sanchez-Mete L, Ferraresi V, Caterino M, et al. Desmoid tumors characteristics, clinical management, active surveillance, and description of our FAP case series. J Clin Med 2020;9(12).

28. Duhil de Bénazé G, Vigan M, Corradini N, et al. Functional analysis of young patients with desmoid-type fibromatosis: Initial surveillance does not jeopardize long term quality of life. Eur J Surg Oncol 2020;46(7):1294–300.

29. Gronchi A, Casali PG, Mariani L, et al. Quality of surgery and outcome in extra-abdominal aggressive fibromatosis: a series of patients surgically treated at a single institution. J Clin Oncol 2003;21(7):1390–7.

30. Crago AM, Denton B, Salas S, et al. A prognostic nomogram for prediction of recurrence in desmoid fibromatosis. Ann Surg 2013;258(2):347–53.

31. Braggio DL, A.; Hernandez, L.; Mercier, K. A patient reported outcomes of treatments for desmoid tumors: an international natural history study. 2021 ASCO Annual Meeting.

32. Bouttefroy SP N, Minard-Colin V, Orbach D, et al. Desmoid type fibromatosis in patients. ESMO Virtual Congress 2020.

33. National clinical-biological prospective cohort of incident cases of aggressive fibromatosis (ALTITUDES) [updated May 13, 2021. ClinicalTrials.gov Identifier: NCT02867033]. Available at: https://clinicaltrials.gov/ct2/show/NCT02867033?recrs=abdf&cond=desmoid&cntry=FR&draw=2&rank=1.

34. Bishop AJ, Landry JP, Roland CL, et al. Certain risk factors for patients with desmoid tumors warrant reconsideration of local therapy strategies. Cancer 2020;126(14):3265–73.

35. Hansmann A, Adolph C, Vogel T, et al. High-dose tamoxifen and sulindac as first-line treatment for desmoid tumors. Cancer 2004;100(3):612–20.

36. Skapek SX, Anderson JR, Hill DA, et al. Safety and efficacy of high-dose tamoxifen and sulindac for desmoid tumor in children: results of a Children's Oncology Group (COG) phase II study. Pediatr Blood Cancer 2013;60(7):1108–12.

37. Fiore M, Colombo C, Radaelli S, et al. Hormonal manipulation with toremifene in sporadic desmold-type fibromatosis. Eur J Cancer 2015;51(18):2800–7.

38. Quast DR, Schneider R, Burdzik E, et al. Long-term outcome of sporadic and FAP-associated desmoid tumors treated with high-dose selective estrogen receptor modulators and sulindac: a single-center long-term observational study in 134 patients. Fam Cancer 2016;15(1):31–40.

39. Azzarelli A, Gronchi A, Bertulli R, et al. Low-dose chemotherapy with methotrexate and vinblastine for patients with advanced aggressive fibromatosis. Cancer 2001;92(5):1259–64.

40. Gega M, Yanagi H, Yoshikawa R, et al. Successful chemotherapeutic modality of doxorubicin plus dacarbazine for the treatment of desmoid tumors in association with familial adenomatous polyposis. J Clin Oncol 2006;24(1):102–5.

41. Heinrich MC, McArthur GA, Demetri GD, et al. Clinical and molecular studies of the effect of imatinib on advanced aggressive fibromatosis (desmoid tumor). J Clin Oncol 2006;24(7):1195–203.

42. Chugh R, Wathen JK, Patel SR, et al. Efficacy of imatinib in aggressive fibromatosis: results of a phase II multicenter Sarcoma Alliance for Research through Collaboration (SARC) trial. Clin Cancer Res 2010;16(19):4884–91.

43. Palassini E, Frezza AM, Mariani L, et al. Long-term efficacy of methotrexate plus vinblastine/vinorelbine in a large series of patients affected by desmoid-type fibromatosis. Cancer J 2017;23(2):86–91.

44. Gounder MM, Mahoney MR, Van Tine BA, et al. Sorafenib for advanced and refractory desmoid tumors. N Engl J Med 2018;379(25):2417–28.

45. Toulmonde M, Pulido M, Ray-Coquard I, et al. Pazopanib or methotrexate-vinblastine combination chemotherapy in adult patients with progressive desmoid tumours (DESMOPAZ): a non-comparative, randomised, open-label, multicentre, phase 2 study. Lancet Oncol 2019;20(9):1263–72.

46. Gounder MM, Lefkowitz RA, Keohan ML, et al. Activity of sorafenib against desmoid tumor/deep fibromatosis. Clin Cancer Res 2011;17(12):4082–90.

47. Kasper B, Gruenwald V, Reichardt P, et al. Imatinib induces sustained progression arrest in RECIST progressive desmoid tumours: final results of a phase II study of the German Interdisciplinary Sarcoma Group (GISG). Eur J Cancer 2017;76:60–7.

48. Szucs Z, Messiou C, Wong HH, et al. Pazopanib, a promising option for the treatment of aggressive fibromatosis. Anticancer Drugs 2017;28(4):421–6.

49. Zheng C, Zhou Y, Wang Y, et al. The activity and safety of anlotinib for patients with extremity desmoid fibromatosis: a retrospective study in a single institution. Drug Des Devel Ther 2020;14:3941–50.

50. Zheng C, Fang J, Wang Y, et al. Efficacy and safety of apatinib for patients with advanced extremity desmoid fibromatosis: a retrospective study. J Cancer Res Clin Oncol 2021;147(7):2127–35.

51. Nishida Y, Hamada S, Urakawa H, et al. Desmoid with biweekly methotrexate and vinblastine shows similar effects to weekly administration: a phase II clinical trial. Cancer Sci 2020;111(11):4187–94.

52. Napolitano A, Provenzano S, Colombo C, et al. Familial adenomatosis polyposis-related desmoid tumours treated with low-dose chemotherapy: results from an international, multi-institutional, retrospective analysis. ESMO Open 2020;5(1).

53. Gennatas S, Chamberlain F, Smrke A, et al. A timely oral option: single-agent vinorelbine in desmoid tumors. Oncologist 2020;25(12):e2013–6.

54. Constantinidou A, Jones RL, Scurr M, et al. Pegylated liposomal doxorubicin, an effective, well-tolerated treatment for refractory aggressive fibromatosis. Eur J Cancer 2009;45(17):2930–4.

55. Garbay D, Le Cesne A, Penel N, et al. Chemotherapy in patients with desmoid tumors: a study from the French Sarcoma Group (FSG). Ann Oncol 2012;23(1):182–6.

56. Shimizu K, Kawashima H, Kawai A, et al. Effectiveness of doxorubicin-based and liposomal doxorubicin chemotherapies for patients with extra-abdominal desmoid-type fibromatosis: a systematic review. Jpn J Clin Oncol 2020;50(11):1274–81.

57. Gounder MM. Notch inhibition in desmoids: "sure it works in practice, but does it work in theory? Cancer 2015;121(22):3933–7.

58. Messersmith WA, Shapiro GI, Cleary JM, et al. A phase I, dose-finding study in patients with advanced solid malignancies of the oral γ-secretase inhibitor PF-03084014. Clin Cancer Res 2015;21(1):60–7.

59. Nirogacestat for adults with desmoid tumor/aggressive fibromatosis (DT/AF) (DeFi) [updated July 27, 2021August 31, 2021]. ClinicalTrials.gov Identifier: NCT03785964]. Available at: https://clinicaltrials.gov/ct2/show/NCT03785964.

60. A study of AL102 in patients with progressing desmoid tumors (RINGSIDE). ClinicalTrials.gov Identifier: NCT04871282]. Available at: https://clinicaltrials.gov/ct2/show/NCT04871282.

61. Keus RB, Nout RA, Blay JY, et al. Results of a phase II pilot study of moderate dose radiotherapy for inoperable desmoid-type fibromatosis–an EORTC STBSG and ROG study (EORTC 62991-22998). Ann Oncol 2013;24(10):2672–6.

62. Gladdy RA, Qin LX, Moraco N, et al. Do radiation-associated soft tissue sarcomas have the same prognosis as sporadic soft tissue sarcomas? J Clin Oncol 2010;28(12):2064–9.

63. Bouhamama A, Lame F, Mastier C, et al. Local control and analgesic efficacy of percutaneous cryoablation for desmoid tumors. Cardiovasc Intervent Radiol 2020;43(1):110–9.

64. Saltiel S, Bize PE, Goetti P, et al. Cryoablation of extra-abdominal desmoid tumors: a single-center experience with literature review. Diagnostics (Basel). 2020;10(8).

65. Kurtz JE, Buy X, Deschamps F, et al. CRYODESMO-O1: a prospective, open phase II study of cryoablation in desmoid tumour patients progressing after medical treatment. Eur J Cancer 2021;143:78–87.

66. Lewis JJ, Boland PJ, Leung DH, et al. The enigma of desmoid tumors. Ann Surg 1999;229(6):866–72.

67. Burtenshaw SM, Cannell AJ, McAlister ED, et al. Toward observation as first-line management in abdominal desmoid tumors. Ann Surg Oncol 2016;23(7):2212–9.

68. Cassidy MR, Lefkowitz RA, Long N, et al. Association of MRI T2 signal intensity with desmoid tumor progression during active observation: a retrospective cohort study. Ann Surg 2020;271(4):748–55.

69. Murahashi Y, Emori M, Shimizu J, et al. The value of the black fiber sign on T1-weighted images for predicting stability of desmoid fibromatosis managed conservatively. Eur Radiol 2020;30(10):5768–76.

70. Gondim Teixeira PA, Biouichi H, Abou Arab W, et al. Evidence-based MR imaging follow-up strategy for desmoid-type fibromatosis. Eur Radiol 2020;30(2):895–902.

71. Crombé A, Kind M, Ray-Coquard I, et al. Progressive desmoid tumor: radiomics compared with conventional response criteria for predicting progression during systemic therapy-a multicenter study by the French Sarcoma Group. AJR Am J Roentgenol 2020;215(6):1539–48.

72. Timbergen MJM, Starmans MPA, Padmos GA, et al. Differential diagnosis and mutation stratification of desmoid-type fibromatosis on MRI using radiomics. Eur J Radiol 2020;131:109266.

73. Newman ET, Lans J, Kim J, et al. PROMIS function scores are lower in patients who underwent more aggressive local treatment for desmoid tumors. Clin Orthop Relat Res 2020;478(3):563–77.

74. Gounder MM, Maddux L, Paty J, et al. Prospective development of a patient-reported outcomes instrument for desmoid tumors or aggressive fibromatosis. Cancer 2020;126(3):531–9.

75. Available at: https://clinicaltrials.gov/ct2/show/NCT04871282.

76. Available at: https://clinicaltrials.gov/ct2/show/NCT03785964.

77. Quality of life of patients with desmoid-type fibromatosis (QUALIFIED) Available at: https://clinicaltrials.gov/ct2/show/NCT04289077?term=quality+of+life&cond=Desmoid&draw=2&rank=1.

Toward Better Understanding and Management of Solitary Fibrous Tumor

Karineh Kazazian, MD, PhD[a], Elizabeth G. Demicco, MD, PhD[b,c],
Marc de Perrot, MD, MSc[a,d], Dirk Strauss, MD[e],
Carol J. Swallow, MD, PhD[a,f],*

KEYWORDS

- Solitary fibrous tumor • NAB2-STAT6 • Risk stratification • Prognostic factors
- Surgery • Therapeutic strategies • Survival

KEY POINTS

- Solitary fibrous tumors (SFTs) are a unique subtype of soft tissue sarcoma, featuring intense vascularity, well-circumscribed margins and a clinical course that is often relatively indolent.
- Description of the characteristic NAB2-STAT6 gene fusion has facilitated accurate diagnosis.
- Optimal management of SFT is focused on complete resection with function preservation.
- Existing risk stratification systems can be used to estimate risk of recurrence following resection; their accuracy is expected to increase with recent improvements in diagnostic accuracy, informing evidence-based management decisions.

DEFINITION AND HISTORICAL PERSPECTIVE

Solitary fibrous tumor (SFT) is a fibroblastic neoplasm characterized by *NGFI-A binding protein 2-signal transducer* and *activator of transcription 6* (*NAB2-STAT6*) gene

[a] Department of Surgery, University of Toronto, Toronto, Canada; [b] Department of Pathology and Laboratory Medicine, Mount Sinai Hospital, 600 University Avenue, Toronto, Ontario M5G 1X5, Canada; [c] Department of Laboratory Medicine and Pathobiology, University of Toronto, Toronto, Canada; [d] Division of Thoracic Surgery, Princess Margaret Cancer Centre/University Health Network, 200 Elizabeth Street, Toronto, Ontario M5G2C4, Canada; [e] Sarcoma Unit, Department of Academic Surgery, Royal Marsden Hospital, Royal Marsden NHS Foundation Trust, Fulham Road, London SW3 6JJ, England; [f] Department of Surgical Oncology, Princess Margaret Cancer Centre/Mount Sinai Hospital, Toronto, Canada
* Corresponding author. Mount Sinai Hospital, Sinai Health System, Room 1225, 600 University Avenue, Toronto, Ontario M5G 1X5, Canada.
E-mail address: Carol.Swallow@sinaihealth.ca

Surg Oncol Clin N Am 31 (2022) 459–483
https://doi.org/10.1016/j.soc.2022.03.009
surgonc.theclinics.com

rearrangements. First recognized in the pleura,[1] SFT was previously referred to by several other names, including hemangiopericytoma (HPC),[2] benign mesothelioma, localized fibrous tumor, subserosal fibroma, and pleural fibroma. SFT is now recognized to occur at all anatomic sites and comprises a histologic spectrum, ranging from "classic" hypocellular fibrous SFT, to hypercellular tumors previously recognized as "hemangiopericytoma," to anaplastic SFT with frank sarcomatous transformation.[3] Historically, SFTs were defined as "benign" or "malignant," based on criteria initially developed for pleural SFT[4]; most series incorporated mitotic activity (>4 mitotic figures/10 high power fields [HPF]) in the definition of malignancy, but inconsistently applied additional tumor characteristics, such as cellularity and nuclear pleomorphism. Moreover, SFT and HPC were treated as different entities with different behavior and diagnostic criteria. In particular, the arbitrary distinction between SFT and HPC, and the relatively nonspecific pattern of tumor vascularity used as a defining feature before the development of specific ancillary studies, resulted in many cases of other sarcomas, such as synovial sarcoma, being misdiagnosed as SFT; this contributed to inconsistency in the correlation between tumor classification and behavior and the false adage that "the behavior of SFT is difficult to predict."

Over the past 2 decades, recognition of the histologic spectrum of SFT, the driving molecular alterations, development of specific diagnostic immunohistochemical and molecular tests, and new risk stratification systems have resulted in improved tumor classification and more accurate prediction of patient outcomes after complete resection.

EPIDEMIOLOGY

SFT is considered a rare soft tissue tumor, accounting for approximately 2% of soft tissue sarcomas treated at a large referral center in one series.[5] A recent Surveillance, Epidemiology, and End Results (SEER) database query showed that the age-adjusted incidence rate for extrameningeal SFTs was 0.61 per 1,000,000 persons per year versus 0.38 for meningeal SFTs.[6,7] Several case series have shown that although these tumors can affect adults aged 20 to 80 years, they are most common in the fifth to seventh decades,[5,7–10] with an equal distribution between men and women.[3,5–7]

SFTs can arise in almost any site of the body, including thorax/pleura, intraabdominally, the central nervous system (CNS)/meninges, extremities/trunk, and head and neck. Around 25% to 30% of cases arise intrathoracically, with pleura being the most common single site. Intraabdominal SFTs (~20%) in the peritoneum, retroperitoneum, and pelvis constitute the largest site-related group in most series of extrapleural SFTs, with the retroperitoneum as the most common intraabdominal site, followed by the pelvis. Approximately 15% of SFTs arise from the CNS, including the meninges, whereas 10% occur in the head and neck[5,8,11]; SFTs of the extracranial head and neck most often arise in the sinonasal tract, orbit, oral cavity, and salivary glands.[12] Tumors in the head and neck and meninges tend to present in younger patients, whereas SFTs arising in deep body cavities (pleura, abdominopelvic area, and retroperitoneum) come to clinical attention in older patients. A further 10% to 20% of SFTs arise in the superficial trunk or soft tissue of the extremities.[13]

There are no known environmental or inherited predisposing risk factors for SFT.

HISTOLOGIC FEATURES

Grossly, SFTs range from less than 1 cm to greater than 40 cm in maximal dimension, with size largely determined by the site and the ability of slow growing tumors to go undetected.[3] Tumors show variable gross appearance ranging from pale and densely

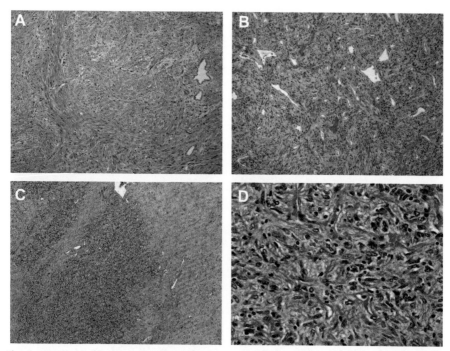

Fig. 1. Histologic features of solitary fibrous tumor (SFT). (*A*) Less cellular SFT comprised of long spindled cells within a densely collagenized and sclerotic-appearing stroma (H&E, 100x). (*B*) Thin-walled, branching vessels are a characteristic feature, although their density may vary. Vessels may be ectatic, compressed, or altered by mural hyalinization (H&E, 100x). (*C*) Alternating cellular and fibrotic or myxoid areas are common in SFTs (H&E, 50x). (*D*) Most SFTs show moderate to scant amounts of palely eosinophilic to amphophilic cytoplasm and irregular ovoid nuclei with slight membrane irregularities, vesicular chromatin, and small, inconspicuous nucleoli (H&E, 400x).

fibrous, to tan and fleshy in cellular tumors, or gelatinous in myxoid tumors. Areas of hemorrhage are common, and necrosis may be seen.

Histologically, SFTs show variable cellular and stromal features. At one end of the spectrum, tumors may be comprised largely of sclerotic, hyalinized collagen fibers with occasional compressed, elongated spindled tumor cells (**Fig. 1**A). Thin-walled vessels are always present, but may be inconspicuous, or altered by stromal hyalinization (**Fig. 1**B). Slightly more cellular tumors may show prominent areas of alternating cellular and hypocellular growth (**Fig. 1**C). Classically, the architecture is described as "haphazard" or "patternless," as tumor cells may be arrayed in short, randomly oriented fascicles, storiform whorls, or nests. Most commonly, the tumor cells are plump, angular to slightly stellate spindled cells with bland oval nuclei with even fine to vesicular chromatin, inconspicuous nucleoli, and slight membrane irregularities (**Fig. 1**D). Some nuclear variability is common, but marked pleomorphism is rare.

On the cellular end of the spectrum, there may be minimal collagenous stroma, and the tumor cells may be more plump and ovoid in appearance, forming nests within a branched, anastomosing vascular network (**Fig. 2**A). Throughout the spectrum of SFT, stromal features may vary, with some tumors showing myxoid changes that may rarely be extensive (**Fig. 2**B). Mitotic activity is usually low. Tumor necrosis is uncommon and must be distinguished from intratumoral hemorrhage. Variants of SFT include lipomatous (fat-forming) SFT[14–16] and giant cell-rich SFT, which

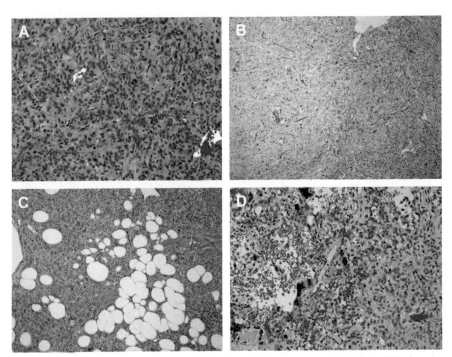

Fig. 2. Spectrum of histologic subtypes of solitary fibrous tumor. (*A*) Cellular SFT showing nests of rounded cells with indistinct cell borders. There is minimal stroma, and tumor nests are delineated by a rich network of compressed, thin-walled blood vessels (H&E, 200x). (*B*) Myxoid SFT. Cellularity is variable, and the stroma is expanded by mucinous material; however, the characteristic haphazard tumor cell arrangement, thin-walled vasculature, and thick collagen bundles remain discernible (H&E, 100x). (*C*) Lipomatous (fat-forming) SFT shows islands of heterologous adipocytic differentiation within an otherwise typical SFT (H&E, 100x). (*D*) Giant cell-rich SFT shows variably prominent multinucleated stromal cells that are often present lining pseudovascular spaces (H&E, 100x).

contains multinucleated, stellate stromal cells that often line pseudovascular spaces in the tissue (**Fig. 2**C–D).[17,18] Anaplastic SFTs have undergone progression to outright sarcoma and usually show areas of recognizable SFTs juxtaposed to a high-grade undifferentiated sarcoma. Heterologous elements have been reported in anaplastic SFTs.[19–21]

Immunohistochemically, the most specific and sensitive diagnostic marker for SFT is nuclear expression of STAT6 (c-terminus), reflecting aberrant expression and localization of the NAB2-STAT6 chimeric protein.[22–25] GRIA2 and ALDH1, discovered in gene profiling studies to be overexpressed in SFTs, have also been proposed as relatively sensitive and specific markers[26,27] but do not seem to show any advantage over STAT6. Stains for CD34 and BCL2 are positive in SFTs but are not specific. SFTs are usually negative for keratins, S100, actin, and desmin, although aberrant expression has been reported. Anaplastic or aggressive SFTs may lose expression of CD34 and STAT6,[28–31] and meningeal SFTs often show only weak or patchy CD34.

MOLECULAR HALLMARKS

SFTs are characterized by a paracentric inversion involving chromosome 12q, resulting in the juxtaposition of the *NAB2* and *STAT6* genes.[23,32–34] More than 20 different fusion types have been reported, involving different exons, introns, or 5′ untranslated regions of these genes. It is thought that the different fusion types may contribute to the phenotypic variability or localization of SFTs, as most of the SFTs arising in the pleura show fusions of *NAB2* exon 4 with *STAT6* exon 2 or 3, whereas in SFTs arising in extrathoracic locations, fusions of *NAB2* exon 5, 6, or 7 to *STAT6* exons 16, 17, or 18 are more common.[35,36] Because of the small size of the chromosomal inversion it is not detectable by most break-apart clinical fluorescence in situ hybridization probes, and the diversity of *NAB2-STAT6* breakpoints requires multiplexed PCR or next-generation sequencing to provide adequate sensitivity (neither method reliably detects intronic fusions). Therefore, demonstration of the *NAB2-STAT6* fusion is not required or routinely recommended for the diagnosis of SFTs. Strong and diffuse nuclear positivity in the absence of cytoplasmic expression on immunohistochemical staining for STAT6 c-terminal epitopes is sensitive and specific for these rearrangements.

Additional mutations have been reported to possibly contribute to SFT progression, including *TP53* mutations or loss in anaplastic SFTs[30,35,37,38] and *TERT* promoter mutations in long-standing tumors diagnosed in older patients.[35,39–41]

Clinical Presentation and Surgical Management

Although the clinical presentation of SFT varies by site (described later), SFTs may also be associated with Doege-Potter paraneoplastic syndrome (up to ~3% of cases), characterized by hypoinsulinaemic hypoglycaemia, due to ectopic secretion of a prohormone of insulinlike growth factor 2 (IGF-2).[42] This paraneoplastic syndrome can occur from SFTs arising at any site but is primarily seen in large peritoneal/pleural tumors[43–45] and resolves following resection.[46] Pleuropulmonary SFTs may also be associated with hypertrophic pulmonary osteoarthropathy, occasionally referred to as Pierre-Marie-Bamberger syndrome, characterized by clubbing of the fingers, hypertrophic skin changes, increased periosteal activity, and synovial effusions.[9,47]

LOCALIZED DISEASE
Extracranial Head and Neck Solitary Fibrous Tumor

SFT of the head and neck represents ~10% of all SFTs[5,12,48] and includes lesions previously described as HPCs, giant cell angiofibromas, and orbital fibrous histiocytoma.[49] A recent series[12] showed that the most prevalent primary site of involvement was the sinonasal tract (30%), followed by the orbit (25%), oral cavity (15%), and the major salivary glands (14%). The median size of SFT at head and neck sites is smaller than at other sites (2.6–2.8 cm[12,50]), with implications for prognostic modeling and clinical nomograms incorporating size.[51] Symptoms of SFT in the head and neck are nonspecific and are related to the presence of a soft tissue mass in the area affected. In the sinonasal tract, SFTs often present with sinus/nasal obstruction and a painless mass, whereas in the orbit the clinical presentation may include an expanding mass in the eyelid or orbit, epiphora, or proptosis. Radiographic features include a solitary well-circumscribed mass that is isodense on plain computed tomography (CT), with marked heterogeneous enhancement on contrast-enhanced CT and MRI.[52,53]

Although complete excision is the mainstay of treatment, the anatomic complexity of the head and neck region may constrain the ability to achieve it, and wide surgical margins are often not feasible. Moreover, endoscopic resections can make margin status difficult to ascertain. In the largest modern series of head and neck SFTs, the rate of histologically positive margins was 67%; it is noteworthy that this did not necessarily correlate with risk of local recurrence (LR), as 52% of cases with positive margins did not recur.[12] LR is common (up to 40%) in head and neck SFTs, whereas metastasis remains relatively rare (6%–12% of cases).[8,50,52,54–56] Recurrence after complete excision is uncommon: in the series by Cox and colleagues,[50] 4 out of 9 cases with positive margins recurred, but no recurrences were noted with negative margins. Several other series do, however, report LR despite negative margins in up to 17%.[12] In one study, median time to recurrence after resection was 10 years, highlighting the need for long-term follow-up for these patients.[12,52]

Central Nervous System Solitary Fibrous Tumor

CNS SFTs are primarily dural based. The majority (70%) are intracranial, whereas 30% are spinal in origin.[57] Overall, SFTs account for 1% to 4% of intracranial tumors.[58,59] Before 2016, SFTs and HPCs in the CNS had been characterized as 2 distinct entities. The identification of the *NAB2-STAT6* fusion as a distinct molecular feature led to the two being combined into one single pathologic entity and classified accordingly.[58,60–62] In the fourth edition of the World Health Organization (WHO) classification of tumors of the CNS, SFTs/HPCs with a classic SFT phenotype were considered grade I, whereas those with an HPC phenotype are classified as grade II or III tumors depending on mitotic count. In the current fifth edition WHO classification of CNS tumors,[13] there is considered to be no distinction between SFT and HPC phenotypes. Instead, grading is based on evidence from more recent series that tumor necrosis is more important in tumor prognostication.[63,64] The fifth edition WHO grading of CNS SFTs defines grade I tumors as those with less than 5 mitotic figures/10 HPF, grade II as those with more than or equal to 5 mitotic figures/10 HPF and grade III as those having both high mitotic activity and tumor necrosis.[13] Grade I CNS SFTs typically cause symptoms through a slow increase in size, either by mass effect and compression of adjacent structures or by increasing intracranial pressure, whereas high-grade II to III SFTs more often present with symptoms of headache, focal neurologic deficits, or seizures caused by mass effect or edema in adjacent brain parenchyma with a shorter duration of symptoms thought to reflect more rapid growth. Mean age at presentation is lower than for SFTs at other sites, more commonly in the fourth and fifth decades, with a slight male predominance.[7,57]

CT features of CNS SFTs are similar to those of SFTs elsewhere, with isoattenuation and avid enhancement after IV contrast administration. In contrast to the bone thickening adjacent to meningiomas, smooth erosion of the skull can be seen adjacent to meningeal SFTs in up to 50% of cases.[65] MRI features include heterogeneous signal intensity on T2-weighted images with intense enhancement on postgadolinium T1-weighted images.

As for all other sarcomas, the recommended treatment of primary localized meningeal SFTs is a wide surgical resection, which is typically challenging in CNS locations, as preservation of neurologic function is also a priority.[66–71] Rates of macroscopic complete resection vary from 49% to 85%. Preoperative embolization may be used in an attempt to improve the chances of complete but safe resection.[59,66] Gross total resection is a prognostic factor that correlates with progression-free survival (PFS) and overall survival (OS), with subtotal resection being associated with increased rates of local "recurrence," metastasis, and reduced PFS.[57,59,66–68,71–73] In the majority (84%) of patients, subtotal resection is followed by adjuvant radiotherapy, with evidence to suggest reduced risk of LR, but no effect on metastasis.[57] In WHO fourth edition grade I CNS SFTs, prognosis is excellent with surgical resection alone, although subtotal resection can result in LR. At the other end of the spectrum, grade III SFTs have higher recurrence rates, more frequent extracranial metastases, and higher mortality rates.[59,66,70,71,74] In a recent systematic review with 368 patients, a 5- and 10-year OS of 79% and 77%, respectively, was described for CNS SFTs.[57]

The reported incidence of extracranial metastases ranges from 13% to 55%; the most common sites include liver, lung, bone, kidney, and peritoneum.[59,67,68,70,74–77] Development of extracranial metastases is most common in patients with high-grade lesions and occurs at 2 to 18 years following resection.[57,66] The median survival for patients with metastatic disease is 4.4 years.[57] In the management of recurrent intracranial SFT, repeat resection with or without adjunctive external beam radiotherapy, radiosurgical intervention, and radiotherapy alone have been described, with a multimodality approach apparently extending time to second recurrence.[72,78] In a recent series of patients who underwent salvage treatment of first LR, 45% experienced a second LR, but patients could achieve long-term survival with a 5-year OS of 89%.[78]

Thoracic/Pleural Solitary Fibrous Tumor

Patients typically present with nonspecific pulmonary symptoms or with an incidental finding of an intrathoracic mass at the time of chest imaging for other reasons. Approximately 40% to 60% of patients are symptomatic, with cough, chest pain, or dyspnea.[42,79–81] Rarely, hemoptysis and obstructive pneumonitis may occur as a result of airway obstruction.[82] Pleuropulmonary tumors can be associated with paraneoplastic syndromes such as hypoglycemia or hypertrophic pulmonary osteoarthropathy in up to ~3% and 20% of cases, respectively.[9,47,83] Pleural SFTs can reach a large size while remaining asymptomatic, with median size in several series ~6 to 10 cm. They can also be associated with pleural effusions.[84] Two-thirds of pleural SFTs arise from the visceral pleura, where the tumor is often attached to the lung by a narrow pedicle, and one-third occur in the parietal, mediastinal, or diaphragmatic pleura where the tumors are often larger, with a broad-based attachment. Chest radiography usually reveals a solitary, well-circumscribed mass located at the periphery of the lung or in fissures. In most cases, CT scan of the thorax shows a solitary, well-circumscribed, hypervascular soft tissue mass of homogenous density, arising from the pleura,[9,85] with larger tumors typically showing displacement rather than invasion of surrounding structures. Contrast enhancement is usually intense and homogenous, although there can be lower density and heterogeneous zones in large tumors due to necrosis or hemorrhage.[9,82,84] MRI can be used to assess relationships with neighboring structures. Pretreatment biopsy is ideal, but not always diagnostic, and resection may be required to finalize the diagnosis.

As with all localized SFTs, complete en bloc resection, preferably with negative margins, is the mainstay of therapy.[9] The tendency of thoracic SFTs to arise from the visceral pleura (60%–80%), and often be pedunculated, facilitates complete resection. Pulmonary wedge resection is the most frequently performed procedure, and this can often be approached through video-assisted thoracic surgery, particularly for tumors less than 10 cm, with the alternative being thoracotomy.[86,87] In SFTs arising from parietal pleura, large sessile lesions, or ipsilateral intrapleural metastases, other resection types, such as lobectomy, pneumonectomy or extrapleural pneumonectomy, chest wall resection, and diaphragm resection en bloc with associated parietal pleural, may be required to achieve negative margins.[81,86,88] Some groups consider angiography and embolization of feeding vessels preoperatively with the purpose of reducing intraoperative bleeding.[89]

Recurrence rates vary based on anatomic and histologic characteristics of resected pleural SFTs (**Table 1**). In one of the most widely validated risk models for pleural SFT that includes both histologic and anatomic parameters, 91% of patients with low-risk

Table 1
Models for risk prediction in pleural slitary fibrous tumors

	Histologic Risk Factors						Anatomic Risk Factors			
	Mitotic figures per 10 high power fields	Hypercellularity	Nuclear Pleomorphism	Tumor Necrosis	Hemorrhage	Stromal/ Vascular Invasion	Tumor Size	Pedunculation	Site	Mib-1 Proliferation Index
England DM et al,[4] 1989	>4	Yes	Yes	Yes	Yes	—	>10 cm	Sessile	Parietal pleural	—
De Perrot M et al,[92] 2002	>4	Yes	Yes	Yes	—	Yes	—	Sessile	—	—
Tapias LC et al., 2015[80]	≥4	Yes	—	Yes	Yes	—	≥10 cm	Sessile	Parietal pleura	—
Diebold M et al.,[130] 2017	≥4	—	—	Yes	—	—	≥10 cm	—	—	≥10%

Malignancy by the criteria of England et al. or De Perrot et al. requires the presence of any one histologic risk factor. A malignant (high-risk) diagnosis according to the Tapias et al. model requires any 3 histologic and/or anatomic risk factors. Diebold et al. found the presence of at least 2 risk factors to be sensitive and specific for poor outcomes.

tumors were alive at 10 years with a 3.5% risk of recurrence at 15 years, compared with 73% 10-year survival and 30% 15-year recurrence risk in patients with high-risk tumors.[90] Reisenauer and colleagues[91] compared risk stratification models proposed by Demicco and colleagues,[8,51] Tapias and colleagues,[80] and de Perrot and colleagues.[92] Tumors that were classified low risk by the modified Demicco, de Perrot (stage 0), or Tapias models had 100%, 100%, and 98% 5-year PFS, respectively, whereas high risk by the modified Demicco, de Perrot (stage 3), or Tapias models had 53%, 80%, and 81% 5-year PFS, respectively.

Reresection of local recurrences usually achieves disease control.[4,81,92] Although LR within the ipsilateral hemithorax is more common, distant recurrences have also been described at a rate of 7%.[4] Extended follow-up is required because of the possibility of late recurrences.[93]

Abdominal/Pelvic/Retroperitoneal Solitary Fibrous Tumor

Intraabdominal SFTs can present as an incidental mass on imaging or a clinically palpable mass, and may cause local pressure symptoms or systemic paraneoplastic symptoms such as hypoglycemia and weight loss. Imaging often shows a large, well-circumscribed solid, vascular tumor, particularly with prominent surrounding feeding vessels. An accurate histologic diagnosis can be established by core needle biopsy.[94] The minority (between 6% and 23%) of intraabdominal SFTs exhibit an aggressive behavior.[5] SFTs account for ~6% of all retroperitoneal sarcomas.[95]

With plentiful surrounding neovascularization, abdominal SFTs may harbor a significant risk of intraoperative bleeding; mitigating preoperative strategies to consider include embolization or preoperative radiotherapy (**Figs. 3** and **4**). The goal is complete resection, with narrowly negative margins and preservation of uninvolved organs and adjacent critical neurovascular structures. An extended resection is not advocated for SFTs, and as tumor borders are readily identified, only clearly involved (encased, adherent, or invaded) organs need to be included in the resection, while adjacent uninvolved organs and structures can be preserved (see **Fig. 3**).[95] This approach is distinct from that recommended for retroperitoneal liposarcoma.[94]

LR and distant metastasis rates 5 years after complete resection have been reported to be 5% and 17%, respectively.[95] Preoperative radiotherapy seems to be associated with a reduced risk of local failure, especially for tumors with a high mitotic count and when microscopically negative margins are not achievable.[10] In cases where surgical resection is not possible due to tumor and/or patient factors, or when resection will be associated with significant morbidity, other options include primary/definitive radiotherapy (see **Fig. 4**) or surveillance alone for asymptomatic patients with no aggressive features on biopsy (**Fig. 5**). Such decisions should be taken in the context of a multidisciplinary tumor board.

Extremity/Trunk Solitary Fibrous Tumor

SFTs of the trunk and extremities, including abdominal wall and bone, account for 10% to 20% of all SFTs.[10,90,96] The most common location reported in several case series is the deep soft tissues of the thigh. Extremity/trunk SFTs are frequently slow growing and generally present as a painless mass that is long-standing, often gradually enlarging over several years. MRI and core needle biopsy should be considered in the diagnostic workup. MRI shows a well-defined solid vascular tumor, often polylobulated and partially encapsulated, that displaces adjacent structures and is isointense or slightly hyperintense on T1 sequences and hyperintense on T2 when compared with muscle. These tumors can be homogeneous or heterogeneous, with signal heterogeneity

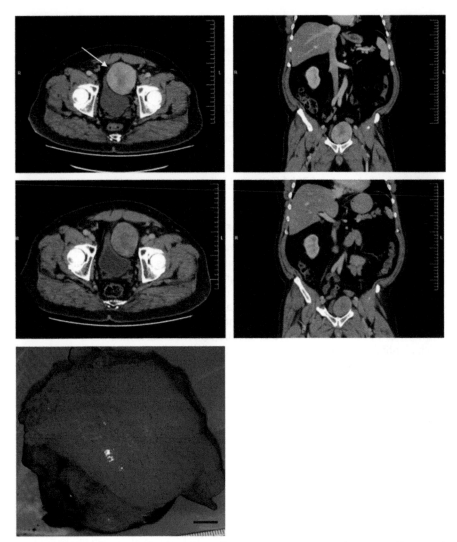

Fig. 3. Radiologic response of pelvic solitary fibrous tumor to preoperative external beam radiation (RT). Baseline CT scans (*top panels*) show a well-circumscribed and intensely vascular tumor, characteristic of SFT. Eight weeks following completion of RT (50 Gy in 25 fractions), CT scans (*middle panels*) show decreased attenuation and a modest decrease in size. Resected specimen following simple excision that included pelvic peritoneal reflection and superior vesical vessels on left side, but preserved other surrounding structures (*bottom panel*). Scale bar, 1 cm.

frequently attributed to necrosis or hemorrhage. Tumors show strong enhancement after gadolinium administration, and a vascular pedicle is often visible.[97,98]

SFTs typically have discrete margins, and surgical excision with microscopically negative margins while preserving limb function, forms the mainstay of treatment.[99] Adequacy of resection margins is generally considered a strong prognostic indicator of local disease control,[10,90] although some series show no impact of margin status on LR or survival.[96,100] The risks of LR and metastasis are lower for extremity SFTs than other extrathoracic SFTs.[96,99–102] In larger series, a 3% to 11% risk of LR and 5% to 20% risk of distant metastasis have been described, with most of the metastases and

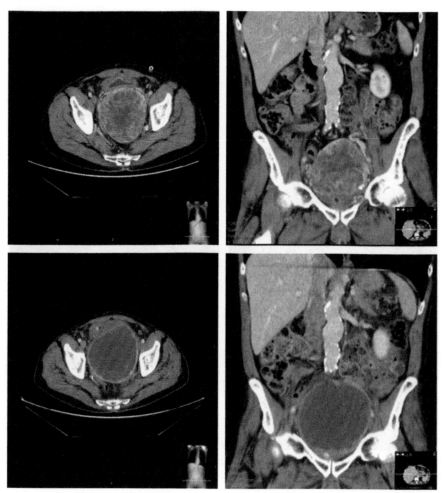

Fig. 4. Solitary fibrous tumor of the pelvis, with prominent intratumoral vascularity and circumferential feeding vessels at baseline (*top panels*), both of which diminished markedly following definitive radiotherapy (*bottom panels*).

local failures detected within the first 2 years, but up to 14 years, after treatment.[5,97–99,103,104] Disease-specific mortality remains low, with disease-specific survival of 86% to 96%.[8,48,96,99] Patients should be considered for local reresection or metastectomy.

NEOADJUVANT AND ADJUVANT THERAPIES
Radiation Therapy

Central nervous system solitary fibrous tumor
Practices with respect to use of radiation therapy (RT) for CNS SFTs vary significantly between centers, and the literature reflects this lack of consensus. There is general agreement that adjuvant RT is indicated following resection of WHO fourth edition grade III CNS SFTs, given the high risk of LR regardless of apparent completeness of resection.[59,78,105,106] Several studies show both improved local control and better recurrence-free survival in patients who received postoperative RT.[59,75,78,105,107]

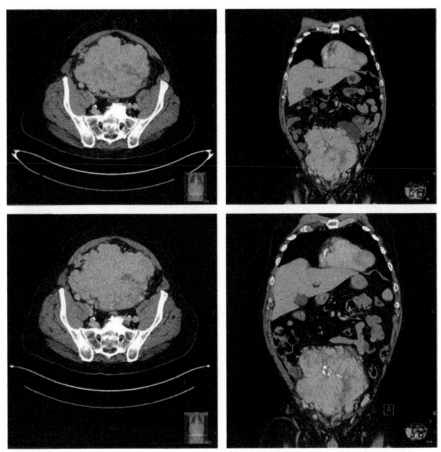

Fig. 5. Solitary fibrous tumor of the pelvis at baseline (*top panels*) and after 4 years of surveillance without any treatment (*bottom panels*), in an asymptomatic patient not willing to undergo active therapy.

However, given the heterogeneous results described in retrospective studies,[75,78,105–108] the role of postoperative RT following grossly complete resection is not entirely clear. Several series report decreased recurrence rates with no survival benefit,[66,71,74,75,106] whereas others report improved survival in addition to decreased LR[7,59,76,105,109] with postoperative adjuvant RT. In cases of grossly incomplete resection, there is some evidence to suggest that the addition of postoperative RT may improve OS, as patients who had RT following subtotal resection compared favorably with patients undergoing R0 resection alone.[105] By contrast, other studies found that OS remained inferior with incomplete resection despite addition of postoperative RT.[75,106] This discrepancy could reflect the fact that postoperative RT fails to prevent recurrences at regional and distant sites, the latter being tied to poor survival outcomes.[73,75,110] In a large series that included data on WHO grade, Lee and colleagues[78] showed significantly better local control and improved PFS in WHO fourth edition grade II and grade III CNS SFT with postoperative RT. The risk of local failure and morbidity of salvage resection in the individual patient with CNS SFTs should be discussed by the multidisciplinary team and should inform the decision regarding adjuvant RT.

Extra-meningeal solitary fibrous tumor

The potential benefit of perioperative radiation therapy in extrameningeal SFTs should be discussed by the multidisciplinary team on a case-by-case basis. A large retrospective study by Haas and colleagues[10] included 549 patients with SFT, 428 (78%) of whom had undergone resection alone while 121 (22%) had surgery plus preoperative or postoperative RT. After propensity score matching, there was a significantly increased rate of local control in the group of patients who received RT ($P = .012$). Nonetheless, no significant OS benefit was observed. Other smaller series have shown similar results.[111–113] There is very little prospective data available regarding outcomes of retroperitoneal SFTs. The initial analysis of the EORTC-sponsored RCT that compared preoperative RT plus surgery with surgery alone for RPS (STRASS) showed no clear benefit in abdominal recurrence-free survival when all histologic types of RPS were considered together, but there was a very limited number of patients with RP SFT included in this study[114] so the applicability of the results to patients with SFT is questionable. Consideration for preoperative RT may be to facilitate negative microscopic margins or even to render resectable tumors that are deemed unresectable or borderline resectable. Preoperative RT can also be considered for tumors that may be difficult to resect upfront due to anatomic constraints or where an adequate dose of RT would be challenging to deliver postoperatively. In addition, in cases where a marginal resection is foreseen and LR would be problematic, there may be a compelling rationale for preoperative RT.

Definitive or palliative radiotherapy can also be considered. In a retrospective series of 40 patients treated with definitive RT ($\sim$60 Gy), there was an objective overall response rate of 67%, with 5-year local control of 81% and 5-year OS of 88%.[115]

Systemic Therapy

Chemotherapy has typically been used in the advanced or metastatic setting for patients with SFT, and the potential role of adjuvant chemotherapy following resection of SFT is unclear. Limited evidence regarding the activity of standard cytotoxic drugs in SFT is available, and no specific clinical trials addressing the value of chemotherapy have been reported for SFT. In advanced disease, several retrospective series with conventional anthracycline-based regimens showed limited activity with overall response rates up to 20% and median PFS of 3 to 5 months.[116–119] In one study, dacarbazine alone or in combination with doxorubicin was evaluated, with 50% of patients showing a partial response, and one patient showing stable disease, by RECIST criteria.[120] In that study, median PFS was 6 months, with 20% of patients still remaining without progression at the 1-year mark.

Recently, several tyrosine kinase inhibitors (TKIs) have been prospectively assessed in patients with advanced SFT who have progressed on prior therapy.[121–123] Pazopanib was assessed in a phase II trial in 36 patients with advanced SFT with aggressive features: an overall response rate (Choi criteria) was achieved in 51%, where 18 patients had partial responses and 9 had stable disease.[122] At a median follow-up of 27 months, median survival was not reached, and a 2-year OS of 73% was reported. In a subsequent phase II trial of pazopanib in patients with metastatic or unresectable SFT with mitotic count less than 4 mitoses per 10 HPF and absence of tumor necrosis or nuclear pleomorphism $\sim$80% of whom had progressed on prior therapies, the overall response rate (Choi criteria) was 58%, with 18/31 patients having a partial response, whereas 12/31 had stable disease.[123] Median PFS was 9.8 months and OS 50 months.

Other TKIs that have been shown to have some activity in SFT are sunitinib, axitinib, and regorafenib.[124–126] In a retrospective series of 31 patients with advanced SFT who received sunitinib, 7% achieved a partial response by RECIST criteria and 48% a partial response by Choi criteria, with a 12-month PFS of 30%.[124] In a phase II study of sunitinib in the treatment of nongastrointestinal stromal tumor sarcomas, durable disease control was achieved in 2 of 3 patients with SFT.[127]

In advanced SFTs, bevacizumab and temozolomide have been evaluated in a retrospective fashion in patients with progression on previous therapy, with 79% of patients showing partial response by Choi criteria and a median PFS of 10 months.[127] Another series showed an overall response rate by RECIST criteria of 21.4% and median PFS and OS of 17 and 45 months, respectively.[128] Further study and additional agents are needed.

CLINICOPATHOLOGIC RISK STRATIFICATION

In general, SFTs are relatively indolent tumors, with 10% to 30% risk of metastasis, depending on the patient population.[3] Although the most aggressive tumors tend to metastasize within the first 5 years after primary presentation, more indolent tumors have been reported, with metastases arising after 10 or even 20 years; long-term follow-up is recommended for patients who are intermediate or high risk for development of metastasis.

Many risk factors have been identified to correlate with metastasis, recurrence, or poor survival in patients with SFT. These risk factors have included mitotic activity, tumor size, tumor cellularity, nuclear pleomorphism, tumor necrosis, patient age, patient sex, tumor site, history of adjuvant radiation therapy, and completeness of resection among others. No single factor taken in isolation provides strong predictive value for risk of recurrence, metastasis, or death. Therefore, several multivariable models have been published for predicting metastatic risk, OS, or disease-free survival in SFTs. Some are site specific, similar to those designed for pleural SFTs (**Table1**),[4,80,82,129,130] meningeal SFTs,[63] or SFTs arising in the orbit,[131] and may take into account site-specific features such as pedunculation of pleural tumors or size restrictions in tumors arising in the head and neck/meninges, whereas others are site agnostic or encompass SFTs of all nonmeningeal sites[8,51,96] or were designed for soft tissue SFTs only.[132]

The most widely used and validated system for risk stratification of SFTs of all nonmeningeal sites (known variously as the [modified] Demicco Score, D-score, or MDACC score; **Table 2**) incorporates mitotic activity, patient age, and tumor size to predict risk of metastasis following curative intent resection of primary tumor arising at any extrameningeal site.[51,90,91,133–135] The modified version of this scoring system includes tumor necrosis as a risk factor and has high specificity to predict tumors at the highest risk of early metastasis, including peritoneal and pleural dissemination, with 61% of patients with high-risk tumors developing metastatic disease by 5 years compared with no metastases in low-risk patients.[90] This model has been validated both for soft tissue SFTs and pleural SFTs, for which it performs similarly to the Tapias model, while offering improved ease of use.[91] The Demicco score is specifically designed to predict metastasis and is not of value for predicting LR; although the model can be used to predict OS, it is not designed for this purpose, and other models may outperform it.

The French Sarcoma group has proposed 3 different models for specifically predicting OS, metastatic risk, and LR (**Table 3**).[96] The Salas system estimates OS and metastatic risk based on mitotic activity and patient age; the model for metastatic risk also includes tumor site (extremity vs other) as a risk factor. Both models have been independently validated.[90,135] Prediction of LR incorporates visceral site, young age, and history of adjuvant radiation and has also been independently validated.[10] Patient

Table 2
Demicco and Modified Demicco Score for prediction of metastatic risk following resection of extrameningeal solitary fibrous tumors

	Demicco et al., 2012		Demicco et al., 2017
		Points	
Patient Age ≥55 y	1		1
Tumor Size			
<5 cm	0		0
5–9.9 cm	1		1
10–14.9 cm	2		2
≥15 cm	3		3
Mitotic Figures/10 High-Power Fields			
0	0		0
1–3	1		1
≥4	2		2
Tumor Necrosis (% of Tumor Volume)			
<10%	—		0
≥10%			1
Risk		**Sum of Points**	
Low risk	0–2		0–3
Intermediate risk	3–4		4–5
High risk	5–6		6–7

follow-up was limited in the patient groups used to design and validate the Demicco and Salas models, and as a result, although both are of great value in the prediction of early metastasis or death, they may underpredict late metastasis and recurrence.

Only one group has published a series of extrameningeal SFTs with median follow-up of greater than 6 years.[135] In this study, Georgiesh and colleagues (2020) found that a model incorporating sex as a predictive feature, with men being at higher risk than women, together with high mitotic rate and the presence of extensive necrosis, was predictive of both early and late local and distant recurrence, with high-risk tumors having a median time to recurrence of 40 months and a 10-year recurrence-free rate of 25%, compared with a 10-year recurrence-free rate of 95% for low-risk tumors (**Table 4**); validation of these findings in an independent patient cohort is required.

For SFT of the meninges, the size and age criteria used to predict risk at other sites are less relevant, and the WHO fifth edition proposes a new grading system for meningeal SFTs based on mitotic activity and presence of tumor necrosis.[13,63,64]

As a caveat for all risk stratification systems, the histologic assessment of mitotic figures, necrosis, nuclear pleomorphism, and tumor cellularity depends on adequate tumor sampling and is prone to subjectivity. Results of the application of different risk stratification systems may vary in a pathologist- or institution-dependent manner. There is also poor concordance between scoring systems as to which specific tumors fall into low-, intermediate-, or high-risk categories.[90,135] Because of this, some investigators have recommended scoring risk in extrameningeal SFTs using multiple systems and determining risk based on concordance of results. Specifically, in one small series of 28 SFTs, Machado and colleagues[136] (2020) found that of patients with tumors classified as high risk by multiple systems (Demicco, Diebold, Salas, and Pasquali) all developed recurrence, whereas patient with tumors classified as

Table 3
Salas models for prediction of overall survival, local recurrence, and metastatic risk following resection of extrameningeal solitary fibrous tumors

	Metastatic Risk	Overall Survival	Local Recurrence
		Points	
Mitotic Figures/10 High-Power Fields >4	1	1	—
Patient Age			
<60	0	0	1
≥60	1	1	0
Site			
Limbs	1	—	0
Viscera	0		1
Other	0		0
No Radiotherapy	—	—	1
Risk		**Sum of Points**	
Very low risk	0	—	0
Low risk	1	0	1
Intermediate risk	2	1	2
High risk	3	2	3

low risk by multiple systems were free of disease. Others have recommended including *TERT* promoter mutation status and/or *TP53* mutational status in risk assessment, particularly for tumors scored as intermediate risk, to provide further evidence of probable aggressive behavior.[39,40,137]

SURVEILLANCE

Continued long-term follow-up is needed for SFTs due to the indolent natural history and possibility of late recurrence many years after surgery.[8,96,100] Surveillance

Table 4
Georgiesh model for prediction of recurrence-free interval following resection of extrameningeal solitary fibrous tumors

	Recurrence (Local or Distant)
	Points
Mitotic Figures/10 High-Power Fields	
≥4	2
Sex	
Male	1
Tumor Necrosis	
Absent	0
<50%	1
≥50%	2
Risk	**Sum of Points**
Low risk	0
Intermediate risk	1–2
High risk	3–5

decisions should incorporate tumor and patient factors and involve estimated risk.[51,96,135] For intermediate- and high-risk tumors, generic NCCN posttreatment guidelines for soft tissue sarcoma recommend imaging every 3 to 4 months for the first 2 years, then every 6 months through year 5, then yearly thereafter. Such imaging would include the primary site and also chest CT. For very low-risk and low-risk tumors, surveillance of the local site every 6 months for 3 years, then yearly thereafter is recommended.

ADVANCED AND METASTATIC DISEASE

Management of patients with SFT who develop locally recurrent or metastatic disease is challenging, as no clearly effective systemic therapies exist. Reresection and/or metastatectomy can lead to improved PFS and should be considered if technically feasible, although this can be challenging especially for tumors in deep spaces such as the epidural space, retroperitoneum, or pelvis.[102,109] Definitive or palliative radiotherapy can also be considered in management strategies, with a retrospective series showing an objective overall response rate of 67% with 5-year local control of 81% and 5-year OS of 88%.[115] Although some chemotherapy agents have efficacy in this disease, objective responses with these agents are uncommon, as noted earlier, and duration of benefit is short.[116,120] Targeted therapies using antiangiogenic agents show efficacy in advanced SFTs and are recommended in patients with progression on prior therapies[121–123,127,138] (see earlier discussion "systemic therapy").

PRINCIPLES OF MULTIDISCIPLINARY CARE

Given the rarity and complex nature of sarcoma diagnosis and management, the authors would recommend management of all sarcomas, including SFTs, at an expert referral center to ensure that provision of care meets internationally agreed standards. Treatment plans should be made in a multidisciplinary setting to optimize oncologic outcomes. Patients can be offered the opportunity to participate in clinical trials and research programs.

CLINICS CARE POINTS

- SFTs can arise at almost any site in the body and are defined by the NAB2-STAT6 gene fusion; review and work-up by an expert sarcoma pathologist is critical.
- Risk stratification models have been developed to accurately predict patient outcomes after complete resection and should be consulted in counselling patients as to best management.
- Complete resection with an emphasis on preservation of function is the mainstay of treatment of SFT, especially for localized disease.
- Perioperative radiotherapy can be considered and should be discussed in a multidisciplinary setting.
- Long-term follow-up is recommended due to the possibility of late recurrence.

DISCLOSURE

The authors have nothing to disclose.

REFERENCES

1. Klemperer P, Rabin CB. Primary neoplasms of the pleura: a report of 5 cases. Arch Pathol 1931;11:385.
2. Stout AP, Murray MR. Hemangiopericytoma: a vascular tumor featuring zimmermann's pericytes. Ann Surg 1942;116(1):26–33.
3. Demicco EG, Fritchie K, Han A. Solitary fibrous tumor. In: Soft tissue and bone tumours World Health organization classification of tumours, vol. 3, 5th edition. Lyon, France: WHO Classification of Tumours Editorial Board IARC Press; 2020. p. 104–8.
4. England DM, Hochholzer L, McCarthy MJ. Localized benign and malignant fibrous tumors of the pleura. A clinicopathologic review of 223 cases. Am J Surg Pathol 1989;13(8):640–58.
5. Gold JS, Antonescu CR, Hajdu C, et al. Clinicopathologic correlates of solitary fibrous tumors. Cancer 2002;94(4):1057–68.
6. Kinslow CJ, Wang TJC. Incidence of extrameningeal solitary fibrous tumors. Cancer 2020;126(17):4067.
7. Kinslow CJ, Bruce SS, Rae AI, et al. Solitary-fibrous tumor/hemangiopericytoma of the central nervous system: a population-based study. J Neurooncol 2018; 138(1):173–82.
8. Demicco EG, Park MS, Araujo DM, et al. Solitary fibrous tumor: a clinicopathological study of 110 cases and proposed risk assessment model. Mod Pathol 2012;25(9):1298–306.
9. Cardillo G, Facciolo F, Cavazzana AO, et al. Localized (solitary) fibrous tumors of the pleura: an analysis of 55 patients. Ann Thorac Surg 2000;70(6):1808–12.
10. Haas RL, Walraven I, Lecointe-Artzner E, et al. Extrameningeal solitary fibrous tumors-surgery alone or surgery plus perioperative radiotherapy: A retrospective study from the global solitary fibrous tumor initiative in collaboration with the Sarcoma Patients EuroNet. Cancer 2020;126(13):3002–12.
11. Hasegawa T, Matsuno Y, Shimoda T, et al. Extrathoracic solitary fibrous tumors: their histological variability and potentially aggressive behavior. Hum Pathol 1999;30(12):1464–73.
12. Smith SC, Gooding WE, Elkins M, et al. Solitary fibrous tumors of the head and neck: a multi-institutional clinicopathologic study. Am J Surg Pathol 2017;41(12): 1642–56.
13. Bouvier C, Demicco EG, Figarella-Branger D, et al. Solitary fibrous tumor. In: Central nervous system tumors. World Health Organization Classification of Tumours 5th edition. WHO Classification of Tumours Editorial Board. Lyon, France:ARC Press; 2021 (in press);vol 6,:01-305.
14. Folpe AL, Devaney K, Weiss SW. Lipomatous hemangiopericytoma: a rare variant of hemangiopericytoma that may be confused with liposarcoma. Am J Surg Pathol 1999;23(10):1201–7.
15. Guillou L, Gebhard S, Coindre JM. Lipomatous hemangiopericytoma: a fat-containing variant of solitary fibrous tumor? Clinicopathologic, immunohistochemical, and ultrastructural analysis of a series in favor of a unifying concept. Hum Pathol 2000;31(9):1108–15.
16. Nielsen GP, Dickersin GR, Provenzal JM, et al. Lipomatous hemangiopericytoma. A histologic, ultrastructural and immunohistochemical study of a unique variant of hemangiopericytoma. Am J Surg Pathol 1995;19(7):748–56.
17. Dei Tos AP, Seregard S, Calonje E, et al. Giant cell angiofibroma. A distinctive orbital tumor in adults. Am J Surg Pathol 1995;19(11):1286–93.

18. Guillou L, Gebhard S, Coindre JM. Orbital and extraorbital giant cell angiofibroma: a giant cell-rich variant of solitary fibrous tumor? Clinicopathologic and immunohistochemical analysis of a series in favor of a unifying concept. Am J Surg Pathol 2000;24(7):971–9.

19. Mosquera JM, Fletcher CD. Expanding the spectrum of malignant progression in solitary fibrous tumors: a study of 8 cases with a discrete anaplastic component–is this dedifferentiated SFT? Am J Surg Pathol 2009;33(9):1314–21.

20. Collini P, Negri T, Barisella M, et al. High-grade sarcomatous overgrowth in solitary fibrous tumors: a clinicopathologic study of 10 cases. Am J Surg Pathol 2012;36(8):1202–15.

21. Thway K, Hayes A, Ieremia E, et al. Heterologous osteosarcomatous and rhabdomyosarcomatous elements in dedifferentiated solitary fibrous tumor: further support for the concept of dedifferentiation in solitary fibrous tumor. Ann Diagn Pathol 2013;17(5):457–63.

22. Doyle LA, Vivero M, Fletcher CD, et al. Nuclear expression of STAT6 distinguishes solitary fibrous tumor from histologic mimics. Mod Pathol 2014;27(3):390–5.

23. Schweizer L, Koelsche C, Sahm F, et al. Meningeal hemangiopericytoma and solitary fibrous tumors carry the NAB2-STAT6 fusion and can be diagnosed by nuclear expression of STAT6 protein. Acta Neuropathol 2013;125(5):651–8.

24. Koelsche C, Schweizer L, Renner M, et al. Nuclear relocation of STAT6 reliably predicts NAB2-STAT6 fusion for the diagnosis of solitary fibrous tumour. Histopathology 2014;65(5):613–22.

25. Demicco EG, Harms PW, Patel RM, et al. Extensive survey of STAT6 expression in a large series of mesenchymal tumors. Am J Clin Pathol 2015;143(5):672–82.

26. Vivero M, Doyle LA, Fletcher CD, et al. GRIA2 is a novel diagnostic marker for solitary fibrous tumour identified through gene expression profiling. Histopathology 2014;65(1):71–80.

27. Bouvier C, Bertucci F, Metellus P, et al. ALDH1 is an immunohistochemical diagnostic marker for solitary fibrous tumours and haemangiopericytomas of the meninges emerging from gene profiling study. Acta Neuropathol Commun 2013;1:10.

28. Schulz B, Altendorf-Hofmann A, Kirchner T, et al. Loss of CD34 and high IGF2 are associated with malignant transformation in solitary fibrous tumors. Pathol Res Pract 2014;210(2):92–7.

29. Dermawan JK, Rubin BP, Kilpatrick SE, et al. CD34-negative solitary fibrous tumor: a clinicopathologic study of 25 cases and comparison with their CD34-positive counterparts. Am J Surg Pathol 2021;45(12):1616–25.

30. Dagrada GP, Spagnuolo RD, Mauro V, et al. Solitary fibrous tumors: loss of chimeric protein expression and genomic instability mark dedifferentiation. Mod Pathol 2015;28(8):1074–83.

31. Schneider N, Hallin M, Thway K. STAT6 Loss in Dedifferentiated Solitary Fibrous Tumor. Int J Surg Pathol 2017;25(1):58–60.

32. Chmielecki J, Crago AM, Rosenberg M, et al. Whole-exome sequencing identifies a recurrent NAB2-STAT6 fusion in solitary fibrous tumors. Nat Genet 2013;45(2):131–2.

33. Mohajeri A, Tayebwa J, Collin A, et al. Comprehensive genetic analysis identifies a pathognomonic NAB2/STAT6 fusion gene, nonrandom secondary genomic imbalances, and a characteristic gene expression profile in solitary fibrous tumor. Genes Chromosomes Cancer 2013;52(10):873–86.

34. Robinson DR, Wu YM, Kalyana-Sundaram S, et al. Identification of recurrent NAB2-STAT6 gene fusions in solitary fibrous tumor by integrative sequencing. Nat Genet 2013;45(2):180–5.

35. Akaike K, Kurisaki-Arakawa A, Hara K, et al. Distinct clinicopathological features of NAB2-STAT6 fusion gene variants in solitary fibrous tumor with emphasis on the acquisition of highly malignant potential. Hum Pathol 2015;46(3):347–56.

36. Barthelmess S, Geddert H, Boltze C, et al. Solitary fibrous tumors/hemangiopericytomas with different variants of the NAB2-STAT6 gene fusion are characterized by specific histomorphology and distinct clinicopathological features. Am J Pathol 2014;184(4):1209–18.

37. Kurisaki-Arakawa A, Akaike K, Hara K, et al. A case of dedifferentiated solitary fibrous tumor in the pelvis with TP53 mutation. Virchows Arch 2014;465(5): 615–21.

38. Subramaniam MM, Lim XY, Venkateswaran K, et al. Dedifferentiated solitary fibrous tumour of the nasal cavity: the first case reported with molecular characterization of a TP53 mutation. Histopathology 2011;59(6):1269–74.

39. Demicco EG, Wani K, Ingram D, et al. TERT promoter mutations in solitary fibrous tumour. Histopathology 2018;73(5):843–51.

40. Bahrami A, Lee S, Schaefer IM, et al. TERT promoter mutations and prognosis in solitary fibrous tumor. Mod Pathol 2016;29(12):1511–22.

41. Lin Y, Seger N, Tsagkozis P, et al. Telomerase promoter mutations and copy number alterations in solitary fibrous tumours. J Clin Pathol 2018;71(9):832–9.

42. Lococo F, Cesario A, Cardillo G, et al. Malignant solitary fibrous tumors of the pleura: retrospective review of a multicenter series. J Thorac Oncol 2012; 7(11):1698–706.

43. Meng W, Zhu HH, Li H, et al. Solitary fibrous tumors of the pleura with Doege-Potter syndrome: a case report and three-decade review of the literature. BMC Res Notes 2014;7:515.

44. Tay CK, Teoh HL, Su S. A common problem in the elderly with an uncommon cause: hypoglycaemia secondary to the Doege-Potter syndrome. BMJ Case Rep 2015;2015;bcr2014207995.

45. Herrmann BL, Saller B, Kiess W, et al. Primary malignant fibrous histiocytoma of the lung: IGF-II producing tumor induces fasting hypoglycemia. Exp Clin Endocrinol Diabetes 2000;108(8):515–8.

46. Ahluwalia N, Attia R, Green A, et al. Doege-Potter Syndrome. Ann R Coll Surg Engl 2015;97(7):e105–7.

47. Rena O, Filosso PL, Papalia E, et al. Solitary fibrous tumour of the pleura: surgical treatment. Eur J Cardiothorac Surg 2001;19(2):185–9.

48. Brunnemann RB, Ro JY, Ordonez NG, et al. Extrapleural solitary fibrous tumor: a clinicopathologic study of 24 cases. Mod Pathol 1999;12(11):1034–42.

49. Furusato E, Valenzuela IA, Fanburg-Smith JC, et al. Orbital solitary fibrous tumor: encompassing terminology for hemangiopericytoma, giant cell angiofibroma, and fibrous histiocytoma of the orbit: reappraisal of 41 cases. Hum Pathol 2011;42(1):120–8.

50. Cox DP, Daniels T, Jordan RC. Solitary fibrous tumor of the head and neck. Oral Surg Oral Med Oral Pathol Oral Radiol Endod 2010;110(1):79–84.

51. Demicco EG, Wagner MJ, Maki RG, et al. Risk assessment in solitary fibrous tumors: validation and refinement of a risk stratification model. Mod Pathol 2017; 30(10):1433–42.

52. Ganly I, Patel SG, Stambuk HE, et al. Solitary fibrous tumors of the head and neck: a clinicopathologic and radiologic review. Arch Otolaryngol Head Neck Surg 2006;132(5):517–25.

53. Liu Y, Li K, Shi H, et al. Solitary fibrous tumours in the extracranial head and neck region: correlation of CT and MR features with pathologic findings. Radiol Med 2014;119(12):910–9.

54. Kao YC, Lin PC, Yen SL, et al. Clinicopathological and genetic heterogeneity of the head and neck solitary fibrous tumours: a comparative histological, immuno-histochemical and molecular study of 36 cases. Histopathology 2016;68(4): 492–501.

55. Bowe SN, Wakely PE Jr, Ozer E. Head and neck solitary fibrous tumors: diag-nostic and therapeutic challenges. Laryngoscope 2012;122(8):1748–55.

56. Kunzel J, Hainz M, Ziebart T, et al. Head and neck solitary fibrous tumors: a rare and challenging entity. Eur Arch Otorhinolaryngol 2016;273(6):1589–98.

57. Giordan E, Marton E, Wennberg AM, et al. A review of solitary fibrous tumor/he-mangiopericytoma tumor and a comparison of risk factors for recurrence, me-tastases, and death among patients with spinal and intracranial tumors. Neurosurg Rev 2021;44(3):1299–312.

58. Bisceglia M, Galliani C, Giannatempo G, et al. Solitary fibrous tumor of the cen-tral nervous system: a 15-year literature survey of 220 cases (August 1996-July 2011). Adv Anat Pathol 2011;18(5):356–92.

59. Schiariti M, Goetz P, El-Maghraby H, et al. Hemangiopericytoma: long-term outcome revisited. Clinical article. J Neurosurg 2011;114(3):747–55.

60. Fritchie KJ, Jin L, Rubin BP, et al. NAB2-STAT6 Gene Fusion in Meningeal He-mangiopericytoma and Solitary Fibrous Tumor. J Neuropathol Exp Neurol 2016;75(3):263–71.

61. Yalcin CE, Tihan T. Solitary Fibrous Tumor/Hemangiopericytoma Dichotomy Re-visited: A Restless Family of Neoplasms in the CNS. Adv Anat Pathol 2016;23(2): 104–11.

62. Zeng L, Wang Y, Wang Y, et al. Analyses of prognosis-related factors of intracra-nial solitary fibrous tumors and hemangiopericytomas help understand the rela-tionship between the two sorts of tumors. J Neurooncol 2017;131(1):153–61.

63. Fritchie K, Jensch K, Moskalev EA, et al. The impact of histopathology and NAB2-STAT6 fusion subtype in classification and grading of meningeal solitary fibrous tumor/hemangiopericytoma. Acta Neuropathol 2019;137(2):307–19.

64. Macagno N, Vogels R, Appay R, et al. Grading of meningeal solitary fibrous tu-mors/hemangiopericytomas: analysis of the prognostic value of the Marseille Grading System in a cohort of 132 patients. Brain Pathol 2019;29(1):18–27.

65. Fargen KM, Opalach KJ, Wakefield D, et al. The central nervous system solitary fibrous tumor: a review of clinical, imaging and pathologic findings among all reported cases from 1996 to 2010. Clin Neurol Neurosurg 2011;113(9):703–10.

66. Kim BS, Kim Y, Kong DS, et al. Clinical outcomes of intracranial solitary fibrous tumor and hemangiopericytoma: analysis according to the 2016 WHO classifi-cation of central nervous system tumors. J Neurosurg 2018;129(6):1384–96.

67. Chen LF, Yang Y, Yu XG, et al. Multimodal treatment and management strategies for intracranial hemangiopericytoma. J Clin Neurosci 2015;22(4):718–25.

68. Damodaran O, Robbins P, Knuckey N, et al. Primary intracranial haemangioper-icytoma: comparison of survival outcomes and metastatic potential in WHO grade II and III variants. J Clin Neurosci 2014;21(8):1310–4.

69. Dufour H, Metellus P, Fuentes S, et al. Meningeal hemangiopericytoma: a retrospective study of 21 patients with special review of postoperative external radiotherapy. Neurosurgery 2001;48(4):756–62 [discussion: 62-3].

70. Ecker RD, Marsh WR, Pollock BE, et al. Hemangiopericytoma in the central nervous system: treatment, pathological features, and long-term follow up in 38 patients. J Neurosurg 2003;98(6):1182–7.

71. Melone AG, D'Elia A, Santoro F, et al. Intracranial hemangiopericytoma–our experience in 30 years: a series of 43 cases and review of the literature. World Neurosurg 2014;81(3–4):556–62.

72. Rutkowski MJ, Bloch O, Jian BJ, et al. Management of recurrent intracranial hemangiopericytoma. J Clin Neurosci 2011;18(11):1500–4.

73. Ghia AJ, Chang EL, Allen PK, et al. Intracranial hemangiopericytoma: patterns of failure and the role of radiation therapy. Neurosurgery 2013;73(4):624–30 [discussion: 30-1].

74. Kim JH, Jung HW, Kim YS, et al. Meningeal hemangiopericytomas: long-term outcome and biological behavior. Surg Neurol 2003;59(1):47–53 [discussion: -4].

75. Rutkowski MJ, Jian BJ, Bloch O, et al. Intracranial hemangiopericytoma: clinical experience and treatment considerations in a modern series of 40 adult patients. Cancer 2012;118(6):1628–36.

76. Soyuer S, Chang EL, Selek U, et al. Intracranial meningeal hemangiopericytoma: the role of radiotherapy: report of 29 cases and review of the literature. Cancer 2004;100(7):1491–7.

77. Ratneswaren T, Hogg FRA, Gallagher MJ, et al. Surveillance for metastatic hemangiopericytoma-solitary fibrous tumors-systematic literature review on incidence, predictors and diagnosis of extra-cranial disease. J Neurooncol 2018; 138(3):447–67.

78. Lee JH, Jeon SH, Park CK, et al. The Role of Postoperative Radiotherapy in Intracranial Solitary Fibrous Tumor/Hemangiopericytoma: A Multi-Institutional Retrospective Study (KROG 18-11). Cancer Res Treat 2022 Jan;54(1):65–74.

79. Sung SH, Chang JW, Kim J, et al. Solitary fibrous tumors of the pleura: surgical outcome and clinical course. Ann Thorac Surg 2005;79(1):303–7.

80. Tapias LF, Mercier O, Ghigna MR, et al. Validation of a scoring system to predict recurrence of resected solitary fibrous tumors of the pleura. Chest 2015;147(1): 216–23.

81. Lahon B, Mercier O, Fadel E, et al. Solitary fibrous tumor of the pleura: outcomes of 157 complete resections in a single center. Ann Thorac Surg 2012;94(2): 394–400.

82. de Perrot M, Kurt AM, Robert JH, et al. Clinical behavior of solitary fibrous tumors of the pleura. Ann Thorac Surg 1999;67(5):1456–9.

83. Briselli M, Mark EJ, Dickersin GR. Solitary fibrous tumors of the pleura: eight new cases and review of 360 cases in the literature. Cancer 1981;47(11):2678–89.

84. Liu CC, Wang HW, Li FY, et al. Solitary fibrous tumors of the pleura: clinicopathological characteristics, immunohistochemical profiles, and surgical outcomes with long-term follow-up. Thorac Cardiovasc Surg 2008;56(5):291–7.

85. Lee KS, Im JG, Choe KO, et al. CT findings in benign fibrous mesothelioma of the pleura: pathologic correlation in nine patients. AJR Am J Roentgenol 1992;158(5):983–6.

86. Zhou C, Li W, Shao J, et al. Thoracic solitary fibrous tumors: an analysis of 70 patients who underwent surgical resection in a single institution. J Cancer Res Clin Oncol 2020;146(5):1245–52.

87. Takahama M, Kushibe K, Kawaguchi T, et al. Video-assisted thoracoscopic surgery is a promising treatment for solitary fibrous tumor of the pleura. Chest 2004; 125(3):1144–7.

88. Harrison-Phipps KM, Nichols FC, Schleck CD, et al. Solitary fibrous tumors of the pleura: results of surgical treatment and long-term prognosis. J Thorac Cardiovasc Surg 2009;138(1):19–25.

89. Aridi T, Tawil A, Hashem M, et al. Unique Presentation and Management Approach of Pleural Solitary Fibrous Tumor. Case Rep Surg 2019;2019:9706825.

90. Demicco EG, Griffin AM, Gladdy RA, et al. Comparison of published risk models for prediction of outcome in patients with extrameningeal solitary fibrous tumour. Histopathology 2019;75(5):723–37.

91. Reisenauer JS, Mneimneh W, Jenkins S, et al. Comparison of Risk Stratification Models to Predict Recurrence and Survival in Pleuropulmonary Solitary Fibrous Tumor. J Thorac Oncol 2018;13(9):1349–62.

92. de Perrot M, Fischer S, Brundler MA, et al. Solitary fibrous tumors of the pleura. Ann Thorac Surg 2002;74(1):285–93.

93. Baldi GG, Stacchiotti S, Mauro V, et al. Solitary fibrous tumor of all sites: outcome of late recurrences in 14 patients. Clin Sarcoma Res 2013;3:4.

94. Swallow CJ, Strauss DC, Bonvalot S, et al. Management of Primary Retroperitoneal Sarcoma (RPS) in the Adult: An Updated Consensus Approach from the Transatlantic Australasian RPS Working Group. Ann Surg Oncol 2021;28: 7873–88.

95. Dingley B, Fiore M, Gronchi A. Personalizing surgical margins in retroperitoneal sarcomas: an update. Expert Rev Anticancer Ther 2019;19(7):613–31.

96. Salas S, Resseguier N, Blay JY, et al. Prediction of local and metastatic recurrence in solitary fibrous tumor: construction of a risk calculator in a multicenter cohort from the French Sarcoma Group (FSG) database. Ann Oncol 2017;28(8): 1979–87.

97. Garcia-Bennett J, Olive CS, Rivas A, et al. Soft tissue solitary fibrous tumor. Imaging findings in a series of nine cases. Skeletal Radiol 2012;41(11):1427–33.

98. Wignall OJ, Moskovic EC, Thway K, et al. Solitary fibrous tumors of the soft tissues: review of the imaging and clinical features with histopathologic correlation. AJR Am J Roentgenol 2010;195(1):W55–62.

99. Espat NJ, Lewis JJ, Leung D, et al. Conventional hemangiopericytoma: modern analysis of outcome. Cancer 2002;95(8):1746–51.

100. Gholami S, Cassidy MR, Kirane A, et al. Size and Location are the Most Important Risk Factors for Malignant Behavior in Resected Solitary Fibrous Tumors. Ann Surg Oncol 2017;24(13):3865–71.

101. Cranshaw IM, Gikas PD, Fisher C, et al. Clinical outcomes of extra-thoracic solitary fibrous tumours. Eur J Surg Oncol 2009;35(9):994–8.

102. Spitz FR, Bouvet M, Pisters PW, et al. Hemangiopericytoma: a 20-year single-institution experience. Ann Surg Oncol 1998;5(4):350–5.

103. Vallat-Decouvelaere AV, Dry SM, Fletcher CD. Atypical and malignant solitary fibrous tumors in extrathoracic locations: evidence of their comparability to intra-thoracic tumors. Am J Surg Pathol 1998;22(12):1501–11.

104. Papathanassiou ZG, Alberghini M, Picci P, et al. Solitary fibrous tumors of the soft tissues: imaging features with histopathologic correlations. Clin Sarcoma Res 2013;3(1):1.

105. Ghia AJ, Allen PK, Mahajan A, et al. Intracranial hemangiopericytoma and the role of radiation therapy: a population based analysis. Neurosurgery 2013; 72(2):203–9.

106. Haas RL, Walraven I, Lecointe-Artzner E, et al. Management of meningeal solitary fibrous tumors/hemangiopericytoma; surgery alone or surgery plus postoperative radiotherapy? Acta Oncol 2021;60(1):35–41.

107. Lee EJ, Kim JH, Park ES, et al. The impact of postoperative radiation therapy on patterns of failure and survival improvement in patients with intracranial hemangiopericytoma. J Neurooncol 2016;127(1):181–90.

108. Zhu H, Duran D, Hua L, et al. Prognostic Factors in Patients with Primary Hemangiopericytomas of the Central Nervous System: A Series of 103 Cases at a Single Institution. World Neurosurg 2016;90:414–9.

109. Guthrie BL, Ebersold MJ, Scheithauer BW, et al. Meningeal hemangiopericytoma: histopathological features, treatment, and long-term follow-up of 44 cases. Neurosurgery 1989;25(4):514–22.

110. Jeon SH, Park SH, Kim JW, et al. Efficacy of adjuvant radiotherapy in the intracranial hemangiopericytoma. J Neurooncol 2018;137(3):567–73.

111. Krengli M, Cena T, Zilli T, et al. Radiotherapy in the treatment of extracranial hemangiopericytoma/solitary fibrous tumor: Study from the Rare Cancer Network. Radiother Oncol 2020;144:114–20.

112. Bishop AJ, Zagars GK, Demicco EG, et al. Soft tissue solitary fibrous tumor: combined surgery and radiation therapy results in excellent local control. Am J Clin Oncol 2018;41(1):81–5.

113. Gao C, Zhang Y, Jing M, et al. Postoperative radiotherapy for the treatment of solitary fibrous tumor with malignant transformation of the pelvic: a rare case report with literature review. Medicine (Baltimore) 2016;95(2):e2433.

114. Bonvalot S, Gronchi A, Le Pechoux C, et al. Preoperative radiotherapy plus surgery versus surgery alone for patients with primary retroperitoneal sarcoma (EORTC-62092: STRASS): a multicentre, open-label, randomised, phase 3 trial. Lancet Oncol 2020;21(10):1366–77.

115. Haas RL, Walraven I, Lecointe-Artzner E, et al. Radiation therapy as sole management for solitary fibrous tumors (SFT): a retrospective study from the global SFT initiative in collaboration with the sarcoma patients euroNet. Int J Radiat Oncol Biol Phys 2018;101(5):1226–33.

116. Stacchiotti S, Libertini M, Negri T, et al. Response to chemotherapy of solitary fibrous tumour: a retrospective study. Eur J Cancer 2013;49(10):2376–83.

117. Constantinidou A, Jones RL, Olmos D, et al. Conventional anthracycline-based chemotherapy has limited efficacy in solitary fibrous tumour. Acta Oncol 2012;51(4):550–4.

118. Levard A, Derbel O, Meeus P, et al. Outcome of patients with advanced solitary fibrous tumors: the Centre Leon Berard experience. BMC Cancer 2013;13:109.

119. Park MS, Ravi V, Conley A, et al. The role of chemotherapy in advanced solitary fibrous tumors: a retrospective analysis. Clin Sarcoma Res 2013;3(1):7.

120. Stacchiotti S, Saponara M, Frapolli R, et al. Patient-derived solitary fibrous tumour xenografts predict high sensitivity to doxorubicin/dacarbazine combination confirmed in the clinic and highlight the potential effectiveness of trabectedin or eribulin against this tumour. Eur J Cancer 2017;76:84–92.

121. Stacchiotti S, Tortoreto M, Baldi GG, et al. Preclinical and clinical evidence of activity of pazopanib in solitary fibrous tumour. Eur J Cancer 2014;50(17):3021–8.

122. Martin-Broto J, Stacchiotti S, Lopez-Pousa A, et al. Pazopanib for treatment of advanced malignant and dedifferentiated solitary fibrous tumour: a multicentre, single-arm, phase 2 trial. Lancet Oncol 2019;20(1):134–44.

123. Martin-Broto J, Cruz J, Penel N, et al. Pazopanib for treatment of typical solitary fibrous tumours: a multicentre, single-arm, phase 2 trial. Lancet Oncol 2020; 21(3):456–66.

124. Stacchiotti S, Negri T, Libertini M, et al. Sunitinib malate in solitary fibrous tumor (SFT). Ann Oncol 2012;23(12):3171–9.

125. Stacchiotti S, Simeone N, Lo Vullo S, et al. Activity of axitinib in progressive advanced solitary fibrous tumour: Results from an exploratory, investigator-driven phase 2 clinical study. Eur J Cancer 2019;106:225–33.

126. Stacchiotti S, Baldi GG, Vullo SL, et al. Regorafenib (R) in advanced solitary fibrous tumor (SFT): Results from an exploratory phase II clinical study. J Clin Oncol 2021;39(15_suppl):11558.

127. George S, Merriam P, Maki RG, et al. Multicenter phase II trial of sunitinib in the treatment of nongastrointestinal stromal tumor sarcomas. J Clin Oncol 2009; 27(19):3154–60.

128. de Lemos ML, Kang I, Schaff K. Efficacy of bevacizumab and temozolomide therapy in locally advanced, recurrent, and metastatic malignant solitary fibrous tumour: A population-based analysis. J Oncol Pharm Pract 2019;25(6):1301–4.

129. Tapias LF, Mino-Kenudson M, Lee H, et al. Risk factor analysis for the recurrence of resected solitary fibrous tumours of the pleura: a 33-year experience and proposal for a scoring system. Eur J Cardiothorac Surg 2013;44(1):111–7.

130. Diebold M, Soltermann A, Hottinger S, et al. Prognostic value of MIB-1 proliferation index in solitary fibrous tumors of the pleura implemented in a new score - a multicenter study. Respir Res 2017;18(1):210.

131. Thompson LDR, Liou SS, Feldman KA. Orbit solitary fibrous tumor: a proposed risk prediction model based on a case series and comprehensive literature review. Head Neck Pathol 2021;15(1):138–52.

132. Pasquali S, Gronchi A, Strauss D, et al. Resectable extra-pleural and extra-meningeal solitary fibrous tumours: a multi-centre prognostic study. Eur J Surg Oncol 2016;42(7):1064–70.

133. Friis RB, Safwat A, Baad-Hansen T, et al. Solitary fibrous tumour: a single institution retrospective study and further validation of a prognostic risk assessment system. Clin Oncol (R Coll Radiol) 2018;30(12):798–804.

134. Ng DWJ, Tan GHC, Soon JJY, et al. The approach to solitary fibrous tumors: are clinicopathological features and nomograms accurate in the prediction of prognosis? Int J Surg Pathol 2018;26(7):600–8.

135. Georgiesh T, Boye K, Bjerkehagen B. A novel risk score to predict early and late recurrence in solitary fibrous tumour. Histopathology 2020;77(1):123–32.

136. Machado I, Morales GN, Cruz J, et al. Solitary fibrous tumor: a case series identifying pathological adverse factors-implications for risk stratification and classification. Virchows Arch 2020;476(4):597–607.

137. Machado I, Nieto Morales MG, Cruz J, et al. Solitary Fibrous Tumor: Integration of Clinical, Morphologic, Immunohistochemical and Molecular Findings in Risk Stratification and Classification May Better Predict Patient outcome. Int J Mol Sci 2021;22(17):9423.

138. Park MS, Patel SR, Ludwig JA, et al. Activity of temozolomide and bevacizumab in the treatment of locally advanced, recurrent, and metastatic hemangiopericytoma and malignant solitary fibrous tumor. Cancer 2011;117(21):4939–47.

Management of Vascular Sarcoma

Aparna Subramaniam, MBBS, MPH[a], Claudia Giani, MD[b],
Andrea Napolitano, MD, PhD[c], Vinod Ravi, MD[a],*, Anna Maria Frezza, MD[b],
Robin L. Jones, MBBS, MRCP, MD[c]

KEYWORDS

- Vascular sarcoma • Hemangioendothelioma • Epithelioid hemangioendothelioma
- Kaposi sarcoma • Angiosarcoma

KEY POINTS

- Vascular sarcomas are extremely rare soft tissue sarcomas characterized by neoplastic cells with a line of differentiation resembling the endothelium of blood vessels.
- There are 3 distinct types of vascular sarcomas: hemangioendothelioma, Kaposi sarcoma, and angiosarcoma, that are heterogeneous in terms of their clinical behavior, biological features, and management approach.
- The diversity of vascular sarcomas needs to be accounted for in the design of clinical trials, in order to produce meaningful results that can be translated to clinical practice.

INTRODUCTION

Vascular sarcomas are soft tissue sarcomas characterized by neoplastic cells with a line of differentiation closely resembling the endothelium of blood vessels. According to the latest World Health Organization classification (**Table 1**),[1] vascular sarcomas include 3 well-characterized sarcoma types, marked by specific epidemiologic, morphologic, and clinical features: hemangioendothelioma, Kaposi sarcoma (KS), and angiosarcoma. Hemangioendothelioma encompasses different variants (epithelioid, kaposiform, retiform, composite, pseudomyogenic) ranging from locally aggressive to malignant disease.

---

[a] Department of Sarcoma Medical Oncology, University of Texas MD Anderson Cancer Center, 1400 Holcombe Blvd, Unit 0450, FC12.3044, Houston, TX 77030, USA; [b] Medical Oncology, Fondazione IRCCS Istituto Nazionale Tumori, Via Giacomo Venezian 1, Milan 20133, Italy; [c] Sarcoma Unit, The Royal Marsden NHS Foundation Trust, 203 Fulham Road, London SW3 6JJ, UK
* Corresponding author.
E-mail address: vravi@mdanderson.org

Surg Oncol Clin N Am 31 (2022) 485–510
https://doi.org/10.1016/j.soc.2022.03.014

The aim of this article is to provide a comprehensive review of the current knowledge on the epidemiologic, biological, and clinical features of vascular sarcomas and a summary of the state-of-the-art for treatment .

EPITHELIOID HEMANGIOENDOTHELIOMA
Epidemiology and Clinical Presentation

Epithelioid hemangioendothelioma (EHE) is an ultrarare vascular sarcoma with an incidence of 0.4 cases per 1,000,000 per year, mostly affecting women and with a peak of incidence in the fourth to fifth decade.[2–5]

Although EHE can occasionally present as an isolated soft tissue mass, predominantly arising at the level of extremities, up to 70% of cases show metastatic disease at the time of diagnosis, with lung, liver, and bone being the most common sites of distant spread.[3,4,6,7]

Most patients with EHE are asymptomatic at presentation, and the initial diagnosis is often incidental. In approximately 50% of cases, symptoms will be reported, either present since diagnosis or developed during time, often in association with disease progression.[8] The most common symptoms reported in the literature include tumor-related pain (40%), weight loss (10%–20%), and fatigue (10%–20%).[3,7,8]

Pathology and Molecular Features

Morphologically, EHE is characterized by epithelioid endothelial cells often organizing in strands and cords set in a collagenous stroma, and expressing endothelial differentiation markers, such as CD31, CD34, factor VIII–related antigen, ERG, and FLI-1.[9] The nuclear expression of Calmodulin Binding Transcription Activator 1 (CAMTA1) is today considered a diagnostic hallmark, being detected in many EHE cases. A histologic grading system based on nuclear pleomorphism, mitotic activity, and necrosis has been proposed, showing a correlation with survival.[10]

The molecular features of EHE are highly distinctive and can play a crucial role in the differential diagnosis with other tumors (ie, angiosarcoma, epithelioid hemangioma, primary or metastatic carcinomas, mesothelioma, and pseudomyogenic hemangioendothelioma [PMHE]), all the more in the context of an unusual clinical scenario.[6] Approximately 90% of all cases are marked by the t(1;3)(p36.3;q25) translocation, that leads to WW Domain Containing Transcription Regulator 1 (WWTR1)–CAMTA1 fusion gene, whereas a minority of cases (10%) are characterized by a t(X;11) (p11;q22) translocation, that leads to fusion of Yes-associated protein 1–Transcription Factor Binding To IGHM Enhancer 3 (TFE3) genes.[11] Rarer genetic fusions, always involving WWTR1 but with different partners, have been recently reported.[12] Given the complexity of EHE pathologic diagnosis, the diagnosis should always be confirmed by a dedicated sarcoma pathologist within sarcoma reference centers or networks. The immunohistochemical detection of CAMTA1 or molecular assessment of WWTR1-CAMTA1 and/or YPA1-TFE3 is strongly recommended.

Natural History and Prognostic Factors

EHE shows low- to intermediate-grade malignancy with a highly variable clinical behavior, ranging from indolent to aggressive life-threatening disease.[3,7] Anecdotal cases of spontaneous regression have also been reported in literature.[13,14] The unpredictable and highly variable behavior is one of the major challenges in the management of this disease. In fact, 3 different clinical patterns of metastatic EHE have been described: naturally stable and slowly progressive disease, both with an indolent

Table 1
World Health Organization classification of vascular sarcomas

Intermediate (Locally Aggressive)	Intermediate (Rarely Metastasizing)	Malignant
• Kaposiform hemangioendothelioma	• Retiform hemangioendothelioma • Composite hemangioendothelioma • Papillary intralymphatic angioendothelioma • Pseudomyogenic hemangioendothelioma • Kaposi sarcoma	• Angiosarcoma • Epithelioid hemangioendothelioma

course, and a rapidly progressive variant, behaving similarly to high-grade soft tissue sarcomas.

Reliable clinical, pathologic, or molecular prognostic factors still need to be validated. Age, gender, tumor primary site, and number of organs involved did not show any impact on survival.[3,4,15] In a retrospective series, overall outcome is known to be poorer in patients with tumor-related symptoms, temperature and serosal involvement, and/or serosal effusion at baseline.[8] Pleural effusion, tumor growth, tumor multifocality or presence of metastases, lymph node involvement, hemoptysis, or more than 2 bones involved are poor prognostic factors.[3,4] Recently, large tumor size (>30 mm) and histologic atypia were confirmed to be significantly associated with a shorter survival.[4,7,15] In a report on pulmonary EHEs, patients with anemia had significantly worse outcome in comparison to those without, with a 1-year overall survival (OS) of 8% and 95%, respectively.[16]

In a retrospective series of 83 patients, the disease-specific survival rate was longer in patients with TFE3-rearranged tumors compared with those with CAMTA1-rearranged tumors, although the difference was not statistically significant. Therefore, the possible prognostic value of the molecular alteration remains uncertain.[4] In a subset of EHE with aggressive behavior, aberrant synaptophysin expression was identified as a potential negative prognostic factor.[15] The prognostic role of inflammatory and hormonal circulating biomarkers is currently under investigation.

Initial Workup and Staging Procedures

The clinical course and the imaging manifestations of EHE are extremely variable (**Fig. 1**). EHE could present as unifocal disease, multifocal single-organ nodules, or systemic metastases with multiorgan involvement. Imaging of the whole body at baseline should include computed tomography (CT) scan and/or MRI to ensure an appropriate whole-body evaluation, including brain, lungs, liver, and bones. In order to properly assess the potential presence of disease in the bones and in the extremities, a whole-body MRI or 18-FDG PET should be considered, depending on what is locally available. The most common pattern of lung EHE at presentation is multiple bilateral ground-glass nodules with or without pleural effusion. On CT, hepatic EHE is seen as multiple peripheral subcapsular nodules, with lower attenuation in comparison to normal hepatic parenchyma and the presence of the target/halo sign. Multiplanar MRI can detect EHE lesions that usually are hypointense on T1- and hyperintense on T2-weighted images. In the postcontrast phase, the lollipop sign (described as

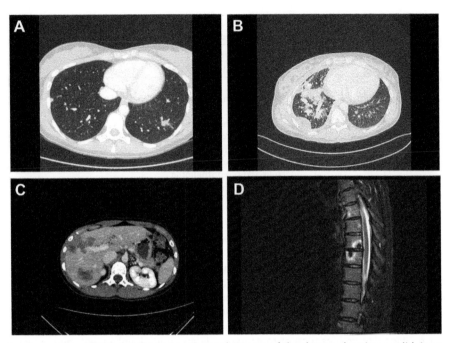

Fig. 1. Imaging of EHE. (*A*) Contrast enhanced CT scan of the thorax, showing a solid, irregular EHE pulmonary nodule. (*B*) Contrast enhanced CT scan of the thorax, showing parenchymal lesions and right-sided pleural effusion (pleural pattern). (*C*) Contrast enhanced CT scan of the abdomen, showing multiple EHE hepatic nodules with irregular profiles, low attenuation and subcapsular retraction. (*D*) Contrast-enhanced STIR MRI, showing EHE bone lesions, with perilesional edema

hepatic or portal vein shaped and ended in the peripheric region, within hypointense nodule) may be seen.[17]

The diagnosis must be confirmed pathologically. In clinical practice, restaging should be performed consistently with the same imaging techniques used at presentation for patients on active surveillance and patients on treatment.[6]

Treatment

Localized disease
Surgical resection is the standard treatment with curative intent for patients with localized, resectable EHE, independent of the primary site (soft tissues, viscera, bone). The standard procedure is an en bloc wide resection with the goal of achieving microscopic negative (R0) margins.[6]

Adjuvant radiation therapy (RT) can be considered in association with surgery in selected cases with R1 margins.[18] Given the very limited activity of conventional chemotherapy in this disease and the absence of data suggesting a potential advantage in survival, neoadjuvant or adjuvant medical treatments are not recommended.

When surgery is not feasible owing to comorbidities or predicted R1-R2 excisions, alternative options may include definitive RT, or ablative procedures, such as chemoembolization or radioembolization and isolated limb perfusion.[6]

Advanced/metastatic disease

Because of EHE's rarity and heterogeneity in clinical behavior, the best treatment approach for patients with advanced EHE is not defined.

As described above, in a significant proportion of patients with EHE with metastases at presentation, prolonged disease stability in the absence of active treatment can be observed, and anecdotal spontaneous regressions have been reported. On this basis, active surveillance is recognized as a reasonable upfront strategy for asymptomatic patients with stable or slowly progressive disease.[19] In this setting, surgical resection can also play a role, particularly for patients with locoregional EHE limited to the liver, showing stability or slow progression over time. In highly selected cases, after multidisciplinary discussion and providing full patient information regarding the absence of definitive supporting data in the literature, liver transplantation can also be offered.

Medical therapies for patients with advanced EHE should be considered mainly for clearly progressive patients. Given the poor prognosis reported in patients with EHE with serosal involvement and/or effusions and/or with systemic symptoms at presentations, recent studies suggest that early initiation of treatment should be considered in this population.[4]

Unfortunately, in advanced EHE, the activity of standard chemotherapy (including standard sarcoma schedules) is very limited. In a recent retrospective series, anthracycline-based regimens and weekly paclitaxel showed limited activity in advanced EHE, consistent with previous studies,[20] with overall response rates (ORR) of 3% and 9%, respectively, and median progression-free survival (m-PFS) of 5.5 and 2.9 months, respectively.[21] Anecdotal responses have been observed with pegylated doxorubicin.[22,23] Other schedules with cytotoxic agents have been used (carboplatin plus etoposide, gemcitabine plus docetaxel, cyclophosphamide plus vinblastine, oral cyclophosphamide, 5-fluorouracil), with stable disease being the best radiological response in most cases.[21]

Better results were described with the use of interferon-alpha, with a reported ORR of 7% and an m-PFS of 8.9 months, suggesting a potential role of immunomodulation in this disease.[21]

In the series from Yousaf and colleagues,[20] celecoxib, a nonsteroidal anti-inflammatory drug, was used in first line or further lines in 6 patients (out of 32 EHE patients), with 4 achieving partial regression as best response.

Given their vascular component and owing to the reported expression of the vascular endothelial growth factor (VEGF) in EHE, antiangiogenic drugs have been also evaluated in both prospective trials and retrospective series. In a phase II trial, including locally advanced or metastatic patients with EHE, the response rate to bevacizumab was 29%, and 57% of patients had stable disease. However, it is not clear that patients enrolled in this trial had evidence of disease progression before study entry. The median PFS and OS were 10 and 36 months, respectively.[24] In a phase II trial evaluating sorafenib in a group of 15 patients with EHE with evidence of progression at the time of trial entry, 2 patients had a partial response and 5 had stable disease, with a 9-month progression-free rate of 31%.[25] Pazopanib, the only antiangiogenic drug currently approved for advanced, soft tissue sarcomas, in the largest retrospective series available, no objective responses were documented, and a short m-PFS of approximately 3 months was reported.[20,21] Case reports describing partial or complete responses have been published.[26,27]

The most encouraging results in the treatment of progressive, advanced EHE are with mammalian target of rapamycin (m-TOR) inhibitors. In a multi-institutional, retrospective series from the Italian Rare Cancer Network including 38 patients with EHE with previous evidence of disease progression, sirolimus showed a significant clinical benefit and prolonged disease control over time, with partial responses and disease stabilizations observed in approximately 11% and 75% of patients, respectively.[28] In the whole population, the m-PFS and m-OS were 13 and 19 months, respectively. Sirolimus efficacy was more evident in the subset of patients without serosal effusions at baseline, both in terms of m-PFS (48 months vs 5 months in patients with baseline serosal effusion) and in m-OS (11 vs 48 months, respectively).[28]

Clinical trials currently ongoing are exploring the potential activity of MEK inhibitors (trametinib)[29] and mitotic inhibitors (eribulin) in EHE.

Outcome and symptoms management

Prognosis prediction remains very difficult in EHE and, although different stratifications based on clinical or histologic features have been attempted,[3] there are currently no validated criteria. In previous studies, the 5-year OS has been reported in the range of 70% to 80%.[3,4,8,15,30] Patients with or without symptoms at baseline or serosal involvement/effusions significantly differ in overall outcome, with reported 5-year OS in the range of 22% to 30% and 70% to 85%, respectively.[3,4,8]

Among the main challenges of this rare condition, the control of tumor-related symptoms, especially pain, is crucial due to its significant impact on quality of life. The cause of tumor-related pain in EHE is only partially understood, but it is known that, in terms of management, it is usually poorly responsive to opioids, whereas it seems sensitive to nonsteroidal anti-inflammatory drugs. There might be a potential relationship between systemic inflammatory process and local nociceptive mechanisms owing to cytokine release from the tumor and tumor interaction with local tissues.[8]

The complexity of this rare disease requires multidisciplinary management and an early team-based outpatient palliative care approach.[31] Further prospective studies are needed to validate clinical prognostic scores, which will allow a better tailored treatment strategy in this disease.

OTHER HEMANGIOENDOTHELIOMAS
Kaposiform Hemangioendothelioma

Kaposiform hemangioendothelioma (KHE) is a rare vascular tumor of intermediate malignancy without tendency to distant metastasis usually diagnosed in infancy or in early childhood.[32] It usually presents as an enlarging firm cutaneous lesion most frequently in the extremities. Noncutaneous deeper lesions (retroperitoneum, mediastinum, bone) have also been described.[32,33] Approximately 70% of patients with KHE develop the so-called Kasabach-Merritt phenomenon (KMP),[32,33] a potentially fatal thrombocytopenia and consumptive coagulopathy with possible microangiopathic hemolytic anemia.[34] Risk factors associated with the development of KMP include younger age, larger lesion size, and lesion associated with deep infiltration or visceral localization.[32,33]

On pathologic review, KHE nodules are composed of spindle endothelial cells aligned to form abnormal lumina expressing both vascular and lymphatic endothelial immunohistochemical markers.[35] No recurrent driver molecular alteration has been identified in KHE samples.

Uncomplicated superficial KHE can be treated with surgical excision, pulse-dye laser, or topical agents. Complicated KHE without KMP is treated with prednisolone, whereas combination treatment with vincristine and prednisolone is recommended for patients with KHE and KMP.[36] More recently, the mTOR inhibitor sirolimus has also been investigated as a potential treatment for KHE.[37]

Pseudomyogenic Hemangioendothelioma

PMHE is a rare intermediate-grade sarcoma with moderately aggressive local behavior and rare distant metastases.[38] PMHE has a male predominance of approximately 5:1 and is more common between the second and third decade of life. It usually presents as multifocal nodules in different tissue planes involving the dermis, subcutis, and bones. The nodules are painful in about half of the patients.[38]

PMHE is characterized by loose fascicles and sheets of plump spindle and epithelioid cells with abundant eosinophilic cytoplasm, and an immunophenotype favoring endothelial differentiation.[38] Recurrent pathogenic translocations involving the *FOSB* gene have been described in PMHE,[39–43] and strong FOSB expression is highly sensitive as a diagnostic marker.[44,45]

Most patients with PMHE are treated with surgery. In unresectable or recurrent cases, occasional responses to chemotherapy and mTOR inhibitors have been described.[46,47] More recently, the multityrosine kinase inhibitor telatinib has also shown activity in a single case of unresectable PMHE.[48]

Retiform Hemangioendothelioma

Retiform hemangioendothelioma (RHE) is an extremely rare intermediate-grade vascular tumor more frequently found in young adults. It usually presents as a solitary gradually growing, exophytic, mass or nodule located in the dermis and subcutaneous tissue in the limbs and trunk. Local recurrences are common, but distant metastases are rare.[49]

Histologically, RHE cases present retiform vessels exhibiting a pattern resembling the rete testis lined by protruding endothelial cells.[49]

Treatment of RHE includes surgical excision for localized disease. The use of radiotherapy and/or chemotherapy has been reported for inoperable and recurrent tumors.[50,51]

Composite Hemangioendothelioma

Composite hemangioendothelioma (CHE) is a very rare vascular neoplasm of intermediate biological potential, characterized by a complex and heterogeneous mixture of benign and different malignant vascular components. It has been reported in patients of any age and usually occurs as a long-standing lesion in the dermis and subcutis of the extremities, although CHEs in visceral sites have been reported.[52,53]

Most CHEs clinically behave in a low-grade manner, with a relatively high rate of local recurrence and rarely nodal and distant metastases. More recently, a variant of aggressive CHE with ectopic expression of neuroendocrine markers, such as synaptophysin, has been reported.[54] Based on molecular studies, this variant might represent a distinct disease, whereas RHE and conventional CHE might represent a morphologic continuum with common genetic abnormalities.[55]

CHE is usually treated surgically when localized, and with radiotherapy and chemotherapy in unresectable, recurrent, and metastatic cases.

ANGIOSARCOMA
Epidemiology and Clinical Presentation

Angiosarcoma is a type of soft tissue sarcoma with an endothelial cell lineage.[56] It is a rare tumor with an age-adjusted incidence rate of 0.1 in 100,000 people per year.[56]

Several etiologic factors have been implicated in the development of angiosarcoma. Cutaneous angiosarcoma of the head and neck region, the most common presentation of angiosarcoma, is thought to be associated with exposure to UV irradiation owing to a dominant presence of the UV mutational signature in the genomic profile.[57,58] Angiosarcoma occurring as a long-term sequela of radiotherapy for other cancers is well

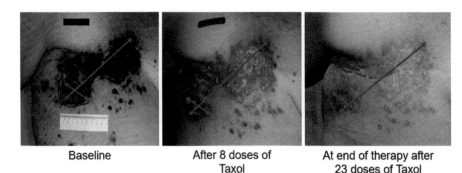

| Baseline | After 8 doses of Taxol | At end of therapy after 23 doses of Taxol |

Fig. 2. Cutaneous angiosarcoma of the chest wall with dark raised lesions at baseline. The lesions show significant clinical response with flattening and fading while the extent of the lesion (*red arrows*) remains the same, making it difficult to characterize response per RE-CIST criteria.

established. Angiosarcoma occurring in the setting of chronic lymphedema is called Stewart Treves syndrome.[59,60] The other reported risk factors include exposure to chemical carcinogens, such as vinyl chloride,[61] thorium dioxide, arsenic,[62] and use of anabolic steroids,[63] particularly in angiosarcoma of the liver. Familial syndromes, such as Li-Fraumeni syndrome, Klippel-Trenaunay syndrome, Maffucci syndrome, and neurofibromatosis type 1, are also associated with angiosarcoma.[64,65]

Angiosarcomas often present with cutaneous lesions, accounting for about 60% of the cases.[66] The other sites of occurrence are breast, organs such as the heart, liver, and spleen (known as visceral angiosarcoma), and bone.[67] About 50% to 80% of the patients present with localized disease, whereas 20% to 45% have metastatic disease at initial presentation.[68] The clinical characteristics of angiosarcoma are dependent on the location of the tumor.[67]

Cutaneous Angiosarcoma

Cutaneous angiosarcoma presents as single (rare) or multiple violaceous nodules on the skin that are sometimes associated with bleeding.[69] These lesions may resemble several other skin conditions, such as rosacea, hemangioma, xanthelasma, facial or eyelid angioedema, and can ulcerate or bleed.[66,69] Multifocality is a hallmark of cutaneous angiosarcoma with tissue infiltration that extends beyond the visible borders of the lesion.[66] These features make it challenging to map the true extent of the tumor, subsequently leading to difficulties in local therapy planning and even assessing response to systemic therapy using conventional radiological response criteria, as seen in **Fig. 2**.

Cutaneous angiosarcoma arising de novo is known as primary angiosarcoma and frequently affects skin of the head and neck region. It has a high rate of local recurrence and can spread to the regional lymph nodes.[66] Cutaneous angiosarcoma can also occur following RT, especially for breast cancer, where a substantial dose of radiation is delivered to the skin. In sharp contrast to primary breast angiosarcoma that affects the breast parenchyma, secondary angiosarcoma primarily affects the skin, and this cutaneous presentation is also referred to as radiation-associated angiosarcoma.

Radiation-associated angiosarcoma has been reported to occur between 2 and 30 years following RT, but the incidence is known to peak at 5 to 10 years.[70]

Visceral Angiosarcoma

Angiosarcomas in the visceral organs usually present as an expanding mass.[68] The most common organs involved are liver, heart, and spleen.[68]

Hepatic angiosarcoma usually presents with nonspecific symptoms, such as right upper quadrant abdominal pain, jaundice, and fatigue. Physical examination findings include jaundice, ascites, and hepatomegaly.[71]

Cardiac angiosarcoma often presents with symptoms such as chest pain, dyspnea, fatigue, cough, and hemoptysis. The right atrium is the most commonly involved site. It often metastasizes to the lung, liver, and brain with many of the patients having metastatic disease at the time of diagnosis.[72]

Angiosarcoma of the spleen is insidious in development. It presents with nonspecific symptoms, such as abdominal pain, fatigue, anorexia, and weight loss.[73]

Diagnosis of visceral angiosarcomas is challenging owing to the nonspecific nature of clinical presentation. It is often diagnosed in the late stages of the disease, resulting in poor patient outcomes. Early biopsy is strongly recommended for prompt diagnosis, as symptoms are often nonspecific.

Soft Tissue Angiosarcoma

Angiosarcoma of the soft tissue involves the extremities, skeletal muscle, retroperitoneum, mesentery, and mediastinum. They present as enlarging lesions, which are often hemorrhagic.[74]

Bone Angiosarcoma

Angiosarcoma of the bone is extremely rare and can present with unifocal or multifocal lesions. The long and short tubular bones, particularly of the lower limbs, are the most common site of tumor. The pelvis, spine, and trunk are the other sites of tumor. Angiosarcomas of the bone are often metastatic at the time of presentation.[75]

Pathology and Molecular Features

Angiosarcomas are predominantly morphologically aggressive lesions with no formal grading system. The separation between well-differentiated and poorly differentiated lesions is not very distinct. The well-differentiated tumor exhibits vasoformative features consisting of vascular channels that are lined by endothelial cells. The poorly differentiated and undifferentiated tumor is marked by predominantly epithelioid or spindle shaped cells, and poorly formed vascular channels.[5]

The typical endothelial markers expressed by angiosarcomas include CD31, CD34, ERG, factor VIII–related antigen, von Willebrand factor, and VEGF.[5,76,77]

Angiosarcoma is genetically complex with mutations reported in multiple different pathways. The most common genes involved are *TP53*, *KRAS*, *PTPRB*, and *PLCG1*.[78–81] The other known mutations are in the *MAPK* and *VEGF* pathway.[58,81] The molecular profiles for primary and secondary angiosarcomas are different. *PIK3CA* and *CIC* mutations are associated with primary breast angiosarcoma.[58,82] Radiation-associated angiosarcomas are associated with an upregulation of *MYC*, *KIT*, *FLT4*, and *RET* genes.[82–87] *KDR* mutations are associated with both primary and secondary angiosarcomas of the breast.[58]

Initial Workup

Contrast-enhanced imaging (CT or MRI) followed by biopsy of the vascular hyperenhancing lesion identified is the preferred approach for establishing the diagnosis (**Fig. 3**). Given the rarity of this entity, this should be carried out within a sarcoma reference center.

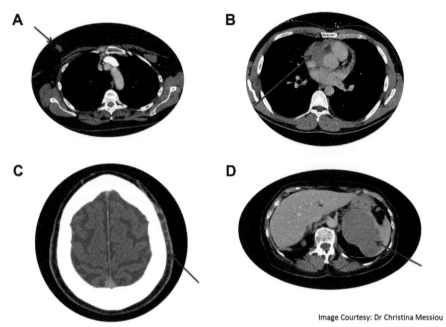

Fig. 3. CT imaging appearance of angiosarcoma of different sites (red arrows). (*A*) Breast angiosarcoma. (*B*) Cardiac angiosarcoma. (*C*) Scalp angiosarcoma. (*D*) Visceral angiosarcoma.

Disease staging should include imaging of the thorax. Brain imaging can be considered, particularly for cardiac angiosarcomas owing to the high prevalence of brain metastases.[88]

Treatment of Angiosarcoma

Angiosarcomas are rare with limited/small clinical trials and no approved therapy to guide treatment. Hence, consultation at a high-volume sarcoma center involving a multidisciplinary approach to treatment is strongly recommended.

Localized disease

Surgical resection with adjuvant radiation is the standard treatment for localized disease. As the tumor is sensitive to chemotherapeutic agents, systemic treatment in the perioperative setting is often used in the treatment of localized angiosarcoma.

Cutaneous angiosarcomas are characterized by the multifocal nature of the lesions. Subclinical satellite lesions make it difficult to achieve long recurrence-free survival even in the setting of margin negative resection. Of the patients who have complete resection for localized disease, 75% will have tumor recurrence and develop metastasis.[89] Except for very small solitary lesions (≤2 cm), neoadjuvant systemic therapy to eliminate microscopic satellite lesions is the standard in most high-volume centers.

Neoadjuvant chemotherapy has shown clinical benefit in retrospective studies. It offers an opportunity to achieve clear surgical margins by reducing tumor size. It can also potentially eliminate micrometastasis and multifocal nests of tumor cells.[90] A multicenter study conducted by the European Organization for Research and Treatment of Cancer included 59 patients with angiosarcoma who received neoadjuvant therapy.[91] The results of this study demonstrated antitumor activity and clinical benefit of various treatments, including chemotherapeutic and antiangiogenic agents. The choice of agent often depends on the location of the primary tumor, histologic features, performance status of the patient, and toxicity profile. Paclitaxel appears to be the first choice for patients with cutaneous angiosarcoma owing to its favorable toxicity profile and excellent clinical outcomes. In an ongoing prospective trial of Oraxol (oral paclitaxel + P-gp inhibitor) for unresectable cutaneous angiosarcoma, 28% of the patients became operable after therapy and received surgical resection.[92] Doxorubicin-based therapies, particularly combination therapy with doxorubicin and ifosfamide, are preferred for patients with noncutaneous angiosarcoma.[90] Combination chemotherapy with gemcitabine and docetaxel is another option, especially for patients with cardiac dysfunction.[90]

Local therapy with surgical resection of the tumor and adjuvant RT is the treatment of curative intent for localized angiosarcoma.[68] Tumor location often dictates the surgical approach. Complete resection with clear margins is the goal, particularly for angiosarcoma of the breast, chest wall, and extremity.[90] Head and neck angiosarcomas often require much wider resection to achieve clear margins and can be disfiguring or not feasible to perform owing to their location. Definitive RT serves as a curative alternative in such cases. Visceral angiosarcomas are often challenging to resect owing to involvement of adjacent structures and early hematogenous spread.[90]

Radiation therapy is mostly used as adjuvant treatment to achieve local control or is reserved for patients unsuitable for surgery.[90] Several retrospective studies have shown that the addition of radiation to surgical resection improves clinical outcomes for cutaneous angiosarcoma. One study in patients with cutaneous angiosarcoma of the head and neck showed a 5-year local control rate of 25% among those who received surgery alone compared with 84% in those who received radiation following surgery.[93] Studies have also demonstrated that the addition of radiation results in significantly longer disease-free survival and OS durations.[89,93,94]

Metastatic disease

Systemic chemotherapeutic agents are the mainstay of treatment of metastatic disease.[90] Although there are no approved therapies for angiosarcoma, agents such as doxorubicin, paclitaxel, and gemcitabine, or targeted therapies have been used in the treatment of metastatic disease. These are used either as single agent or in combination schedules.[91] Multiagent chemotherapy is associated with better response rates and duration of response compared with single agents and should be considered in patients based on performance status and comorbidities. **Table 2** lists the commonly used systemic agents that have demonstrated clinical activity in angiosarcoma.

Anthracycline based. The activity of doxorubicin-based regimens in angiosarcoma is mainly obtained from small retrospective studies or pooled studies with several soft tissue sarcomas. The response rate is around 29% with an m-PFS ranging between 3 and 3.7 months for doxorubicin and 4.2 and 5 months for liposomal doxorubicin.[95–97] The combination of doxorubicin plus ifosfamide has better durability of response with an m-PFS of 5.4 months.[97]

Taxanes. Several studies have demonstrated that angiosarcoma, especially the cutaneous subtype, is sensitive to single-agent paclitaxel. The ANGIOTAX trial showed a response rate of 19% at 4 months, whereas the paclitaxel arm of the ANGIOTAX II trial showed a response rate of 46% at 4 months.[98,99] The response rate with single-agent paclitaxel is considerably variable, ranging from 19% to 89%. Single-agent paclitaxel

Table 2
Summary of clinical activity of systemic therapy agents used in the treatment of angiosarcoma

	Study	Design (N)	Therapeutic Agents	Overall Response Rate, %	Median PFS, mo	Median OS, mo
Doxorubicin based	Young et al,[95] 2014	Pooled analysis (108)	Doxorubicin/doxorubicin (liposomal)/doxorubicin + ifosfamide	25	4.9	9.9
	Italiano et al,[96] 2011	Retrospective (42)	Doxorubicin	29	3.0	5.5
	Fury et al,[97] 2004	Retrospective (12)	Doxorubicin	—	3.7	—
	Fury et al,[97] 2004	Retrospective (11)	Doxorubicin (liposomal)	—	4.2	—
	Fury et al,[97] 2004	Retrospective (7)	Doxorubicin + ifosfamide	—	5.4	—
Taxanes	Ray-Coquard et al,[99] 2015	Randomized (24)	Paclitaxel	46	6.6	19.5
	Ray-Coquard et al,[99] 2015	Randomized (25)	Paclitaxel + bevacizumab	28	6.6	15.9
	Bui et al,[110] 2018	Randomized (16)	Paclitaxel + bevacizumab	45	5.16	16.0
	Penel et al,[98] 2008	Prospective (30)	Paclitaxel	19	4.0	8.0
	Fata et al,[111] 1999	Prospective (9)	Paclitaxel	89		
	Apice et al,[112] 2016	Prospective and Retrospective (18)	Paclitaxel	35	4.6	18.6
	Italiano et al,[96] 2011	Retrospective (75)	Paclitaxel	53	5.8	10.3
	Fury, 2004[97]	Retrospective (41)	Paclitaxel	—	4.	—
	Nagano et al,[113] 2007	Retrospective (9)	Docetaxel	67	—	—
Gemcitabine based	Stachiotti et al,[100] 2012	Retrospective (25)	Gemcitabine	64	7	17
	Dickson et al,[114] 2015	Prospective (5)	Gemcitabine + docetaxel + bevacizumab	60	—	—
	Kim et al,[115] 2019	Retrospective (2)	Gemcitabine + docetaxel	50	—	—
	Fury et al,[97] 2004	Retrospective (11)	Gemcitabine	—	2.2	—
Targeted therapies	Mehren et al,[116] 2019	Prospective (29)	Pazopanib	3	3.3	16.1

Jones et al,[103] 2019	Randomized (53)	Pazopanib	13	4.3	8.7
Jones et al,[103] 2019	Randomized (61)	Pazopanib + TRC105	5	4.2	—
Kollar et al,[27] 2016	Retrospective (40)	Pazopanib	20	3.0	9.9
Kim et al,[115] 2019	Retrospective (9)	Pazopanib	0	—	—
Ray-Coquard et al,[101] 2012	Prospective (41)	Sorafenib	17	—	—
Maki et al,[102] 2009	Prospective (37)	Sorafenib	14	3.8	14.9
Agulnik et al,[24] 2013	Prospective (23)	Bevacizumab	9	3.0	—
Immunotherapy agents Florou et al,[106] 2019	Retrospective (7)	Pembrolizumab/ pembrolizumab + axitinib/AGEN1884	71	—	—
Wagner et al,[105] 2021	Prospective (16)	Nivolumab + ipilimumab	25	—	—

has comparable efficacy to doxorubicin in angiosarcoma, and for many patients, it is preferred owing to its more favorable toxicity profile.

Gemcitabine based. Gemcitabine is an effective agent in the treatment of angiosarcoma, both as a single agent and in combination with taxanes. In a retrospective study, it has shown a response rate of 64% with an m-PFS of 7 months.[100]

Targeted therapies. Anti-VEGF antibody bevacizumab had a response rate of 9% in a phase II trial.[24] In combination with paclitaxel, the addition of bevacizumab did not improve either response rate or m-PFS in angiosarcoma. Two prospective trials with sorafenib have shown a response rate ranging between 14% and 17%.[101,102] The m-PFS was 3.8 months.[102] Pazopanib is approved for advanced, pretreated soft tissue sarcomas and is often used to treat angiosarcoma. The outcomes have not been promising, with 1 prospective trial showing a response rate of 3%, whereas the TAPPAS trial showed a 5% response rate in the pazopanib arm and no clinical benefit with the addition of an antiendoglin antibody to pazopanib.[103] Radiological responses were reported in 3 of the 20 patients with angiosarcoma included in the phase II trial of brivanib in advanced solid tumors.[104]

Immunotherapy. The immune microenvironment of angiosarcoma is not very well understood, and the role of immunotherapy in the treatment of angiosarcoma is currently being explored.[58] A phase II trial of ipilimumab and nivolumab in unresectable angiosarcoma has shown a response rate of 25% with a 60% response rate in the cutaneous angiosarcoma subset.[105] A retrospective study of 7 patients, with a predominant cutaneous angiosarcoma patient population using several immunotherapy agents, demonstrated a response rate of 75%.[106]

Prognosis

Angiosarcomas are highly malignant and aggressive with a high rate of recurrence and propensity to metastasize.[67,68] They have a high mortality with an overall 5-year survival of about 26%.[56,68] The prognosis varies depending on several factors. Patients with localized disease have a median OS that ranges between 24 and 60 months depending on the location of the tumor. However, prognosis is very poor for patients with metastatic disease, with a median OS of 8 to 11 months.[107] The important factors associated with poor prognosis include size of the tumor (>5 cm), location of the tumor (liver, heart, retroperitoneum), and metastatic disease at the time of diagnosis.[108,109]

KAPOSI SARCOMA
Introduction

KS is a multicentric vascular tumor initially described by Moritz Kaposi,[117] an Austro-Hungarian physician and dermatologist, in 1872. Infection with the Kaposi sarcoma-related herpesvirus (KSHV), also known as human herpesvirus 8, was identified during the human AIDS epidemic of the 1990s as the key pathogenic event of KS.[118,119]

Clinical Presentation

KS can present in several distinct populations with different incidences and a variety of clinical courses. Five main forms are now recognized, which reflect the uneven global distribution of KSHV infection prevalence, as well as different types of impaired host immunity.[120]

1. *Classic or sporadic KS*: Rare disease occurring more frequently in elderly men of regions with high KSHV prevalence (Mediterranean, Eastern Europe, Middle

East). It typically presents on the lower extremities, and it is characterized by a rela-tively indolent course.[121]

2. *Endemic (African) KS*: Occurring with high incidence (from 1 to 6 cases per 1000 person-years) in the pediatric and young adult population in sub-Saharan Africa, primarily presenting as an aggressive disease with diffuse lymphadenopathy.[122,123]

3. *Epidemic (or AIDS-related) KS*: Clinically variable form of KS generally affecting men who have sex with men (MSM) with severe immunodeficiency secondary to AIDS. In fact, KS represents one of the AIDS-defining cancers. In this population, the prevalence of KS was reported in the early 1990s to be 20,000 times higher than in the general population.[124] The incidence of epidemic KS has dramatically decreased since the introduction of combined anti-retroviral therapy (cART).[125]

4. *Iatrogenic KS*: Occurring in individuals with iatrogenic immunodeficiency, such as that seen in organ transplant recipients. In this population, KS risk peaks in the first 2 years posttransplant and represents up to 5% of all diagnosed malignancies, with an incidence between 50 and 500 times higher than in the general population.[126,127]

5. *KS in MSM without human immunodeficiency virus (HIV) infection*: Clinical features in common with classical KS but occurs in younger MSM patients who are not immunocompromised by HIV, possibly owing to higher transmission rates of KSHV in this population.[128]

In all forms of KS, cutaneous lesions usually present as multiple, pigmented, raised or flat, painless lesions. Occasionally, KS can also present in the form of exophytic, ulcerated nodules. In AIDS-related KS, oral and visceral lesions can frequently occur.[120]

Diagnosis

In most Western countries, the diagnosis of KS is confirmed by pathologic assess-ment. This is more challenging in some areas of Africa, where the diagnosis is often clinical and potentially associated with inappropriate treatments.[129]

Histologic features characteristic of KS can include vascular proliferation in the dermis, vessels without an endothelium, and diffuse spindle cell proliferation. Immu-nohistochemical markers usually show a combined immunophenotype of vascular endothelial, lymphatic endothelial, and mesenchymal cells. Analysis of KSHV antigens or, more recently, of KSHV DNA can also be used to confirm the diagnosis.[120]

Treatment

Treatment of KS varies based on cause and extent of disease. All patients with AIDS-related KS and iatrogenic KS, in which immunosuppression is potentially reversible, should respectively receive cART and either a reduced dose of immunosuppressive drugs or undergo conversion of calcineurin inhibitors to mTOR inhibitors.[120,130] These treatments are associated with rare complications, represented by graft rejection for transplanted patients and KS–immune reconstitution inflammatory syndrome (KS-IRIS) for patients with AIDS-related KS. KS-IRIS refers to a potentially life-threatening clinical worsening of KS following cART-mediated reconstitution of the im-mune system that often requires prompt initiation of systemic therapy.[131]

Treatments directed at the tumors are necessary in patients with classic KS, endemic KS, KS in MSM without HIV infection, and in those cases of AIDS-related and iatrogenic KS in whom bolstering the immune system is insufficient in causing regression of the disease.[130] In all these cases, treatments largely depend on whether the disease is limited and only localized to the skin, or if it affects the skin extensively, visceral sites, or the nodes. For AIDS-related KS, CD4 cell count and global performance status also provide information that can guide a stage-stratified treatment approach.[132]

For limited, asymptomatic cutaneous disease, initial observation is recommended if aesthetically acceptable. Local excision, cryotherapy, radiotherapy, intralesional chemotherapy with vinca alkaloids or topical treatments with imiquimod or alitretinoin are recommended in symptomatic or aesthetically unacceptable cases. There are no randomized clinical trials comparing these different modalities.[133]

In the case of progressive or metastatic disease, the recommended first-line agents are pegylated liposomal doxorubicin[134,135] and paclitaxel.[136] A randomized clinical trial showed that these 2 drugs had comparable response rates and survival rates; however, liposomal doxorubicin was better tolerated than paclitaxel.[137] For this reason, liposomal anthracyclines are favored in high-income settings, whereas paclitaxel, which is more affordable, is usually considered the first-line treatment in countries with lower incomes. Recently, a noninferiority trial in patients with advanced AIDS-related KS in low- and middle-income countries compared cART with intravenous paclitaxel (the control arm) to cART with intravenous bleomycin and vincristine or oral etoposide (the investigational arms). Noninferiority of either investigational intervention was not shown.[138]

Subsequent treatments with limited prospective evidence of efficacy include antiangiogenic and immunomodulatory agents, for example, bevacizumab[139] and pomalidomide,[140] the tyrosine kinase inhibitor imatinib,[141] other single-agent chemotherapeutic regimens, such as low-dose etoposide,[142] or the proteasome inhibitor bortezomib.[143] Given the viral cause of KS and the prominent role of the immune system in its pathogenesis, several trials are currently exploring the efficacy of immune checkpoint inhibitors in patients with KS,[144] and positive outcomes have been reported in limited case series.[145,146] In particular, the PD-1 inhibitor pembrolizumab has been evaluated in a phase 1 trial in patients with HIV-related malignancies, including KS,[147] and 2 phase II trials assessing its efficacy in KS are ongoing (NCT03469804 and NCT02595866). The preliminary results of the KAPKEY study (NCT03469804) presented at ESMO 2020 reported disease control in 12 of the 16 treated patients.[148] Additional promising immunotherapies that are being evaluated in patients with KS include the combination of the CTLA-4 inhibitor ipilimumab + the PD-1 inhibitor nivolumab (NCT03219671 and NCT02408861).

Prognosis

The prognosis of patients with KS largely depends on the subtype of KS, the extent of disease, and the presence of comorbidities.

In most cases, classical KS has an indolent biologic behavior and does not seem to significantly impact the mortality.[149]

Endemic KS is considered a more aggressive variant, although prospective prognostic data are limited. In a recent analysis on a combined cohort of patients with classical and endemic KS, the endemic variant was associated with a shorter time to systemic treatment initiation compared with classical variant, but with similar response rates and duration of response.[150]

The prognosis of AIDS-related KS depends on tumor extent, severity of immunosuppression, and presence of other systemic HIV-associated illness.[151,152] Mortality of this variant of KS has dramatically decreased over time following the introduction of cART. For example, the percentage of patients surviving 24 months after diagnosis has risen from 35% in 1996 to 2000 to 81% in 2001 to 2006. Among patients diagnosed in the last decades, survival rates are higher in patients with higher CD4 cell count at KS diagnosis.[153]

In patients with iatrogenic KS, the prognosis is often dependent on their underlying condition and their ability to tolerate a reduction in immunosuppression. In the case of liver and kidney transplant recipients, the development of KS does not appear to have a significant impact on the outcomes.[154,155]

SUMMARY

Vascular sarcomas are a group of soft tissue sarcomas grouped under the same umbrella by the same line of differentiation of the neoplastic cells but encompassing several sarcoma types that are very different in terms of clinical behavior, biological features, and treatment approach. Because of this heterogeneity, and as most of these sarcomas are exceedingly rare, it is crucial that vascular sarcomas are treated in sarcoma reference centers or networks, in order to ensure optimal management. Their diversity also needs to be taken into account in the design of clinical trials, in order to produce meaningful results that can be consistently translated into everyday clinical practice.

CLINICS CARE POINTS

- Vascular sarcomas are heterogeneous in their clinical behavior, biological features, and management approach.
- Active surveillance is recognized as a reasonable upfront strategy for asymptomatic patients with stable or slowly progressive epithelioid hemangioendothelioma.
- Mammalian target of rapamycin inhibitors have shown significant clinical benefit and prolonged disease control in the treatment of progressive, advanced epithelioid hemangioendothelioma.
- Cutaneous angiosarcomas are characterized by the multifocal nature of the lesions, making it difficult to achieve long recurrence-free survival even in the setting of margin negative resection.
- Several systemic and targeted therapies have been used in the treatment of metastatic angiosarcoma, and the response rates and progression-free survival are highly variable.
- In Kaposi sarcoma where bolstering the immune system is not sufficient, treatment largely depends on whether the disease is limited and only localized to the skin, or if it affects the skin extensively, visceral sites, or the nodes.

DISCLOSURE

A. Napolitano reports financial support for an educational course from PharmaMar. V. Ravi reports grant funding to his institution in relation to clinical trial support from Athenex, Tracon, Novartis; personal fees for consulting from Daiichi Sankyo, Guidepoint, GLG; royalties from UpToDate. A. M. Frezza reports research support to her institution from Advenchen Laboratories, Amgen Dompe, Arog Pharmaceuticals, Bayer, Blueprint Medicines, Daiichi Sankyo Pharma, Deciphera, Eli Lilly & Co, Epizyme, GlaxoSmithKline, Karyopharm Therapeutics, Novartis, Pfizer, PharmaMar, SpringWorks Therapeutics; R. L. Jones reports grants and research support from Merck Sharp and Dohme Corp, GlaxoSmithKline; consultation fees from Adaptimmune Therapeutics PLC, Astex Pharmaceuticals, Athenex, Bayer, Boehringer Ingelheim, Blueprint Medicines, Clinigen Group, Eisai Co Ltd, Epizyme, Daiichi Sankyo, Deciphera, Immune Design, Immunicum, Karma Oncology, Lilly, Merck Sharp and Dohme Corp, Mundipharma, PharmaMar, SpringWorks Therapeutics, SynOx Therapeutics, Tracon

Pharmaceuticals, UpToDate. A. Subramaniam and C. Giani have no conflicts of interest to report.

REFERENCES

1. Stacchiotti S, Frezza AM, Blay JY, et al. Ultra-rare sarcomas: a consensus paper from the Connective Tissue Oncology Society community of experts on the incidence threshold and the list of entities. Cancer 2021;127(16):2934–42.

2. de Pinieux G, Karanian M, Le Loarer F, et al. Nationwide incidence of sarcomas and connective tissue tumors of intermediate malignancy over four years using an expert pathology review network. PLoS One 2021;16(2):e0246958.

3. Lau K, Massad M, Pollak C, et al. Clinical patterns and outcome in epithelioid hemangioendothelioma with or without pulmonary involvement: insights from an internet registry in the study of a rare cancer. Chest 2011;140(5):1312–8.

4. Rosenbaum E, Jadeja B, Xu B, et al. Prognostic stratification of clinical and molecular epithelioid hemangioendothelioma subsets. Mod Pathol 2020;33(4): 591–602.

5. Antonescu C. Malignant vascular tumors–an update. Mod Pathol 2014;27(Suppl 1):S30–8.

6. Stacchiotti S, Miah AB, Frezza AM, et al. Epithelioid hemangioendothelioma, an ultra-rare cancer: a consensus paper from the community of experts. ESMO Open 2021;6(3):100170.

7. Shiba S, Imaoka H, Shioji K, et al. Clinical characteristics of Japanese patients with epithelioid hemangioendothelioma: a multicenter retrospective study. BMC Cancer 2018;18(1):993.

8. Frezza AM, Napolitano A, Miceli R, et al. Clinical prognostic factors in advanced epithelioid haemangioendothelioma: a retrospective case series analysis within the Italian Rare Cancers Network. ESMO Open 2021;6(2):100083.

9. Rossi S, Orvieto E, Furlanetto A, et al. Utility of the immunohistochemical detection of FLI-1 expression in round cell and vascular neoplasm using a monoclonal antibody. Mod Pathol 2004;17(5):547–52.

10. Righi A, Sbaraglia M, Gambarotti M, et al. Primary vascular tumors of bone: a monoinstitutional morphologic and molecular analysis of 427 cases with emphasis on epithelioid variants. Am J Surg Pathol 2020;44(9):1192–203.

11. Errani C, Zhang L, Sung YS, et al. A novel WWTR1-CAMTA1 gene fusion is a consistent abnormality in epithelioid hemangioendothelioma of different anatomic sites. Genes Chromosomes Cancer 2011;50(8):644–53.

12. Suurmeijer AJH, Dickson BC, Swanson D, et al. Variant WWTR1 gene fusions in epithelioid hemangioendothelioma-a genetic subset associated with cardiac involvement. Genes Chromosomes Cancer 2020;59(7):389–95.

13. Kitaichi M, Nagai S, Nishimura K, et al. Pulmonary epithelioid haemangioendothelioma in 21 patients, including three with partial spontaneous regression. Eur Respir J 1998;12(1):89–96.

14. Otrock ZK, Al-Kutoubi A, Kattar MM, et al. Spontaneous complete regression of hepatic epithelioid haemangioendothelioma. Lancet Oncol 2006;7(5):439–41.

15. Shibayama T, Makise N, Motoi T, et al. Clinicopathologic characterization of epithelioid hemangioendothelioma in a series of 62 cases: a proposal of risk stratification and identification of a synaptophysin-positive aggressive subset. Am J Surg Pathol 2021;45(5):616–26.

16. Bagan P, Hassan M, Le Pimpec Barthes F, et al. Prognostic factors and surgical indications of pulmonary epithelioid hemangioendothelioma: a review of the literature. Ann Thorac Surg 2006;82(6):2010–3.
17. Epelboym Y, Engelkemier DR, Thomas-Chausse F, et al. Imaging findings in epithelioid hemangioendothelioma. Clin Imaging 2019;58:59–65.
18. Sardaro A, Bardoscia L, Petruzzelli MF, et al. Epithelioid hemangioendothelioma: an overview and update on a rare vascular tumor. Oncol Rev 2014;8(2):259.
19. Tong D, Constantinidou A, Engelmann B, et al. The role of local therapy in multifocal epithelioid haemangioendothelioma. Anticancer Res 2019;39(9):4891–6.
20. Yousaf N, Maruzzo M, Judson I, et al. Systemic treatment options for epithelioid haemangioendothelioma: the Royal Marsden Hospital experience. Anticancer Res 2015;35(1):473–80.
21. Frezza AM, Ravi V, Lo Vullo S, et al. Systemic therapies in advanced epithelioid haemangioendothelioma: a retrospective international case series from the World Sarcoma Network and a review of literature. Cancer Med 2021;10(8): 2645–59.
22. Kelly H, O'Neil BH. Response of epithelioid haemangioendothelioma to liposomal doxorubicin. Lancet Oncol 2005;6(10):813–5.
23. Grenader T, Vernea F, Reinus C, et al. Malignant epithelioid hemangioendothelioma of the liver successfully treated with pegylated liposomal doxorubicin. J Clin Oncol 2011;29(25):e722–4.
24. Agulnik M, Yarber JL, Okuno SH, et al. An open-label, multicenter, phase II study of bevacizumab for the treatment of angiosarcoma and epithelioid hemangioendotheliomas. Ann Oncol 2013;24(1):257–63.
25. Chevreau C, Le Cesne A, Ray-Coquard I, et al. Sorafenib in patients with progressive epithelioid hemangioendothelioma: a phase 2 study by the French Sarcoma Group (GSF/GETO). Cancer 2013;119(14):2639–44.
26. Semenisty V, Naroditsky I, Keidar Z, et al. Pazopanib for metastatic pulmonary epithelioid hemangioendothelioma-a suitable treatment option: case report and review of anti-angiogenic treatment options. BMC Cancer 2015;15:402.
27. Kollar A, Jones RL, Stacchiotti S, et al. Pazopanib in advanced vascular sarcomas: an EORTC Soft Tissue and Bone Sarcoma Group (STBSG) retrospective analysis. Acta Oncol 2017;56(1):88–92.
28. Stacchiotti S, Provenzano S, Dagrada G, et al. Sirolimus in advanced epithelioid hemangioendothelioma: a retrospective case-series analysis from the Italian Rare Cancer Network database. Ann Surg Oncol 2016;23(9):2735–44.
29. Schuetze S, Ballman KV, Ganjoo KN, et al. P10015/SARC033: a phase 2 trial of trametinib in patients with advanced epithelioid hemangioendothelioma (EHE). J Clin Oncol 2021;39(15_suppl):11503.
30. Gronchi A, Miah AB, Dei Tos AP, et al. Soft tissue and visceral sarcomas: ESMO-EURACAN-GENTURIS clinical practice guidelines for diagnosis, treatment and follow-up*. Ann Oncol 2021;32(11):1348–65.
31. Zimmermann C, Ryan S, Hannon B, et al. Team-based outpatient early palliative care: a complex cancer intervention. BMJ Support Palliat Care 2019. https://doi.org/10.1136/bmjspcare-2019-001903.
32. Croteau SE, Liang MG, Kozakewich HP, et al. Kaposiform hemangioendothelioma: atypical features and risks of Kasabach-Merritt phenomenon in 107 referrals. J Pediatr 2013;162(1):142–7.
33. Ji Y, Yang K, Peng S, et al. Kaposiform haemangioendothelioma: clinical features, complications and risk factors for Kasabach-Merritt phenomenon. Br J Dermatol 2018;179(2):457–63.

34. Kasabach HH, Merritt KK. Capillary hemangioma with extensive purpura: report of a case. Am J Dis Child 1940;59(5):1063–70.

35. Lyons LL, North PE, Mac-Moune Lai F, et al. Kaposiform hemangioendothelioma: a study of 33 cases emphasizing its pathologic, immunophenotypic, and biologic uniqueness from juvenile hemangioma. Am J Surg Pathol 2004; 28(5):559–68.

36. Drolet BA, Trenor CC 3rd, Brandao LR, et al. Consensus-derived practice standards plan for complicated Kaposiform hemangioendothelioma. J Pediatr 2013; 163(1):285–91.

37. Ji Y, Chen S, Xiang B, et al. Sirolimus for the treatment of progressive kaposiform hemangioendothelioma: a multicenter retrospective study. Int J Cancer 2017; 141(4):848–55.

38. Hornick JL, Fletcher CD. Pseudomyogenic hemangioendothelioma: a distinctive, often multicentric tumor with indolent behavior. Am J Surg Pathol 2011; 35(2):190–201.

39. Trombetta D, Magnusson L, von Steyern FV, et al. Translocation t(7;19)(q22;q13)-a recurrent chromosome aberration in pseudomyogenic hemangioendothelioma? Cancer Genet 2011;204(4):211–5.

40. Agaram NP, Zhang L, Cotzia P, et al. Expanding the spectrum of genetic alterations in pseudomyogenic hemangioendothelioma with recurrent novel ACTB-FOSB gene fusions. Am J Surg Pathol 2018;42(12):1653–61.

41. Bridge JA, Sumegi J, Royce T, et al. A novel CLTC-FOSB gene fusion in pseudomyogenic hemangioendothelioma of bone. Genes Chromosomes Cancer 2021;60(1):38–42.

42. Hakar MH, White K, Hansford BG, et al. Novel EGFL7-FOSB fusion in pseudomyogenic haemangioendothelioma with widely metastatic disease. Histopathology 2021;79(5):888–91.

43. Murshed KA, Torres-Mora J, ElSayed AM, et al. Pseudomyogenic hemangioendothelioma of bone with rare WWTR1-FOSB fusion gene: case report and literature review. Clin Case Rep 2021;9(3):1494–9.

44. Sugita S, Hirano H, Kikuchi N, et al. Diagnostic utility of FOSB immunohistochemistry in pseudomyogenic hemangioendothelioma and its histological mimics. Diagn Pathol 2016;11(1):75.

45. Hung YP, Fletcher CD, Hornick JL. FOSB is a useful diagnostic marker for pseudomyogenic hemangioendothelioma. Am J Surg Pathol 2017;41(5):596–606.

46. Joseph J, Wang WL, Patnana M, et al. Cytotoxic and targeted therapy for treatment of pseudomyogenic hemangioendothelioma. Clin Sarcoma Res 2015;5:22.

47. Ozeki M, Nozawa A, Kanda K, et al. Everolimus for treatment of pseudomyogenic hemangioendothelioma. J Pediatr Hematol Oncol 2017;39(6):e328–31.

48. van IDGP, Sleijfer S, Gelderblom H, et al. Telatinib is an effective targeted therapy for pseudomyogenic hemangioendothelioma. Clin Cancer Res 2018;24(11): 2678–87.

49. Calonje E, Fletcher CD, Wilson-Jones E, et al. Retiform hemangioendothelioma. A distinctive form of low-grade angiosarcoma delineated in a series of 15 cases. Am J Surg Pathol 1994;18(2):115–25.

50. Colmenero I, Hoeger PH. Vascular tumours in infants. Part II: vascular tumours of intermediate malignancy [corrected] and malignant tumours. Br J Dermatol 2014;171(3):474–84.

51. Hirsh AZ, Yan W, Wei L, et al. Unresectable retiform hemangioendothelioma treated with external beam radiation therapy and chemotherapy: a case report

and review of the literature. Sarcoma 2010;2010. https://doi.org/10.1155/2010/75624690.

52. Nayler SJ, Rubin BP, Calonje E, et al. Composite hemangioendothelioma: a complex, low-grade vascular lesion mimicking angiosarcoma. Am J Surg Pathol 2000;24(3):352–61.

53. Shang Leen SL, Fisher C, Thway K. Composite hemangioendothelioma: clinical and histologic features of an enigmatic entity. Adv Anat Pathol 2015;22(4):254–9.

54. Perry KD, Al-Lbraheemi A, Rubin BP, et al. Composite hemangioendothelioma with neuroendocrine marker expression: an aggressive variant. Mod Pathol 2017;30(10):1512.

55. Antonescu CR, Dickson BC, Sung YS, et al. Recurrent YAP1 and MAML2 gene rearrangements in retiform and composite hemangioendothelioma. Am J Surg Pathol 2020;44(12):1677–84.

56. Khan JA, Maki RG, Ravi V. Pathologic angiogenesis of malignant vascular sarcomas: implications for treatment. J Clin Oncol 2018;36(2):194–201.

57. Stenback F. Cellular injury and cell proliferation in skin carcinogenesis by UV light. Oncology 1975;31(2):61–75.

58. Painter CA, Jain E, Tomson BN, et al. The Angiosarcoma Project: enabling genomic and clinical discoveries in a rare cancer through patient-partnered research. Nat Med 2020;26(2):181–7.

59. Huang J, Mackillop WJ. Increased risk of soft tissue sarcoma after radiotherapy in women with breast carcinoma. Cancer 2001;92(1):172–80.

60. Pereira ES, Moraes ET, Siqueira DM, et al. Stewart Treves syndrome. An Bras Dermatol 2015;90(3 Suppl 1):229–31.

61. Makk L, Creech JL, Whelan JG Jr, et al. Liver damage and angiosarcoma in vinyl chloride workers. A systematic detection program. JAMA 1974;230(1):64–8.

62. Centeno JA, Mullick FG, Martinez L, et al. Pathology related to chronic arsenic exposure. Environ Health Perspect 2002;110(Suppl 5):883–6.

63. Daneshmend TK, Bradfield JW. Hepatic angiosarcoma associated with androgenic-anabolic steroids. Lancet 1979;2(8154):1249.

64. Ploegmakers MJ, Pruszczynski M, De Rooy J, et al. Angiosarcoma with malignant peripheral nerve sheath tumour developing in a patient with Klippel-Trenaunay-Weber syndrome. Sarcoma 2005;9(3–4):137–40.

65. Calvete O, Martinez P, Garcia-Pavia P, et al. A mutation in the POT1 gene is responsible for cardiac angiosarcoma in TP53-negative Li-Fraumeni-like families. Nat Commun 2015;6:8383.

66. Shustef E, Kazlouskaya V, Prieto VG, et al. Cutaneous angiosarcoma: a current update. J Clin Pathol 2017;70(11):917–25.

67. Ravi V, Patel S. Vascular sarcomas. Curr Oncol Rep 2013;15(4):347–55.

68. Young RJ, Brown NJ, Reed MW, et al. Angiosarcoma. Lancet Oncol 2010;11(10):983–91.

69. Shon W, Billings SD. Cutaneous malignant vascular neoplasms. Clin Lab Med 2017;37(3):633–46.

70. Mery CM, George S, Bertagnolli MM, et al. Secondary sarcomas after radiotherapy for breast cancer: sustained risk and poor survival. Cancer 2009;115(18):4055–63.

71. Chaudhary P, Bhadana U, Singh RA, et al. Primary hepatic angiosarcoma. Eur J Surg Oncol 2015;41(9):1137–43.

72. Look Hong NJ, Pandalai PK, Hornick JL, et al. Cardiac angiosarcoma management and outcomes: 20-year single-institution experience. Ann Surg Oncol 2012;19(8):2707–15.

73. Li R, Li M, Zhang LF, et al. Clinical characteristics and prognostic factors of primary splenic angiosarcoma: a retrospective clinical analysis from China. Cell Physiol Biochem 2018;49(5):1959–69.

74. Meis-Kindblom JM, Kindblom LG. Angiosarcoma of soft tissue: a study of 80 cases. Am J Surg Pathol 1998;22(6):683–97.

75. Verbeke SL, Bertoni F, Bacchini P, et al. Distinct histological features characterize primary angiosarcoma of bone. Histopathology 2011;58(2):254–64.

76. Miettinen M, Lindenmayer AE, Chaubal A. Endothelial cell markers CD31, CD34, and BNH9 antibody to H- and Y-antigens–evaluation of their specificity and sensitivity in the diagnosis of vascular tumors and comparison with von Willebrand factor. Mod Pathol 1994;7(1):82–90.

77. Sullivan HC, Edgar MA, Cohen C, et al. The utility of ERG, CD31 and CD34 in the cytological diagnosis of angiosarcoma: an analysis of 25 cases. J Clin Pathol 2015;68(1):44–50.

78. Behjati S, Tarpey PS, Sheldon H, et al. Recurrent PTPRB and PLCG1 mutations in angiosarcoma. Nat Genet 2014;46(4):376–9.

79. Italiano A, Chen CL, Thomas R, et al. Alterations of the p53 and PIK3CA/AKT/mTOR pathways in angiosarcomas: a pattern distinct from other sarcomas with complex genomics. Cancer 2012;118(23):5878–87.

80. Naka N, Tomita Y, Nakanishi H, et al. Mutations of p53 tumor-suppressor gene in angiosarcoma. Int J Cancer 1997;71(6):952–5.

81. Murali R, Chandramohan R, Moller I, et al. Targeted massively parallel sequencing of angiosarcomas reveals frequent activation of the mitogen activated protein kinase pathway. Oncotarget 2015;6(34):36041–52.

82. Huang SC, Zhang L, Sung YS, et al. Recurrent CIC gene abnormalities in angiosarcomas: a molecular study of 120 cases with concurrent investigation of PLCG1, KDR, MYC, and FLT4 gene alterations. Am J Surg Pathol 2016;40(5):645–55.

83. Fernandez AP, Sun Y, Tubbs RR, et al. FISH for MYC amplification and anti-MYC immunohistochemistry: useful diagnostic tools in the assessment of secondary angiosarcoma and atypical vascular proliferations. J Cutan Pathol 2012;39(2):234–42.

84. Manner J, Radlwimmer B, Hohenberger P, et al. MYC high level gene amplification is a distinctive feature of angiosarcomas after irradiation or chronic lymphedema. Am J Pathol 2010;176(1):34–9.

85. Mentzel T, Schildhaus HU, Palmedo G, et al. Postradiation cutaneous angiosarcoma after treatment of breast carcinoma is characterized by MYC amplification in contrast to atypical vascular lesions after radiotherapy and control cases: clinicopathological, immunohistochemical and molecular analysis of 66 cases. Mod Pathol 2012;25(1):75–85.

86. Shon W, Sukov WR, Jenkins SM, et al. MYC amplification and overexpression in primary cutaneous angiosarcoma: a fluorescence in-situ hybridization and immunohistochemical study. Mod Pathol 2014;27(4):509–15.

87. Requena C, Rubio L, Lavernia J, et al. Immunohistochemical and fluorescence in situ hybridization analysis of MYC in a series of 17 cutaneous angiosarcomas: a single-center study. Am J Dermatopathol 2018;40(5):349–54.

88. Bishop AJ, Zheng J, Subramaniam A, et al. High terminal hemorrhage risk from cardiac angiosarcoma brain metastases warrants frequent brain imaging and early intervention. Int J Radiat Oncol Biol Phys 2021;111(3):e314.

89. Mark RJ, Poen JC, Tran LM, et al. Angiosarcoma. A report of 67 patients and a review of the literature. Cancer 1996;77(11):2400–6.

90. Chen TW, Burns J, Jones RL, et al. Optimal clinical management and the molecular biology of angiosarcomas. Cancers (Basel) 2020;12(11). https://doi.org/10.3390/cancers1211332191.

91. Constantinidou A, Sauve N, Stacchiotti S, et al. Evaluation of the use and efficacy of (neo)adjuvant chemotherapy in angiosarcoma: a multicentre study. ESMO Open 2020;5(4). https://doi.org/10.1136/esmoopen-2020-000787105.

92. Ravi V, Wagner M, Chen TW-W, et al. A phase II study of oraxol in the treatment of unresectable cutaneous angiosarcoma. J Clin Oncol 2020;38(15_suppl):11517.

93. Guadagnolo BA, Zagars GK, Araujo D, et al. Outcomes after definitive treatment for cutaneous angiosarcoma of the face and scalp. Head Neck 2011;33(5):661–7.

94. Pawlik TM, Paulino AF, McGinn CJ, et al. Cutaneous angiosarcoma of the scalp: a multidisciplinary approach. Cancer 2003;98(8):1716–26.

95. Young RJ, Natukunda A, Litiere S, et al. First-line anthracycline-based chemotherapy for angiosarcoma and other soft tissue sarcoma subtypes: pooled analysis of eleven European Organisation for Research and Treatment of Cancer Soft Tissue and Bone Sarcoma Group trials. Eur J Cancer 2014;50(18):3178–86.

96. Italiano A, Cioffi A, Penel N, et al. Comparison of doxorubicin and weekly paclitaxel efficacy in metastatic angiosarcomas. Cancer 2012;118(13):3330–6.

97. Fury MG, Antonescu CR, Van Zee KJ, et al. A 14-year retrospective review of angiosarcoma: clinical characteristics, prognostic factors, and treatment outcomes with surgery and chemotherapy. Cancer J 2005;11(3):241–7.

98. Penel N, Bui BN, Bay JO, et al. Phase II trial of weekly paclitaxel for unresectable angiosarcoma: the ANGIOTAX Study. J Clin Oncol 2008;26(32):5269–74.

99. Ray-Coquard IL, Domont J, Tresch-Bruneel E, et al. Paclitaxel given once per week with or without bevacizumab in patients with advanced angiosarcoma: a randomized phase II trial. J Clin Oncol 2015;33(25):2797–802.

100. Stacchiotti S, Palassini E, Sanfilippo R, et al. Gemcitabine in advanced angiosarcoma: a retrospective case series analysis from the Italian Rare Cancer Network. Ann Oncol 2012;23(2):501–8.

101. Ray-Coquard I, Italiano A, Bompas E, et al. Sorafenib for patients with advanced angiosarcoma: a phase II trial from the French Sarcoma Group (GSF/GETO). Oncologist 2012;17(2):260–6.

102. Maki RG, D'Adamo DR, Keohan ML, et al. Phase II study of sorafenib in patients with metastatic or recurrent sarcomas. J Clin Oncol 2009;27(19):3133–40.

103. Jones RL, Ravi V, Brohl AS, et al. Results of the TAPPAS trial: an adaptive enrichment phase III trial of TRC105 and pazopanib (P) versus pazopanib alone in patients with advanced angiosarcoma (AS). Ann Oncol 2019;30:v683.

104. Jones RL, Ratain MJ, O'Dwyer PJ, et al. Phase II randomised discontinuation trial of brivanib in patients with advanced solid tumours. Eur J Cancer 2019;120:132–9.

105. Wagner MJ, Othus M, Patel SP, et al. Multicenter phase II trial (SWOG S1609, cohort 51) of ipilimumab and nivolumab in metastatic or unresectable angiosarcoma: a substudy of dual anti-CTLA-4 and anti-PD-1 blockade in rare tumors

(DART). J Immunother Cancer 2021;9(8). https://doi.org/10.1136/jitc-2021-002990109.

106. Florou V, Rosenberg AE, Wieder E, et al. Angiosarcoma patients treated with immune checkpoint inhibitors: a case series of seven patients from a single institution. J Immunother Cancer 2019;7(1):213.

107. Albores-Saavedra J, Schwartz AM, Henson DE, et al. Cutaneous angiosarcoma. Analysis of 434 cases from the Surveillance, Epidemiology, and End Results Program, 1973-2007. Ann Diagn Pathol 2011;15(2):93–7.

108. Shin JY, Roh SG, Lee NH, et al. Predisposing factors for poor prognosis of angiosarcoma of the scalp and face: systematic review and meta-analysis. Head Neck 2017;39(2):380–6.

109. Weidema ME, Flucke UE, van der Graaf WTA, et al. Prognostic factors in a large nationwide cohort of histologically confirmed primary and secondary angiosarcomas. Cancers (Basel) 2019;11(11). https://doi.org/10.3390/cancers11111780150.

110. Bui N, Kamat N, Ravi V, et al. A multicenter phase II study of Q3 week or weekly paclitaxel in combination with bevacizumab for the treatment of metastatic or unresectable angiosarcoma. Rare Tumors 2018;10. 2036361318771771.

111. Fata F, O'Reilly E, Ilson D, et al. Paclitaxel in the treatment of patients with angiosarcoma of the scalp or face. Cancer 1999;86(10):2034–7.

112. Apice G, Pizzolorusso A, Di Maio M, et al. Confirmed activity and tolerability of weekly paclitaxel in the treatment of advanced angiosarcoma. Sarcoma 2016; 2016:6862090.

113. Nagano T, Yamada Y, Ikeda T, et al. Docetaxel: a therapeutic option in the treatment of cutaneous angiosarcoma: report of 9 patients. Cancer 2007;110(3): 648–51.

114. Dickson MA, D'Adamo DR, Keohan ML, et al. Phase II trial of gemcitabine and docetaxel with bevacizumab in soft tissue sarcoma. Sarcoma 2015;2015: 532478.

115. Kim JH, Park HS, Heo SJ, et al. Differences in the efficacies of pazopanib and gemcitabine/docetaxel as second-line treatments for metastatic soft tissue sarcoma. Oncology 2019;96(2):59–69.

116. Mehren MV, Litwin S, Ravi V, et al. Multicenter phase II trial of pazopanib (P) in patients with angiosarcoma (AS). J Clin Oncol 2019;37(15_suppl):11039.

117. Kaposi. Idiopathisches multiples Pigmentsarkom der Haut. Archiv für Dermatologie und Syphilis 1872;4(2):265–73.

118. Chang Y, Cesarman E, Pessin MS, et al. Identification of herpesvirus-like DNA sequences in AIDS-associated Kaposi's sarcoma. Science 1994;266(5192): 1865–9.

119. Flore O, Rafii S, Ely S, et al. Transformation of primary human endothelial cells by Kaposi's sarcoma-associated herpesvirus. Nature 1998;394(6693):588–92.

120. Cesarman E, Damania B, Krown SE, et al. Kaposi sarcoma. Nat Rev Dis Primers 2019;5(1):9.

121. Iscovich J, Boffetta P, Franceschi S, et al. Classic Kaposi sarcoma: epidemiology and risk factors. Cancer 2000;88(3):500–17.

122. Cook-Mozaffari P, Newton R, Beral V, et al. The geographical distribution of Kaposi's sarcoma and of lymphomas in Africa before the AIDS epidemic. Br J Cancer 1998;78(11):1521–8.

123. Parkin DM, Sitas F, Chirenje M, et al. Part I: cancer in indigenous Africans–burden, distribution, and trends. Lancet Oncol 2008;9(7):683–92.

124. Beral V, Peterman TA, Berkelman RL, et al. Kaposi's sarcoma among persons with AIDS: a sexually transmitted infection? Lancet 1990;335(8682):123–8.

125. Armstrong AW, Lam KH, Chase EP. Epidemiology of classic and AIDS-related Kaposi's sarcoma in the USA: incidence, survival, and geographical distribution from 1975 to 2005. Epidemiol Infect 2013;141(1):200–6.

126. Mendez JC, Paya CV. Kaposi's sarcoma and transplantation. Herpes 2000;7(1): 18–23.

127. Grulich AE, Vajdic CM. The epidemiology of cancers in human immunodeficiency virus infection and after organ transplantation. Semin Oncol 2015; 42(2):247–57.

128. Denis D, Seta V, Regnier-Rosencher E, et al. A fifth subtype of Kaposi's sarcoma, classic Kaposi's sarcoma in men who have sex with men: a cohort study in Paris. J Eur Acad Dermatol Venereol 2018;32(8):1377–84.

129. Amerson E, Woodruff CM, Forrestel A, et al. Accuracy of clinical suspicion and pathologic diagnosis of Kaposi sarcoma in East Africa. J Acquir Immune Defic Syndr 2016;71(3):295–301.

130. Delyon J, Rabate C, Euvrard S, et al. Management of Kaposi sarcoma after solid organ transplantation: a European retrospective study. J Am Acad Dermatol 2019;81(2):448–55.

131. Letang E, Lewis JJ, Bower M, et al. Immune reconstitution inflammatory syndrome associated with Kaposi sarcoma: higher incidence and mortality in Africa than in the UK. AIDS 2013;27(10):1603–13.

132. Bower M, Dalla Pria A, Coyle C, et al. Prospective stage-stratified approach to AIDS-related Kaposi's sarcoma. J Clin Oncol 2014;32(5):409–14.

133. Lebbe C, Garbe C, Stratigos AJ, et al. Diagnosis and treatment of Kaposi's sarcoma: European consensus-based interdisciplinary guideline (EDF/EADO/ EORTC). Eur J Cancer 2019;114:117–27.

134. Northfelt DW, Dezube BJ, Thommes JA, et al. Pegylated-liposomal doxorubicin versus doxorubicin, bleomycin, and vincristine in the treatment of AIDS-related Kaposi's sarcoma: results of a randomized phase III clinical trial. J Clin Oncol 1998;16(7):2445–51.

135. Stewart S, Jablonowski H, Goebel FD, et al. Randomized comparative trial of pegylated liposomal doxorubicin versus bleomycin and vincristine in the treatment of AIDS-related Kaposi's sarcoma. International Pegylated Liposomal Doxorubicin Study Group. J Clin Oncol 1998;16(2):683–91.

136. Gill PS, Tulpule A, Espina BM, et al. Paclitaxel is safe and effective in the treatment of advanced AIDS-related Kaposi's sarcoma. J Clin Oncol 1999;17(6): 1876–83.

137. Cianfrocca M, Lee S, Von Roenn J, et al. Randomized trial of paclitaxel versus pegylated liposomal doxorubicin for advanced human immunodeficiency virus-associated Kaposi sarcoma: evidence of symptom palliation from chemotherapy. Cancer 2010;116(16):3969–77.

138. Krown SE, Moser CB, MacPhail P, et al. Treatment of advanced AIDS-associated Kaposi sarcoma in resource-limited settings: a three-arm, open-label, randomised, non-inferiority trial. Lancet 2020;395(10231):1195–207.

139. Uldrick TS, Wyvill KM, Kumar P, et al. Phase II study of bevacizumab in patients with HIV-associated Kaposi's sarcoma receiving antiretroviral therapy. J Clin Oncol 2012;30(13):1476–83.

140. Polizzotto MN, Uldrick TS, Wyvill KM, et al. Pomalidomide for symptomatic Kaposi's sarcoma in people with and without hiv infection: a phase I/II study. J Clin Oncol 2016;34(34):4125–31.

141. Koon HB, Krown SE, Lee JY, et al. Phase II trial of imatinib in AIDS-associated Kaposi's sarcoma: AIDS Malignancy Consortium Protocol 042. J Clin Oncol 2014;32(5):402–8.

142. Evans SR, Krown SE, Testa MA, et al. Phase II evaluation of low-dose oral etoposide for the treatment of relapsed or progressive AIDS-related Kaposi's sarcoma: an AIDS Clinical Trials Group clinical study. J Clin Oncol 2002;20(15): 3236–41.

143. Reid EG, Suazo A, Lensing SY, et al. Pilot Trial AMC-063: safety and efficacy of bortezomib in AIDS-associated Kaposi sarcoma. Clin Cancer Res 2020;26(3): 558–65.

144. Garcia A, Nelson K, Patel V. Emerging therapies for rare cutaneous cancers: a systematic review. Cancer Treat Rev 2021;100:102266.

145. Galanina N, Goodman AM, Cohen PR, et al. Successful treatment of HIV-associated Kaposi sarcoma with immune checkpoint blockade. Cancer Immunol Res 2018;6(10):1129–35.

146. Delyon J, Bizot A, Battistella M, et al. PD-1 blockade with nivolumab in endemic Kaposi sarcoma. Ann Oncol 2018;29(4):1067–9.

147. Uldrick TS, Goncalves PH, Abdul-Hay M, et al. Assessment of the safety of pembrolizumab in patients with HIV and advanced cancer-a phase 1 study. JAMA Oncol 2019;5(9):1332–9.

148. Delyon J, Resche-Rigon M, Renaud M, et al. PD1 blockade with pembrolizumab in classic and endemic Kaposi sarcoma: a multicenter phase II study. Ann Oncol 2020;31:S732.

149. Franceschi S, Arniani S, Balzi D, et al. Survival of classic Kaposi's sarcoma and risk of second cancer. Br J Cancer 1996;74(11):1812–4.

150. Benajiba L, Lambert J, La Selva R, et al. Systemic treatment initiation in classical and endemic Kaposi's sarcoma: risk factors and global multi-state modelling in a monocentric cohort study. Cancers (Basel) 2021;13(11). https://doi.org/10.3390/cancers13112519.

151. Krown SE, Testa MA, Huang J. AIDS-related Kaposi's sarcoma: prospective validation of the AIDS Clinical Trials Group staging classification. AIDS Clinical Trials Group Oncology Committee. J Clin Oncol 1997;15(9):3085–92.

152. Nasti G, Talamini R, Antinori A, et al. AIDS-related Kaposi's sarcoma: evaluation of potential new prognostic factors and assessment of the AIDS Clinical Trial Group Staging System in the Haart Era–the Italian Cooperative Group on AIDS and Tumors and the Italian Cohort of Patients Naive From Antiretrovirals. J Clin Oncol 2003;21(15):2876–82.

153. Lodi S, Guiguet M, Costagliola D, et al. Kaposi sarcoma incidence and survival among HIV-infected homosexual men after HIV seroconversion. J Natl Cancer Inst 2010;102(11):784–92.

154. Einollahi B, Lessan-Pezeshki M, Nourbala MH, et al. Kaposi's sarcoma following living donor kidney transplantation: review of 7,939 recipients. Int Urol Nephrol 2009;41(3):679–85.

155. Taborelli M, Piselli P, Ettorre GM, et al. Survival after the diagnosis of de novo malignancy in liver transplant recipients. Int J Cancer 2019;144(2):232–9.

Management of Skin Sarcomas

Valentina Messina, MD[a,1], Brandon Cope, MD[b,1], Emily Z. Keung, MD, AM[b],
Marco Fiore, MD, FACS, FEBSh[a,*]

KEYWORDS

- Angiosarcoma • Atypical fibroxanthoma • Dermatofibrosarcoma protuberans
- DFSP • Leiomyosarcoma • Pleomorphic dermal sarcoma • Skin sarcoma
- Stewart-Treves

KEY POINTS

- Skin sarcomas are a subset of soft tissue sarcomas that are superficial by definition and usually small in size. Although these are generally favorable prognostic factors, skin sarcomas are often underrecognized and misdiagnosed at presentation.
- Careful attention to clinical history and physical examination at presentation and performing either a core needle or punch biopsy are crucial for diagnosis and appropriate management of skin sarcomas.
- Dermatofibrosarcoma protuberans is among the most frequent skin sarcomas with overall good prognosis, with the exception of the fibrosarcomatous variant. Risk of local recurrence following wide resection is low.
- Cutaneous angiosarcoma is an aggressive tumor, with high rate of local recurrence and distant metastasis. It may also arise in the context of chronic lymphedema (Stewart-Treves syndrome).
- Atypical fibroxanthoma, pleomorphic dermal sarcoma, and cutaneous leiomyosarcoma are other common skin sarcomas. Overall, these have good prognosis, provided initial surgery is performed with negative margins.

INTRODUCTION

Skin sarcomas are a peculiar subset of soft tissue sarcomas (STS). They are superficial by definition, and usually small in size in comparison with other STS arising in deeper extremity/truncal or retroperitoneal/abdominal sites. Both small size and superficial presentation are generally favorable prognostic factors with respect to both local

[a] Sarcoma Service - Department of Surgery, Fondazione IRCCS Istituto Nazionale dei Tumori, Via Venezian, 1, Milan 20133, Italy; [b] Department of Surgical Oncology, The University of Texas MD Anderson Cancer Center, 1515 Holcombe Boulevard, Unit 1484, Houston, TX, 77030, USA
[1] authors contributed equally.
* Corresponding author.
E-mail address: marco.fiore@istitutotumori.mi.it

Surg Oncol Clin N Am 31 (2022) 511–525
https://doi.org/10.1016/j.soc.2022.03.010
1055-3207/22/© 2022 Elsevier Inc. All rights reserved.

control and overall survival (OS). Surgery is therefore the mainstay of treatment, although some histologic types warrant multidisciplinary management. Because of their rarity, however, cutaneous sarcomas are often underrecognized and misdiagnosed. Providers should maintain a high level of suspicion as early recognition and appropriate management of cutaneous sarcomas at initial patient presentation is critically important to achieve optimal oncologic outcomes.

Here, the epidemiology, clinical presentation, management, and surveillance of 4 of the most common cutaneous sarcomas are reviewed: dermatofibrosarcoma protuberans (DFSP), leiomyosarcoma (limited to the dermal presentation), angiosarcoma (limited to sporadic dermal presentation), and atypical fibroxanthoma (AFX)/pleomorphic dermal sarcoma (PDS) (**Table 1**).

DERMATOFIBROSARCOMA PROTUBERANS
Epidemiology and Clinical Presentation

DFSP is a rare, low- to intermediate-grade malignant sarcoma that can be locally aggressive but rarely metastasizes. Although accounting for less than 1% of all STS, DFSP represents one of the most common skin sarcomas.[1] DFSP most often occurs in the third to fifth decades of life but has been described in all age groups. It most commonly affects the trunk and proximal extremities, groin, axilla, and pubic region (~90% of cases), the head and neck (10%–15% of cases), and rarely the distal extremities.

At presentation, DFSP is often unsuspected and misdiagnosed (**Fig. 1**). Early lesions may appear as skin-colored dermal plaques. They are typically slow-growing (over years), small, firm, painless, and fixed in the skin. Subcutaneous thickening or atrophic nonprotuberant skin lesion may also occur. At later stages, protuberant, indurated, reddish-blue or violaceous nodules develop within the lesion. Advanced DFSP can invade underlying fascia and muscle and rarely even periosteum and bone. Importantly in the case of nodular lesions, a biopsy should target the nodule rather than the surrounding plaque. Children more commonly have nonprotruding lesions resembling a morphea plaque or, in congenital cases, an atrophic plaque or vascular malformation.

OS for patients with DFSP is high, with sarcoma-specific death of 2.8% at 10 years. Although local recurrence is ~4% at 10 years following wide local excision (WLE) with negative microscopic margins (R0),[2] local recurrence occurs in up to 20% to 50% of cases following resection with inadequate margins.[3,4] Conversely, DFSP rarely metastasizes (2% at 10 years),[2] unless a fibrosarcomatous component is detected. Fibrosarcomatous variant (FS-DFSP) is found in roughly 5% of cases; and 10% to 15% of cases determine distant metastasis.

Diagnosis and Pathology

The diagnosis of DFSP is confirmed by biopsy (either core needle biopsy [CNB] of nodular lesions or punch biopsy of plaques, which should include subcutaneous tissue). Histologically, DFSP presents as a storiform or fascicular proliferation often with an infiltrative growth pattern, characterized by tentacle-like projections that extend from the dermis into the subcutaneous tissue for considerable distances. Among DFSP histologic variants (myxoid, pigmented, giant cell, giant cell fibroblastoma, granular cell, sclerotic and fibrosarcomatous), only FS-DFSP exhibits an increased risk of local and distant recurrence compared with other variants. FS-DFSP is characterized by significantly increased mitotic activity and is considered an intermediate-grade sarcoma.

Table 1
Clinical features of cutaneous sarcomas

	DFSP	AS	AFX/PDS	LMS
Growth pattern	Exophytic, large plaque with multiple superficial nodules	Multifocal skip lesions	Nodular or polypoid dermal lesions, often ulcerated	Papules, nodules, or plaques. Occasionally with irregular or ulcerative surface
Color	Pink, violaceous, reddish-brown (changing over time)	Bruiselike lesion that mimics a hemangioma, hematomas, dermatosis, rosacea, or mycosis	Erythematous macules	Skin-colored, erythematous, or blue
Size	1–5 cm at diagnosis	1–5 cm	PDS: 2.5 cm AFX: <2 cm	0.3–3 cm
Anatomic site	Proximal Extremities (30%–40%) Trunk (40%–50%) Head and neck (10%–15%)	Scalp, head and neck (60%)	Scalp, face	Extremities (50%–85%)
Evolution	Slow-growth (years), evolution from plaque to nodular	Low rates of local control, high recurrence rates, high rate of metastasis	Rapidly growing	Slow-growth
Pain	No	Yes	No	Uncommonly
Margins	Well-circumscribed when nodular, plaques can have irregular margins	Irregular margin	Well-circumscribed	Irregular/asymmetric or well-circumscribed
Peak of Incidence	Adults between the 3rd and 5th decades of life	Elderly male patients	Elderly, male, Caucasian patients	Adults between the 5th and 8th decades of life

Abbreviations: AS, angiosarcoma; AFX, atypical fibroxanthoma; DFSP, dermatofibrosarcoma protuberans; LMS, leiomyosarcoma; PDS, pleomorphic dermal sarcoma.

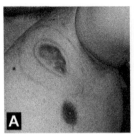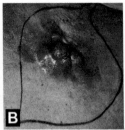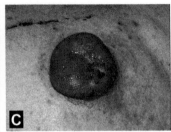

Fig. 1. Clinical presentations of dermatofibrosarcoma: (*A*) plaque lesion; (*B*) plaque lesion with initial nodular evolution; (*C*) fibrosarcomatous variant with nodular growth. (*Courtesy of* Marco Fiore.)

Molecularly, DFSP is characterized by cytogenetic features, including a chromosomal translocation between chromosomes 17 and 22 [t(17;22) (q11; q13.1)] or supernumerary ring chromosomes containing sequences from chromosomes 17 and 22[5] that result in fusion of the platelet-derived growth factor-beta (PDGFB) and collagen type 1A1 genes in nearly 90% of cases.[2] The COL1A1-PDGFB fusion gene results in growth factor activity stimulating the proliferation of tumor cells. Fluorescence *in situ* hybridization for COL1A1−PDGFB may be helpful in diagnosis.

Imaging

Preoperative imaging should include MRI to ascertain the extent of tumor involvement. Because lymphatic and hematogenous dissemination is rare, an extensive staging workup is not routinely indicated. Nonetheless, a chest computed tomography (CT) should be performed to assess for pulmonary metastasis in patients with prolonged history of and/or locally advanced or recurrent DFSP and in all cases of FS-DFSP. A preoperative chest radiograph (CXR) is enough in the other cases.

Treatment

Surgery

Surgery is the treatment of choice for localized DFSP. Complete resection with negative margins at the time of initial therapy is the standard of treatment. Because irregular and deep extensions are often present microscopically beyond what is clinically apparent, WLE with 2 to 4 cm margins is recommended whenever feasible.[6] Excision of the deep fascia is indicated, as it acts as a barrier between anatomic compartments. Complex wound closure involving tissue undermining or reconstruction by means of skin graft, locoregional flap, or after skin expander insertion is often necessary; in such cases, surgical reconstruction can be delayed until all margins are confirmed negative.

In cases of positive microscopic margins (R1) following initial resection, most guidelines recommend reresection. Given the low risk of distant relapse, however, active surveillance after R1 resection with subsequent resection at the time of local recurrence may be reasonable.[7,8] In cases of FS-DFSP, an R0 resection should be ensured with reresection performed after R1 margins when technically feasible.[9,10]

Limited data in the dermatologic literature suggest that Mohs micrographic surgery (MMS) may be noninferior to surgical resection, although this technique is rarely adopted in sarcoma centers.

Radiation therapy

In North America, the use of radiation therapy (RT) has been reported in limited series following positive margin resection or after planned marginal excision in critical anatomic sites in the adjuvant setting or for definitive or palliative treatment in cases with no reasonable surgical approach.[11] In contrast, adjuvant RT is usually not recommended in European guidelines in the management of DFSP.[8]

Imatinib

Systemic therapy using imatinib is approved in Europe for inoperable DFSP, locally advanced recurrent disease, and metastatic DFSP. Imatinib has inhibitor activity against the protein product of the COL1A1-PDGFB gene fusion, with an observed response rate of ~50%.[9] In one series, patients with advanced DFSP treated with imatinib achieved a 5-year progression-free survival (PFS) of 58% and 5-year OS of 64%. Patients with FS-DFSP and metastatic disease had worse PFS and OS: 5-year PFS rate was 93% for classic DFSP and 33% for FS-DFSP. The best overall responses were 68% partial responses (including 8 FS-DFSP, but the responses were shorter than for classic DFSP), 19% stable disease, and 13% progressive disease.

Imatinib may also have a role in the neoadjuvant setting,[12] particularly in locally advanced cases when resection may be facilitated by tumor downstaging.

Follow-up

Despite the good prognosis of patients with DFSP after R0 (and even R1) resection, local recurrence may occur years after surgery. Long-term surveillance is recommended with follow-up every 6 months for the first 5 years and then annually.[9] Examination of the primary site and surrounding skin should be performed at each visit. If local recurrence is suspected, a biopsy should be performed. Ultrasound imaging can be performed on the primary site, and for patients with high-risk features, the lungs can be imaged (CXR or CT scan). In a series of 357 patients, 61.7% of recurrences were discovered on patient self-examination; only 3.7% were detected at clinical surveillance. All metastatic recurrences were identified by imaging after patients presented with symptomatic disease.[9,13] Therefore, consideration should be given to individualize follow-up schedules based on risk factors.

ANGIOSARCOMA
Primary Cutaneous Angiosarcoma

Epidemiology and clinical presentation

Angiosarcoma is a rare tumor that arises from vascular or lymphatic endothelial cells, primarily affects elderly male patients, and can arise at any site.[14] Cutaneous lesions are most common, followed by angiosarcoma of the breast, deep soft tissues, visceral organs, and bone. Although most angiosarcomas are sporadic, suggested risk factors include chronic lymphedema, immunosuppression, radiotherapy, foreign material, and various clinical syndromes. Angiosarcoma is aggressive with low rates of local control, high recurrence rates, and a high rate of metastasis. Five-year OS is 10% to 40% in most studies.

Here, sporadic primary cutaneous angiosarcoma of the head, neck, scalp, and breast and secondary angiosarcoma associated with chronic lymphedema (Stewart-Treves syndrome) are discussed. Radiation-induced and visceral angiosarcoma are discussed in a separate article in this work.

Diagnosis and pathology

Diagnosis of angiosarcoma requires careful patient assessment including a thorough history and physical examination (H&P) (**Fig. 2A**). Patients are often initially misdiagnosed, given the relatively benign-appearing bruiselike lesion that mimics a

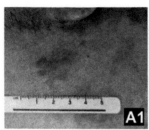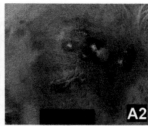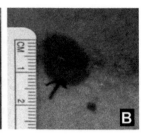

Fig. 2. Clinical presentations of primary cutaneous angiosarcoma: (*A1, A2*) cutaneous and (*B*) breast angiosarcoma. (*From* [*A1, A2*] Bernstein JM, Irish JC, Brown DH, et al. Survival outcomes for cutaneous angiosarcoma of the scalp versus face. Head Neck. 2017;39(6):1205 to 1211. [*B*] Moon IJ, Kim YJ, Won CH, et al. Clinicopathological and survival analyses of primary cutaneous angiosarcoma in an Asian population: prognostic value of the clinical features of skin lesions. Int J Dermatol. 2020;59(5):582 to 589.)

hemangioma.[15] For cases involving the scalp, there may be a delay in presentation and diagnosis due to overlying hair.

Diagnosis is confirmed by tissue biopsy, typically in the form of punch biopsy. Specific attention should be paid to tumor grade and size, features associated with prognosis, as well as mitotic index, necrosis, and depth.[15,16] Histopathologic findings can range from benign hemangioma-like structures to poorly differentiated dermal tumors, making it difficult to reach a definitive diagnosis in some cases. Skip lesions are a hallmark of angiosarcoma in which lesions are separated by areas free of tumor cells. Angiosarcoma may also be present beyond what is visibly apparent. These features contribute to a high rate of local recurrence, even among patients who undergo an R0 resection. Whenever feasible, mapping biopsies may be helpful to assess tumor extent before curative resection or preoperative treatments.

Imaging
Imaging should be performed preoperatively, using CT or MRI of the primary site along with a chest CT to assess for metastasis. Abdominal/pelvic CT should also be performed with imaging of the central nervous system as clinically indicated. Identification of metastatic disease, which is present in 10% to 25% of patients at diagnosis, should prompt early multidisciplinary discourse.

Treatment
Recommended approaches to definitive management vary in the literature. Given the high recurrence rates in nonmetastatic angiosarcoma, there remains debate on extent of surgery and utilization of single-modal versus multimodal therapy. All patients should be offered multidisciplinary evaluation. Most studies assert that surgery combined with RT is the optimal approach to achieve local control.[17] For patients with high-risk, locally advanced or metastatic disease, chemotherapy in combination with RT has also been associated with favorable short-term OS.

Primary Breast Angiosarcoma

Epidemiology and clinical presentation
Established recommendations for primary breast angiosarcoma are limited due to their rarity although many of the principles of diagnosis, staging, and treatment are similar as earlier. In a review from the Mayo Clinic of only 25 primary breast sarcomas compiled over 90 years, 6 were primary breast angiosarcoma[18] and were associated with far worse OS compared with other histologic subtypes. Primary breast

angiosarcoma affects women in the fifth or sixth decade of life.[16] Typically a firm, well-defined, unilateral, and rapidly growing breast mass is found, which can cause blue or purple discoloration of the overlying skin, reflecting hemorrhage or vascularity of the lesion (**Fig. 2**B). The disease process may also involve the cutaneous layer resulting in skin thickening.

Imaging
Mammography may demonstrate a nonspiculated dense mass without microcalcifications but performs poorly in most cases and may miss cutaneous lesions. Fine-needle aspiration (FNA) is poorly diagnostic; CNB is preferred. Breast MRI is the gold standard of imaging and demonstrates that primary breast angiosarcoma is often more extensive than appreciable on physical examination. Because of their hypervascularity, angiosarcoma typically has low signal intensity on T1-weighted images and high signal intensity on T2.

Treatment
Surgery. Simple mastectomy with adjuvant RT is typically recommended for localized primary breast angiosarcoma in most, if not all, cases over breast-conserving surgery. More extensive resections should be performed when adjacent tissues (ie, chest wall) are involved.[19] Because of their infiltrative spiculae and high probability of local recurrence, margins up to 3 cm have been proposed. Clear excision margin and tumor size are the 2 most important factors associated with survival.[20,21]

The axilla should be routinely evaluated with axial imaging preoperatively and axillary/nodal surgery considered only in highly selective circumstances, such as extension of primary tumor into the axilla, or in the rare case of nodal only metastasis. Otherwise, there are no indications for routine sentinel lymph node biopsy (SLNB) or lymphadenectomy.[22] When nodal involvement is present, one should consider the diagnosis of a metaplastic carcinoma even in the presence of a pure spindle-cell neoplasm. Unfortunately, when nodal involvement is present, distant metastasis is often also present, and lymphadenectomy confers no survival benefit.

Radiation therapy. Adjuvant RT has been associated with lower rates of local recurrence for primary breast angiosarcoma in some, but not all, studies.[19,20] In one study, local recurrence occurred in 34% of patients after mastectomy alone compared with 13% after mastectomy and RT, although this difference was not statistically significant. In another series, adjuvant RT was associated with better cause-specific survival (91% vs 50%).[20]

Stewart-Treves Syndrome

Epidemiology and clinical presentation
Secondary angiosarcoma presenting in the setting of chronic lymphedema, known as Stewart-Treves syndrome, is a rare entity first described in 1948: 6 cases of angiosarcoma in patients who developed lymphedema following radical mastectomy for breast cancer were reported.[23] In a series of 6919 patients with breast cancer, cumulative incidence of secondary angiosarcoma 10, 20, and 30 years after treatment were 0.2%, 0.4%, and 0.8%, respectively. Of 11 posttreatment sarcomas, 2 were attributed to Stewart-Treves syndrome and 9 were secondary to radiation.[24] Although the underlying cause for the development of angiosarcoma remains unknown, vascular endothelial growth factor–initiated cytokines released due to lymphatic blockage has been hypothesized.[25]

Although typically affecting the upper extremity in the setting of postmastectomy lymphedema, secondary angiosarcoma can also arise in other chronic (primary or secondary) lymphedema conditions of both upper and lower extremities (congenital/idiopathic lymphedema; posttraumatic or secondary to filariasis), as well as the abdominal wall (lymphedema postlymphadenectomy for penile carcinoma).[26]

The clinical progression of postmastectomy edema results in chronic swelling from the arm to the hand, resulting in diminished function and worsened lymphatic and venous drainage. Brawny edema develops with atrophy of the skin, and cellulitis commonly develops with skin breakdown, chronic ulceration, and drainage. Over the years, a purplish-red, subdermal, macular, or polypoid lesion finally appears. Angiosarcoma develops as a solitary tumor, followed by similar satellite areas sometimes confluent in larger lesions (**Fig. 3**A). Median latency since lymphedema onset is 11 years (range 4–44 years).[25]

Prognosis is generally poor given the high metastatic risk. Despite aggressive surgical amputation and multimodal treatment, 5-year OS is 10% to 40%.[25–27] Mean survival after diagnosis is approximately 20 months with untreated survival of about 5 to 8 months.[28] A high index of suspicion is paramount, as delay in diagnosis negatively

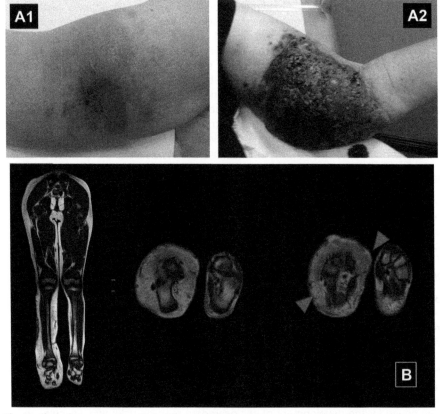

Fig. 3. Clinical presentation (*A1, A2*) and MRI (*B*) of Stewart-Treves syndrome involving the upper and lower extremity. ([*A1*] *From* Vojtíšek R, Sukovská E, Kylarová M, et al. Stewart-Treves syndrome: Case report and literature review. Rep Pract Oncol Radiother. 2020;25(6):934 to 938. [*A2*] *From* Gottlieb R, Serang R, Chi D, Menco H. Stewart-Treves syndrome. Radiol Case Rep. 2012;7(4):693. [*B*] *Courtesy of* Marco Fiore.)

affects survival. Woodward and colleagues[27] found that long-term survivors had an average time of 5.6 weeks between onset of lesions and amputation compared with an average of 24 weeks for nonsurvivors. Close follow-up of all patients with chronic lymphedema of the arm following mastectomy is recommended, and early recognition of suspicious lesions may be the key to longer survival.

Diagnosis and pathology

An H&P and tissue biopsy (CNB) are required for diagnosis. The patient's surgical history and history of chronic lymphedema should be elicited. The timing and discovery of the lesion may be incorrectly attributed to a trivial trauma that never healed and continually worsened.

Imaging

Staging workup consists of CT of the chest/abdomen/pelvis with MRI of the involved extremity (**Fig. 3**B). Early referral to an experienced multidisciplinary team at a tertiary center is paramount.

Treatment

Surgery and RT are typically recommended for resectable disease. RT may improve local disease control but does not affect OS.[29] Grobmyer and colleagues reported that initial amputation, disarticulation, or WLE with 3 cm margins, all provided better survival than did RT or regional chemotherapy. There was a high rate of conversion to amputation following inadequate WLE.[28]

Isolated limb perfusion (ILP) has also been evaluated for AS of the extremities, offering a potential for limb salvage. In a prospective study consisting of locally advanced angiosarcoma in the extremities, Huis in 't Veld and colleagues[30] determined that 59% of patients had a complete response after ILP with high-dose melphalan and tumor necrosis factor alpha. In total, 13 of the 39 patients enrolled and required further surgical intervention following ILP with a trend toward improved OS. Subsequent case studies have been conducted with varied results.[31]

Metastatic disease should preclude the use of surgical therapy except for highly selective palliative situations.[28]

Systemic therapy for angiosarcoma. The role of systemic therapy for localized angiosarcoma in general remains unclear and should be discussed after thorough individual risk assessment.[21,25,29,32] However, many chemotherapeutic regimens demonstrate activity in angiosarcoma. See Subramaniam and colleagues' article, "Management of Vascular Sarcoma," in this issue for further information regarding systemic therapy for angiosarcoma.

Follow-up for angiosarcoma

In general, patients with primary cutaneous and breast angiosarcoma and Stewart-Treves syndrome require life-long surveillance on completion of treatment. For both primary cutaneous and breast angiosarcoma, recurrence is most likely in the first 6 months following surgery.[25–27] Follow-up with appropriate imaging should occur at least every 3 months for the first 2 years and every 6 months thereafter until year 5 and annually thereafter.

ATYPICAL FIBROXANTHOMA/PLEOMORPHIC DERMAL SARCOMA
Epidemiology and Clinical Presentation

AFX and PDS represent 2 malignancies with overlapping clinical and histologic features.[33,34] Both are tumors of atypical spindle cells that present as rapidly growing, often ulcerated, nodular or polypoid dermal lesions on chronically sun-damaged skin (**Fig. 4**A, B), arising predominantly on the head and face of elderly Caucasian patients with higher male incidence.[33]

AFX and PDS differ in their propensity to invade and metastasize. AFX are lesions confined to the dermis, rarely recur locally following resection, and have good prognosis. PDS are invasive with infiltration of subcutis and deep soft tissues and have modest local recurrence and metastatic rates (both 5%–25%),[35] although prognosis is still overall favorable.[33,36]

Diagnosis and Pathology

The diagnosis of AFX/PDS requires an H&P and punch biopsy but are diagnoses of exclusion.[35,36] AFX/PDS may initially seem as small erythematous macules on the skin of the head and neck 2 to 12 months before a phase of rapid growth in the weeks to months, leading up to clinical presentation with ulceration and crusting in most cases.[37] PDS lesions may be slightly more diffuse and occasionally polypoid nodular-like growth with median tumor size of 2.5 cm compared with AFX lesions that are generally less than 2 cm.[33,34]

AFX and PDS share similar immunohistochemistry profiles, staining positively for vimentin, CD10, and p53, and both are closely linked to ultraviolet-induced TERT

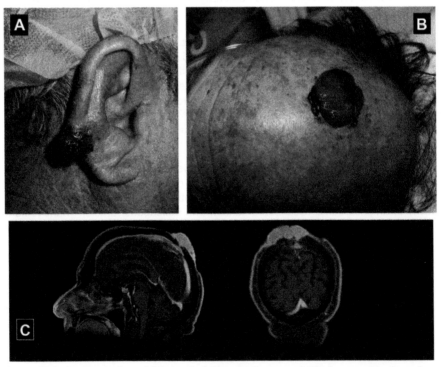

Fig. 4. Clinical presentation of (*A*) atypical fibroxanthoma and (*B*) pleomorphic dermal sarcoma (PDS). (*C*) MRI showing cranial invasion by PDS. ([*A*] *From* Mentzel T, Requena L, Brenn T. Atypical Fibroxanthoma Revisited. Surg Pathol Clin. 2017;10(2):319 to 335. [*B*] *From* Tardío JC, Pinedo F, Aramburu JA, et al. Pleomorphic dermal sarcoma: a more aggressive neoplasm than previously estimated. Journal of Cutaneous Pathology. 2016;43(2):101 to 112. [*C*] *Courtesy of* Marco Fiore.)

promoter and TP53 gene mutations.[38] Complex cytogenetic changes have been described in cases of PDS but not in AFX.[1,34]

Imaging

Although staging imaging is not routinely recommended for AFX, patients with PDS should be staged preoperatively. CT or MRI of the primary site along with either CT of the chest/abdomen/pelvis or whole-body PET-CT to assess for metastasis should be performed. In recurrent disease of the scalp, preoperative imaging should be explicitly aimed to exclude bone invasion.

Treatment

Surgery

The primary treatment of AFX/PDS is surgical resection. For AFX, WLE with 1 cm margins down to subcutaneous tissue is generally associated with low recurrence rates. Optimal management of PDS is less clear given the paucity of available data; however, extirpation with complete tumor margin control is paramount due to its greater propensity to recur and metastasize. Surgical resection of AFX/PDS occurring on the scalp should be aggressive, particularly in obtaining negative deep margins, as there may be limited ability to achieve local control if bone invasion is present at the time of local recurrence (**Fig. 4**C). The role of SLNB in management and clinical outcomes of AFX/PDS are unclear given the lack of available data.[36]

MMS has also been reported in the treatment of AFX,[37,39] with reports of similar local control rates compared with WLE.

Radiation therapy

RT has been described in treating AFX/PDS in the setting of unresectable, locally recurrent, or regionally metastatic disease.[36]

Systemic therapy

There are currently no standard-of-care systemic therapies for AFX/PDS, although several studies have reported potential efficacy of anti-PD1 therapy in PDS.[40]

Follow-up

Follow-up after surgical resection should occur every 3 to 6 months for 2 years then every 6 months up to 5 years. Imaging, including the previous surgical site and as clinically indicated comprehensibly, should be performed at regular intervals.

CUTANEOUS LEIOMYOSARCOMA
Epidemiology and Clinical Presentation

Cutaneous leiomyosarcoma is a rare smooth muscle neoplasm, most commonly involving the extremities (50%–85%) and affecting men in the fifth to eighth decade of life, although pediatrics cases have been described. Cutaneous leiomyosarcomas include 2 subtypes: dermal and subcutaneous leiomyosarcoma. Dermal leiomyosarcoma originates from arrector pili muscle, whereas subcutaneous leiomyosarcoma originates from smooth muscular fascicles in subcutaneous tissue and from the wall of subcutaneous vessels. Cutaneous leiomyosarcomas can vary in appearance, presenting as irregular, asymmetrical, painful nodules, or plaques that may bleed or ulcerate or as solitary, erythematous, or brownish well-circumscribed dermal nodules (**Fig. 5**). Their size ranges from 0.3 to 3 cm in diameter; subcutaneous leiomyosarcoma lesions are often larger at presentation.

Estimated rates of OS for cutaneous leiomyosarcoma at 5 and 10 years are 64% and 46%, respectively.[41] Local recurrences may occur in 6% of dermal tumors and

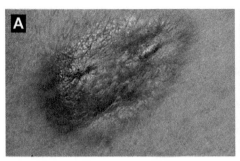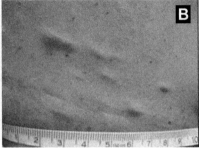

Fig. 5. Clinical presentation of cutaneous leiomyosarcoma. (*From* [A] Yamada S, Guo X, Yoshizawa M, et al. Primary desmoplastic cutaneous leiomyosarcoma associated with high MIB-1 labeling index: a teaching case giving rise to diagnostic difficulties on a small biopsy specimen. Pathol Res Pract. 2011;207(11):728 to 732. [B] Fondriest SA, Gowdy JM, Goyal M, Sheridan KC, Wasdahl DA. Concurrent renal-cell carcinoma and cutaneous leiomyomas: A case of HLRCC. Radiol Case Rep. 2015;10(1):962.)

18% of subcutaneous leiomyosarcoma.[42] Dermal leiomyosarcoma rarely metastasizes (12% of cases) and has a very low mortality, whereas the subcutaneous leiomyosarcoma is associated with higher rates of metastasis (27%–63% of cases) and higher mortality (25%–41%).[43]

Imaging

CT of the chest/abdomen/pelvis or PET/CT (scalp to toes) should be performed in patients with subcutaneous leiomyosarcoma to exclude an unknown primary leiomyosarcoma at another site (such as a vascular leiomyosarcoma) with a cutaneous metastasis. MRI is used to evaluate the extent of leiomyosarcoma and for surgical planning.

Diagnosis and Pathology

Diagnosis of cutaneous leiomyosarcoma is made by CNB or punch biopsy, although excisional biopsy for small lesions less than 3 cm is acceptable. Dermal and subcutaneous leiomyosarcoma share histopathologic features (spindled cells with smooth muscle phenotype, variable rate of nuclear pleomorphism, presence of mitoses).[5] However, the former has significantly better prognosis due to its lower metastatic potential.[41,44,45]

Treatment

An R0 resection is the mainstay treatment of cutaneous leiomyosarcoma with resection margins of greater than or equal to 1 cm considered adequate and is associated with low rates of local recurrence.[43,44] Plastic reconstruction may be required. Adjuvant therapies usually are not required for lesions smaller than 5 cm.[46]

Follow-up

Dermal leiomyosarcoma is a low-risk tumor with little metastatic risk. In contrast, subcutaneous leiomyosarcoma should be surveilled as a high-risk STS due to its propensity for local recurrence and distant metastasis. For both, follow-up is recommended for at least 5 years. Some recommend complete skin examination every 3 months for 3 years after resection, then every 6 months for the next 2 years, and then yearly for up to 10 years. For patients with subcutaneous leiomyosarcoma, a chest CT is advised every 6 to 12 months together with MRI of the primary tumor site.[46]

SUMMARY

Although skin sarcomas generally have good overall prognosis, patients with these rare tumors benefit from evaluation and management by multidisciplinary expert teams. Knowledge of histology-specific behavior will guide appropriate multimodal management. Early recognition and diagnosis are crucial to avoid treatment delay that can impair both local disease control and eventual cosmetic results, as well as sarcoma-specific survival in high-risk presentations.

DISCLOSURE

All authors–none.

REFERENCES

1. Mentzel T. Cutaneous mesenchymal tumours: an update. Pathology 2014;46(2): 149–59.
2. Fiore M, Miceli R, Mussi C, et al. Dermatofibrosarcoma protuberans treated at a single institution: a surgical disease with a high cure rate. J Clin Oncol 2005; 23(30):7669–75.
3. Goldblum JR, Reith JD, Weiss SW. Sarcomas arising in dermatofibrosarcoma protuberans: a reappraisal of biologic behavior in eighteen cases treated by wide local excision with extended clinical follow up. Am J Surg Pathol 2000; 24(8):1125–30.
4. Mendenhall WM, Zlotecki RA, Scarborough MT. Dermatofibrosarcoma. Protuberans Cancer 2004;101(11):2503–8.
5. WHO Classification of Tumours Editorial Board. Soft tissue and bone tumours. Lyon (France): International Agency for Research on Cancer; 2020. (WHO classification of tumours series, 5th ed.; vol. 3; 100-103). https://publications.iarc.fr/ 588. Soft Tissue and Bone Tumours 2020.
6. Website. Website. 13. National Comprehensive Cancer Network. Dermatofibrosarcoma Protuberans (Version 1.2020). Avaiable at: http://www.nccn.org/ professionals/physician_gls/pdf/dermatofibrosarcomaprotuberans.pdf. Accessed Sept 10, 2021.
7. Decanter G, Stoeckle E, Honore C, et al. Watch and wait approach for re-excision after unplanned yet macroscopically complete excision of extremity and superficial truncal soft tissue sarcoma is safe and does not affect metastatic risk or amputation rate. Ann Surg Oncol 2019;26(11):3526–34.
8. Gronchi A, Miah AB, Dei Tos AP, et al. Soft tissue and visceral sarcomas: ESMO-EURACAN-GENTURIS Clinical Practice Guidelines for diagnosis, treatment and follow-up. Ann Oncol 2021;32(11):1348–65.
9. Saiag P, Grob J-J, Lebbe C, et al. Diagnosis and treatment of dermatofibrosarcoma protuberans. European consensus-based interdisciplinary guideline. Eur J Cancer 2015;51(17):2604–8.
10. van Houdt WJ. Margins in DFSP Reconsidered: Primum Non Nocere. Ann Surg Oncol 2020;27(3):634–6.
11. Ballo MT, Zagars GK, Pisters P, et al. The role of radiation therapy in the management of dermatofibrosarcoma protuberans. Int J Radiat Oncol Biol Phys 1998; 40(4):823–7.
12. Ugurel S, Mentzel T, Utikal J, et al. Neoadjuvant imatinib in advanced primary or locally recurrent dermatofibrosarcoma protuberans: a multicenter phase II De-COG trial with long-term follow-up. Clin Cancer Res 2014;20(2):499–510.

13. Huis In 't Veld EA, van Coevorden F, et al. Outcome after surgical treatment of dermatofibrosarcoma protuberans: Is clinical follow-up always indicated? Cancer 2019;125(5):735–41.
14. Albores-Saavedra J, Schwartz AM, Henson DE, et al. Cutaneous angiosarcoma. Analysis of 434 cases from the Surveillance, Epidemiology, and End Results Program, 1973-2007. Ann Diagn Pathol 2011;15(2):93–7.
15. Pawlik TM, Paulino AF, McGinn CJ, et al. Cutaneous angiosarcoma of the scalp: a multidisciplinary approach. Cancer 2003;98(8):1716–26.
16. Lim SZ, Ong KW, Tan BKT, et al. Sarcoma of the breast: an update on a rare entity. J Clin Pathol 2016;69(5):373–81.
17. Guadagnolo BA, Zagars GK, Araujo D, et al. Outcomes after definitive treatment for cutaneous angiosarcoma of the face and scalp. Head Neck 2011;33(5):661–7.
18. Adem C, Reynolds C, Ingle JN, et al. Primary breast sarcoma: clinicopathologic series from the Mayo Clinic and review of the literature. Br J Cancer 2004;91(2):237–41.
19. Abraham JA, Hornicek FJ, Kaufman AM, et al. Treatment and outcome of 82 patients with angiosarcoma. Ann Surg Oncol 2007;14(6):1953–67.
20. McGowan TS, Cummings BJ, O'Sullivan B, et al. An analysis of 78 breast sarcoma patients without distant metastases at presentation. Int J Radiat Oncol Biol Phys 2000;46(2):383–90.
21. Fields RC, Aft RL, Gillanders WE, et al. Treatment and outcomes of patients with primary breast sarcoma. Am J Surg 2008;196(4):559–61.
22. Gutman H, Pollock RE, Ross MI, et al. Sarcoma of the breast: implications for extent of therapy. The M. D. Anderson experience. Surgery 1994;116(3):505–9.
23. Stewart FW, Treves N. Lymphangiosarcoma in postmastectomy lymphedema; a report of six cases in elephantiasis chirurgica. Cancer 1948;1(1):64–81.
24. Taghian A, de Vathaire F, Terrier P, et al. Long-term risk of sarcoma following radiation treatment for breast cancer. Int J Radiat Oncol Biol Phys 1991;21(2):361–7.
25. Brady MS, Garfein CF, Petrek JA, et al. Post-treatment sarcoma in breast cancer patients. Ann Surg Oncol 1994;1(1):66–72.
26. Berebichez-Fridman R, Deutsch YE, Joyal TM, et al. Stewart-treves syndrome: a case report and review of the literature. Case Rep Oncol 2016;9(1):205–11.
27. Woodward AH, Ivins JC, Soule EH. Lymphangiosarcoma arising in chronic lymphedematous extremities. Cancer 1972;30(2):562–72.
28. Grobmyer SR, Daly JM, Glotzbach RE, et al. Role of surgery in the management of postmastectomy extremity angiosarcoma (Stewart-Treves syndrome). J Surg Oncol 2000;73(3):182–8.
29. Kaufmann T, Chu F, Kaufman R. Post-mastectomy lymphangiosarcoma (Stewart-Treves syndrome): report of two long-term survivals. Br J Radiol 1991;64(765):857–60.
30. Huis In 't Veld EA, Grünhagen DJ, et al. Isolated limb perfusion for locally advanced angiosarcoma in extremities: A multi-centre study. Eur J Cancer 2017;85:114–21.
31. Lans TE, de Wilt JHW, van Geel AN, et al. Isolated limb perfusion with tumor necrosis factor and melphalan for nonresectable sSewart-Treves lymphangiosarcoma. Ann Surg Oncol 2002;9(10):1004–9.
32. Bousquet G, Confavreux C, Magné N, et al. Outcome and prognostic factors in breast sarcoma: a multicenter study from the rare cancer network. Radiother Oncol 2007;85(3):355–61.

33. Miller K, Goodlad JR, Brenn T. Pleomorphic dermal sarcoma: adverse histologic features predict aggressive behavior and allow distinction from atypical fibroxanthoma. Am J Surg Pathol 2012;36(9):1317–26.
34. Beer TW, Drury P, Heenan PJ. Atypical fibroxanthoma: a histological and immunohistochemical review of 171 cases. Am J Dermatopathol 2010;32(6):533–40.
35. Cesinaro AM, Gallo G, Tramontozzi S, et al. Atypical fibroxanthoma and pleomorphic dermal sarcoma: a reappraisal. J Cutan Pathol 2021;48(2):207–10.
36. Soleymani T, Tyler Hollmig S. Conception and management of a poorly understood spectrum of dermatologic neoplasms: atypical fibroxanthoma, pleomorphic dermal sarcoma, and undifferentiated pleomorphic sarcoma. Curr Treat Options Oncol 2017;18(8):50.
37. Ang GC, Roenigk RK, Otley CC, et al. More than 2 decades of treating atypical fibroxanthoma at mayo clinic: what have we learned from 91 patients? Dermatol Surg 2009;35(5):765–72.
38. Griewank KG, Schilling B, Murali R, et al. TERT promoter mutations are frequent in atypical fibroxanthomas and pleomorphic dermal sarcomas. Mod Pathol 2014; 27(4):502–8.
39. Phelan PS, Rosman IS, Council ML. Atypical Fibroxanthoma: the washington university experience. Dermatol Surg 2019;45(12):1450–8.
40. Klein S, Quaas A, Noh K-W, et al. Integrative analysis of pleomorphic dermal sarcomas reveals fibroblastic differentiation and susceptibility to immunotherapy. Clin Cancer Res 2020;26(21):5638–45.
41. Svarvar C, Böhling T, Berlin O, et al. Clinical course of nonvisceral soft tissue leiomyosarcoma in 225 patients from the Scandinavian Sarcoma Group. Cancer 2007;109(2):282–91.
42. Massi D, Franchi A, Alos L, et al. Primary cutaneous leiomyosarcoma: clinicopathological analysis of 36 cases. Histopathology 2010;56(2):251–62.
43. Wong GN, Webb A, Gyorki D, et al. Cutaneous leiomyosarcoma: dermal and subcutaneous. Australas J Dermatol 2020;61(3):243–9.
44. Wellings EP, Tibbo ME, Rose PS, et al. Treatment outcome of superficial leiomyosarcoma. J Surg Oncol 2021;123(1):127–32.
45. Kraft S, Fletcher CDM. Atypical intradermal smooth muscle neoplasms: clinicopathologic analysis of 84 cases and a reappraisal of cutaneous "leiomyosarcoma. Am J Surg Pathol 2011;35(4):599–607.
46. Zacher M, Heppt MV, Brinker TJ, et al. Primary leiomyosarcoma of the skin: a comprehensive review on diagnosis and treatment. Med Oncol 2018;35(10):135.

Leiomyosarcoma
Current Clinical Management and Future Horizons

Nicolas Devaud, MD[a], Olga Vornicova, MD[b],
Albiruni R. Abdul Razak, MB, BCh[b], Korosh Khalili, MD[c],
Elizabeth G. Demicco, MD, PhD[d], Cristina Mitric, MD[b,e],
Marcus Q. Bernardini, MD, MSc[b,e], Rebecca A. Gladdy, MD, PhD[b,f],*

KEYWORDS

- Leiomyosarcoma • Soft tissue sarcoma • Uterine sarcoma • Retroperitoneum
- Vascular origin • Systemic treatment • Metastasis

KEY POINTS

- Leiomyosarcomas (LMSs) are soft tissue tumors with metastatic potential that arise from smooth muscle fibers, and are derived from organs and venous structures in the pelvis and retroperitoneum.
- Uterine leiomyosarcoma is the most frequent site followed by retroperitoneal LMS.
- Surgery is the main curative treatment, which may involve a multivisceral resection and/or major vascular reconstruction.
- The high rates of metastatic failure that occur after surgical resection has prompted investigation of neoadjuvant systemic treatment strategies, with a current international phase III RCT under recruitment.
- The benefit of adjuvant treatment after surgery is limited.

[a] Instituto Oncologico Fundacion Arturo Lopez Perez (FALP), Santiago, Chile; [b] Princess Margaret Cancer Centre, University Health Network, Toronto, Ontario, Canada; [c] Joint Department of Medical Imaging, University of Toronto, Toronto, Ontario, Canada; [d] Department of Laboratory Medicine and Pathobiology, Sinai Health System, University of Toronto, Toronto, Ontario, Canada; [e] Department of Obstetrics and Gynaecology, University of Toronto, Toronto, Ontario, Canada; [f] Division of General Surgery, Sinai Health System, University of Toronto, Toronto, Ontario, Canada
* Corresponding author. 600 University Avenue, Suite 1225, Toronto, Ontario M5G 1X5, Canada.
E-mail address: Rebecca.gladdy@sinaihealth.ca
Twitter: @GladdyLab (R.A.G.)

Surg Oncol Clin N Am 31 (2022) 527–546
https://doi.org/10.1016/j.soc.2022.03.011
1055-3207/22/© 2022 Elsevier Inc. All rights reserved.

surgonc.theclinics.com

INTRODUCTION

Leiomyosarcomas (LMSs) are soft tissue tumors that develop primarily from smooth muscle in visceral organs, such as the uterus or the gastrointestinal tract, and nonvisceral structures, such as large to mid-sized veins and/or dermal pilar smooth muscle in the extremities or trunk. Their behavior has a range of outcomes, primarily based on grade, with a predilection for the development of metastasis.[1] LMSs constitute between 15% and 20% of all newly diagnosed soft tissue tumors in adults.[2]

In this review, the clinical and pathologic characteristics of LMS are described, followed by clinical considerations for the most common sites of disease: retroperitoneum and uterus. Because the development of metastasis is a common challenge, a state-of-the-art review on systemic agents is presented. Finally, future directions for advancing patient care through translational research is discussed.

CLINICAL CHARACTERISTICS OF LEIOMYOSARCOMA

The incidence of LMS increases with age, with a peak at 70 years of age. Uterine LMS (uLMS), however, occurs at a younger age with an increasing incidence at 30 years of age and a peak at 50 years of age, within the perimenopausal age group.[3] Overall, the incidence of LMS by sex varies depending on tumor location. Retroperitoneal leiomyosarcomas (RP-LMSs), particularly of the inferior vena cava (IVC), occur with a higher incidence in women,[4,5] whereas cutaneous and other LMS sites, have a slight male predominance.[6]

Ninety percent of all LMSs arise from intra-abdominal organs, such as the uterus and venous structures of the retroperitoneum (RP-LMS). LMSs account for the third most common soft tissue sarcoma (STS) after gastrointestinal stromal tumor (GIST) and liposarcoma and is the predominant sarcoma arising from large blood vessels. Within intra-abdominal LMS, uLMSs have a higher incidence compared with other RP-LMSs, with an estimated incidence of 0.64 cases per 100,000 women. They are the most common type of uterine sarcomas and account for the single largest site-specific group of LMSs.[7]

RP-LMSs account for the second most common intra-abdominal type of LMS, arising predominantly from vascular smooth muscle, such as midsize vessels including renal veins, iliac or gonadal vessels, or the IVC proper. LMS may also originate from smooth muscle of the gastrointestinal tract, but are less frequent than GIST (ratio of 1:10).[8] RP-LMSs are generally asymptomatic at presentation, although for a minority of patients, their diagnosis is defined by a veno-occlusive episode such as a deep venous thrombosis (DVT).

Extra-abdominal LMSs include tumors that develop in extremities (**Fig. 1**), superficial trunk, and head and neck structures, which account for less than 10% of LMS sites.[9] There is also a subgroup of cutaneous LMSs that originate in the dermis from the arrectores pilorum muscles of the hair follicles and from the smooth muscle surrounding sweat glands, which show a more benign tumor biology compared with deeper sites and may be referred to as "atypical intradermal smooth muscle neoplasms" when confined to the dermis to reflect their minimal metastatic risk.[9,10]

LMS can present as primary disease only or with synchronous metastases, which occurs in 20% of patients and is associated with a 5-year disease-specific survival of approximately 20%.[11] Metastatic disease is also the most common pattern of failure after curative intent treatment for both intra-abdominal and extra-abdominal LMS.[12] Recent data from expert sarcoma centers in Europe and North America report an 8-year crude cumulative incidence (CCI) for distant metastases of 50% in patients with primary retroperitoneal sarcoma (RPS) with LMS, in stark contrast to less than

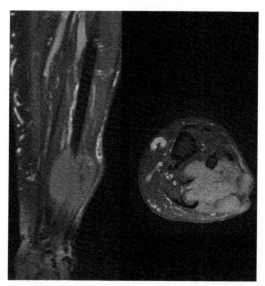

Fig. 1. Deep lower extremity LMS. Coronal and cross-section MRI with LMS involving deep and superficial left lateral compartments of leg.

10% for local recurrence after curative intent treatment.[1] The most frequent sites for first metastases are lung (49%), followed by liver (19%), soft tissue (14%), and bone (5%).[12] Lymph node involvement is exceedingly uncommon (2.7%).[13] Therefore, regional lymphadenectomy as standard of care is generally not indicated, unless clinically evident or radiologically concerning nodal disease is encountered.

Finally, there are genetic predispositions associated with LMS, such as retinoblastoma and Li-Fraumeni Syndrome (LFS). Patients with retinoblastoma have a cumulative risk of 13.1% of developing secondary sarcomas after radiation therapy which are predominately LMS.[14] Patients with LFS have a lifetime LMS incidence of 7% to 8%, which occurs at a median age of 44 years. Exposure to radiation also may increase the risk of developing LMS in these patients; however, most of these are sporadic cases.

PATHOLOGIC AND MOLECULAR CHARACTERISTICS OF LEIOMYOSARCOMA

LMSs are tumors of smooth muscle differentiation, and well-differentiated tumors show typical architecture of smooth muscle with broad fascicles of plump spindle cells intersecting at right angles (**Fig. 2**).[5] Tumors may show varying degrees of hyalinization. Neoplastic spindle cells contain abundant brightly eosinophilic fibrillary cytoplasm, with distinct cell borders and cigar-shaped nuclei. Conventional LMSs also often contain scattered "monster cells" with markedly pleomorphic and hyperchromatic nuclei. More poorly differentiated tumors may show more haphazard fascicular architecture, loss of cytoplasmic eosinophilia, or may become markedly pleomorphic, with loss of histologic evidence of smooth muscle differentiation. Epithelioid and myxoid variants of LMS tend to behave more aggressively, and most commonly arise in the uterus. Rarely, heterologous elements such as fat or bone formation may be seen.

Diagnostic immunohistochemical studies are useful to confirm the diagnosis of LMS in ambiguous cases; generally, at least patchy expression of at least 2 of the following muscle markers are used to confirm smooth muscle differentiation: desmin, smooth muscle actin, muscle actin HHF-35, h-caldesmon, smooth muscle myosin, or calponin

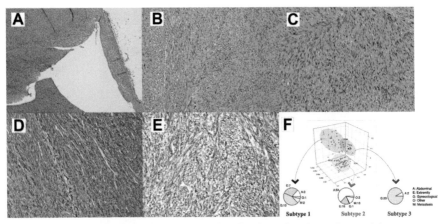

Fig. 2. Histopathologic characterization and molecular subtyping of LMS. (*A*) Low-power view showing a subcutaneous LMS arising in the wall of a small vein (at left) (hematoxylin-eosin [H&E], original magnification ×50). (*B*) Higher-power view of conventional LMS showing intersecting fascicles of brightly eosinophilic spindle cells with abundant cytoplasm and elongated ovoid nuclei. A mitotic figure is visible at center (H&E, original magnification ×100). (*C*) High-power image of conventional LMS showing intersecting fascicles of brightly eosinophilic spindle cells with abundant cytoplasm and elongated, blunt-ended ovoid nuclei (H&E, original magnification ×200). (*D*) Conventional LMS showing diffuse expression of h-caldesmon (original magnification ×100). (*E*) Conventional LMS showing diffuse expression of smooth muscle actin (original magnification ×100). (*F*) Three molecular subtypes of LMS arise following principal components analysis of transcriptomes with anatomic differences.[16]

(see **Fig. 2**). Immunohistochemical assessment should always be performed on the most well-differentiated appearing area of the tumor, as pleomorphic or dedifferentiated areas may lose all expression of myogenic markers. Keratin and epithelial membrane antigen are seen in up to 40% of these tumors, particularly in high-grade tumors, but is not LMS-specific.[5] Estrogen receptor (ER) and progesterone receptor (PR) expression may be seen in uLMS as well as some nonuterine retroperitoneal LMS arising in women, and rarely in extremity tumors of both sexes, but is often lost in high-grade disease. In some cases, the strong and diffuse expression of ER and PR in well-differentiated smooth muscle tumors of the abdomen/pelvis can be used to help support a diagnosis of leiomyoma of gynecologic origin versus a well-differentiated soft tissue LMS.

Tumor grade for extrauterine LMS should be scored according to the French Federation of Cancer Centers Sarcoma Group system (Federation Nationale des Centers de Lutte Contre le Cancer [FNCLCC]). The FNCLCC system categorizes tumors based on the mitotic rate, extent of necrosis, and degree of differentiation.[15] Pathologic assessment should be performed by an expert in soft tissue sarcomas, as this diagnosis can be complex and access to ancillary molecular testing may be required to secure the correct diagnosis.

LMS has been subject to comprehensive molecular profiling, including whole genome sequencing, RNA transcriptomes, and methylation profiling.[16–18] Overall, it is appreciated to be a genomically unstable tumor with evidence of complex genomic rearrangements, such as chromothripsis, followed by whole genome doubling. Mutations and dysregulation of key tumor suppressors such as TP53, RB1 are early in the molecular evolution of LMS and thus are commonly detected (>90%) with next generation sequencing. Recently, mutational signature analysis, which examines the processes that drive tumor progression, suggest that LMS may be enriched for defects in homologous recombination (Mut sig 3). Further studies are warranted to validate how prevalent this finding is, but suggests that DNA repair inhibitors may have clinical promise. Finally, comprehensive expression analysis by RNA sequencing by multiple independent efforts has identified 3 molecular subtypes, which are associated with disease outcome, and other disease features such as site and immune involvement[16,17,19,20] (see **Fig. 2**).

- Subtype I LMS: represents a less differentiated form of LMS and partially overlaps in a subset of patients with undifferentiated pleomorphic sarcoma
- Subtype II LMS: expresses most genes associated with smooth muscle differentiation (conventional LMS subtype) with better oncologic outcomes and primarily occurs in the retroperitoneum
- Subtype III LMS: is the only subtype that displays a preference for a specific anatomic site and is more likely to be from the uterus

Ongoing molecular profiling efforts are under way to address what the clinical utility of these subgroups are, along with the development of novel drug therapy that specifically targets DNA damage pathways and/or cell cycle regulation.

RETROPERITONEAL LEIOMYOSARCOMA
Diagnostic Workup

Intra-abdominal/retroperitoneal leiomyosarcomas are characterized by an expansive, non-infiltrative growth pattern.[21] Diagnosis in many patients is incidental after abdominal imaging (computed tomography [CT], MRI), or can be suspected by symptoms related to major venous obstruction, including DVT or collateral abdominal venous circulation.

Intra-abdominal/RP-LMSs most commonly originate from major retroperitoneal or deep pelvic veins such as the IVC; gonadal, renal, and iliac veins; or smaller mesenteric tributaries. They are also commonly seen arising from the gastrointestinal tract, bladder, or the prostate or adrenal glands. Tumors arising from large vessels may be intraluminal, extraluminal, or a combination of both. Cross-sectional imaging is necessary to provide a detailed evaluation of the size and local extent of the tumor and to define if any metastatic disease is present. Initial investigation should include CT of the chest/abdominal/pelvis and, when appropriate, a dedicated MRI. Intravenous contrast should be administered, as they commonly exhibit avid enhancement in the venous phase but with heterogeneity due to internal hemorrhage, necrosis, or cystic changes. Calcification is uncommon.[22]

Common sites of metastasis include lung, liver, soft tissues, and bones. Lymph node metastases are uncommon but should be evaluated in preoperative imaging. Intracranial metastases are exceedingly rare and thus brain imaging is usually only warranted if focal neurologic signs are present. For retroperitoneal tumors, MRI is not as useful as CT scan in defining the vascular relationships of the tumor with major vessels in the abdomen due to its lower spatial resolution and propensity to motion artifact. It is, however, better than CT in depicting tumor relationship to adjacent organs in the pelvis and also to differentiate intravascular tumor from bland thrombus.

The use of PET-CT for disease staging in RP-LMS is not yet considered standard of care; however, several studies have explored the complementary role of fluorodeoxyglucose PET-CT in the grading of STS. Benz and colleagues[23] analyzed 120 patients with 12 different subtypes. Their study revealed a significant relationship between the standard uptake value (SUV) at maximum SUV (SUVmax) of a lesion and the histologic grade given by the 3-tiered FNCLCC system when using a cutoff of 6.6 g/mL.

Finally, a complete diagnostic assessment requires a percutaneous biopsy, if technically feasible, as this establishes the diagnosis of LMS in most cases. Core needle biopsy of RPS is safe and does not adversely affect oncologic outcome, as recently demonstrated by several expert institutes.[24,25] The risk of needle tract seeding is approximately 0.5%.[25] A coaxial technique should be used, as it diminishes the risk of seeding. Also, the peritoneum should not be traversed if feasible. Multiple cores, preferably 5 to 10, should be obtained of the area of the tumor that appears highest grade and viable (enhancing) on imaging. Laparoscopic or open incisional biopsy should not be performed because the sample may not be representative of the higher tumor grade because of the lack of 3-dimensional image guidance. Future planes of dissection may also be altered during the incisional biopsy, or peritoneal contamination may occur,[26] and this approach is strongly discouraged.

Multidisciplinary Care in Retroperitoneal Leiomyosarcoma

Once the diagnosis of LMS of the retroperitoneum is established, patients should be evaluated by an expert sarcoma multidisciplinary team (MDT) consisting of medical, radiation, and surgical oncology. Following diagnostic imaging and pathology review, patients with this rare disease warrant a multidisciplinary discussion of care. Currently, the standard of care for resectable RP-LMS is upfront surgery, although high postoperative rates of distant metastasis has engaged the community to consider the role of neoadjuvant chemotherapy, as described later in this article. In patients with primary disease deemed borderline or unresectable, a discussion about the use of chemotherapy and/or radiation therapy should occur by the sarcoma MDT.

Although there has been a paucity of data on the utility of preoperative chemotherapy for primary RP STS,[21] this approach hypothetically may reduce distant microscopic disease and allow for completion of cytotoxic drug regimens, which may be difficult to complete after major surgery. A recently published collaborative study of 13 major sarcoma centers, exploring the benefit of neoadjuvant chemotherapy in primary RP STS has shown promising results.[27] This retrospective study included 158 patients with a median number of 3 chemotherapy cycles based on anthracycline regimens. Using RECIST criteria for tumor response, patients with partial response and stable disease (SD) after chemotherapy had significantly better overall survival (OS) compared with those with progressive disease (PD). At 5 years, OS was 26% (95% confidence interval [CI], 13%–54%) for patients with PD, 56% (95% CI, 39%–81%) for those with a partial response, and 58% (95% CI, 45%–73%) for those with SD. After comparing by histology and type of chemotherapy, the subgroup analysis showed a higher partial response rate in LMS treated with anthracycline and dacarbazine (partial response = 37%). These results suggest that there is an enhanced response with doxorubicin-based chemotherapy in combination with dacarbazine, rather than ifosfamide.[28] Further development of histology-based chemotherapy drug combinations is ongoing.

To address the utility of neoadjuvant chemotherapy for resectable RP-LMS, an open-label multicenter, randomized phase III trial, STRASS 2, sponsored by the European Organisation for Research and Treatment of Cancer (EORTC) has recently opened (NCT04031677). It is currently recruiting patients in the EU and Canada with plans to open in Australia, Japan, and possibly the United States. This trial was specifically designed to investigate whether preoperative chemotherapy improves the prognosis of patients with high-risk RP–dedifferentiated liposarcoma (DD-LPS) or RP-LMS (G1-G3) followed by curative intent surgery (**Fig. 3**). Patients who meet

Schema

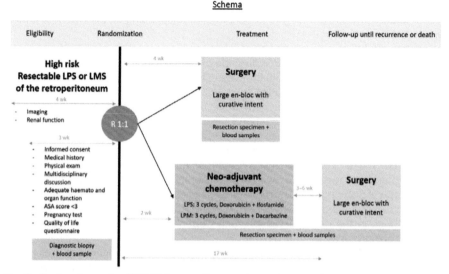

Fig. 3. Study schema for STRASS 2: neoadjuvant chemotherapy plus surgery versus surgery only for resectable LMS of the retroperitoneum.

inclusion criteria will be randomized to the standard arm (upfront en bloc curative intent surgery within 4 weeks after randomization) or the experimental arm. The experimental arm consists of 3 cycles of neoadjuvant anthracycline-based chemotherapy starting within 2 weeks after randomization. Combination therapy will be histotype-directed with dacarbazine or ifosfamide for LMS or DD-LPS, respectively.

Whether there is a benefit to adding neoadjuvant radiation therapy to this patient population was recently addressed by the phase-3 randomized clinical trial, STRASS.[29] Unlike STRASS 2, this study included most major sarcoma types, in which 14% (38 of 266) were RP-LMS. Overall, the 3-year analysis showed no statistically significant difference in abdominal recurrence-free survival (ARFS) for all histology types; 58.7% (95% CI 49.5–66.7) in the surgery group and 60.4% (51.4–68.2) in the radiotherapy plus surgery group. Importantly, post hoc analyses of ARFS demonstrated no significant difference for RP-LMS.[29] Given the increasing data that there is a lower incidence of local recurrence in RP-LMS (8-year CCI <10%),[1] along with randomized data from the STRASS trial, these data have been interpreted that neoadjuvant radiation for resectable primary RP-LMS is unlikely to provide benefit.

Surgical Treatment

Surgery is the mainstay for curative intent treatment in LMS. For intra-abdominal/retroperitoneal lesions, this usually consists of a multivisceral resection of adjacent organs with the goal of achieving an en bloc R0 resection. Curative intent multivisceral surgery for primary RP-LMS can be planned in 3 clinical settings: (1) resectable disease, (2) borderline resectable, and (3) primary tumor with synchronous oligometastatic disease.

Multivisceral surgery for retroperitoneal and pelvic LMS generally includes resection and possible reconstruction of major vascular structures, such as the IVC, renal veins. or iliac vessels, determined by the vascular origin of these tumors. Overall, the goal is to achieve a complete resection, which may require either partial resection followed by primary vascular closure repair or a complete segmental resection with a biological or polytetrafluoroethylene (PTFE) graft reconstruction, depending on the extent of tumor involvement.

Because the IVC is a common site of origin, en bloc resection of these tumors requires resection and possible reconstruction of the IVC and other major venous tributaries, depending on the location, intravascular tumor extent, and collateral venous drainage at the time of surgery (**Fig. 4**). In IVC-LMS, tumor location has been previously described based on the segment of IVC involved and distance to the main iliac confluence, renal veins, and retrohepatic segment of the IVC.[30] The complexity and risk of this reconstruction increases as the retrohepatic segment of the IVC is included in the resection, particularly when major hepatic veins or the right atrium of the heart are involved. These highly challenging resections may require a hepatic mobilization, including major liver resection or even extracorporeal bypass circulation. Thus, preoperative surgical planning with appropriate surgical expertise is key to achieve optimal oncologic resection and mitigate perioperative morbidity and mortality.[30–34] RP-LMS also can arise in the gonadal vessels, and depending on their location, a kidney-sparing procedure may be feasible (**Fig. 5**).

Borderline resectability is often defined by the proximity or involvement of major vascular structures that may not be possible to resect or reconstruct, along with the extent of other viscera that would require resection to achieve a grossly negative result. For borderline resectable disease, an initial neoadjuvant systemic treatment approach, followed by neoadjuvant radiation therapy, or trimodal approach, may aid in defining patients who will succumb early to metastatic disease, while also providing the opportunity to potentially cytoreduce technically challenging tumors, which may result in less morbid procedures. Although radiation therapy does not appear to help with local control rates based on the STRASS data, its utility here is potentially facilitating resectability.

The role of curative intent surgery for RP-LMS in the setting of synchronous oligometastases is a matter of debate. The role of surgery applies most commonly to lung metastases; however, similar principles could be extrapolated to limited hepatic, soft tissue, and/or rarely isolated bone metastases. When analyzing prognostic factors involved in the survival benefit of surgery for oligometastasis, timing of metastases (synchronous vs metachronous), progression-free interval, number of lesions, and complete metastases resection, are prognostic, with the caveat of patient selection in these retrospective studies.[35,36]

Surveillance

RP-LMSs, as previously discussed, demonstrate a high rate of metastatic recurrence.[1,12,37] This pattern of recurrence can be exclusively metastatic, or local and metastatic after many years following resection. Late local and distant recurrences (5–10 years after diagnosis) may occur in 27% and 9%, respectively, in RP-LMS.[12] Clinical follow-up must therefore include a CT series of chest, abdomen, and pelvis for the remainder of the patient's life, as late recurrences of more than 25 years have been documented. In most expert centers, follow-up intervals for RP-LMS is cross-sectional imaging every 4 months for 2 years after surgery, every 6 months between 2 and 5 years postoperatively, and then yearly.[21]

UTERINE LEIOMYOSARCOMA

uLMS is an aggressive tumor arising from smooth muscle and is the most common site of disease. Although it accounts for only 1% to 2% of uterine malignancies, it

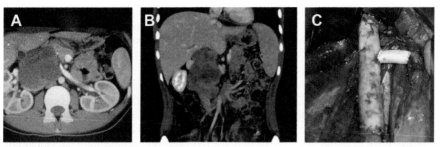

Fig. 4. IVC-LMS resection with major vascular reconstruction. (*A*) Cross-sectional and (*B*) coronal CT scan of grade 2 IVC-LMS involving IVC and right renal vein. (*C*) En bloc resection including IVC reconstruction with cadaveric aortic graft and left renal vein reimplantation with PTFE graft.

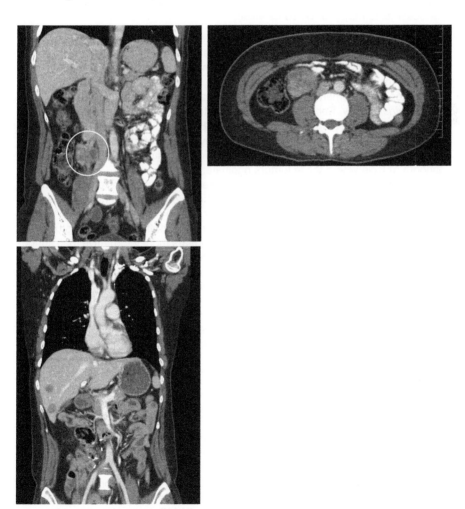

Fig. 5. Gonadal vein LMS. A grade 3 LMS was resected en bloc with a mid-ureteric repair (top left coronal image, top right axial image). Hepatic metastasis developed within the first postoperative year (bottom left coronal image).

has a poor prognosis, with overall 5-year survival ranging from 15% to 65%.[38–40] Women with uLMS should be clinically managed in specialty centers with expertise in gynecology oncology and sarcoma; however, unfortunately these referrals often occur postoperatively after hysterectomy or myomectomy for presumed benign uterine leiomyomas.[41]

Preoperative Assessment

uLMS is challenging to diagnose preoperatively given its radiologic resemblance to benign uterine leiomyomas, low utilization of preoperative biopsy for diagnosis, and sampling error in those few tumors that are biopsied preoperatively. This distinction between leiomyoma and LMS is important to make, as en bloc hysterectomy is the surgical standard of care for uLMS, whereas procedures such as morcellation and myomectomy are strictly reserved for leiomyomas. Although there is currently no clinical or serologic test to confidently distinguish between the 2 pathologies, certain clinical assessments may provide some value.

1. *Clinical features.* Although both benign and malignant entities can present with uterine bleeding, a uterine mass, or pelvic pain, new or growing fibroids in postmenopausal women who are not using hormonal replacement therapy are concerning for malignancy.[38,41] Rapid fibroid growth or large uterine size in premenopausal women do not correlate with an increased risk of malignancy.[39,41]
2. *Endometrial biopsy.* Sampling of the endometrium has limited value, as sensitivity and specificities were found to be of 35% to 80% and 30% to 65%, respectively, with no difference between office biopsy and curettage as a sampling method,[39,41,42] which is likely because of difficulty in sampling the deeper uterine smooth muscle where these tumors originate.
3. *Laboratory markers.* Several markers have been investigated to discern between LMS and leiomyomas. None are clinically effective. Lactate dehydrogenase is a nonspecific marker, as it has been previously shown to have a sensitivity of 47% to 74% and specificity of 85% to 100% at various cutoff values in one study.[43]
4. *MRI.* In terms of imaging, MRI with contrast appears more informative than sonography and CT. Sensitivity and specificity were reported as 77% to 96%[39]; however, the generalizability of such results is limited. Valuable findings include dark and homogeneous mass in T2-weighted images having a high negative predictive value for LMS, presence of calcifications associated with fibroids, and ill-defined margins associated with LMS[41] (**Fig. 6**).
5. *Morcellation.* Leiomyomas are a common reason for gynecologic surgery, and morcellation has allowed women with enlarged fibroids to benefit from minimally invasive surgery.[41] The low incidence of LMS diagnosis in presumed benign leiomyomas is estimated at 0.007% to 0.2%,[39–41] and this is because of limitations in preoperative assessment tools, as there is genetic evidence that most uLMSs arise independently of fibroids.[39,41] If LMS diagnosis occurred after myomectomy, hysterectomy is necessary to complete surgical management.[44]

Subsequent to a "black box" warning issued by the Food and Drug Administration in 2014 regarding electromechanical morcellator devices, this practice changed throughout North America and varies between gynecologic departments from no morcellation at all to carefully selected patients to in-bag only morcellation.[39] This concern is related to risk of occult malignancy dissemination, as well as increased rates of recurrence and decreased survival.[39,40,45] As such, if LMS diagnosis occurs after morcellation, National Comprehensive Cancer Network (NCCN) guidelines recommend imaging and to consider reexploration surgery.[44]

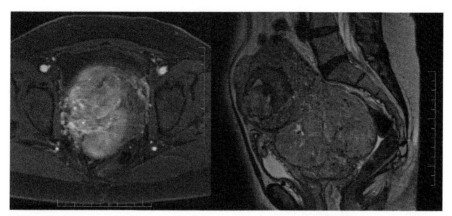

Fig. 6. MRI features of uterine mass concerning for LMS. A large heterogenous uterine mass demonstrates irregular boarders on axial T1 images with enhancement (left) and greater than 50% T2 signal on sagittal images (right). Right pelvic sidewall extension and suspicious posterior bladder involvement are present.

There are no studies looking at survival and recurrence rates in LMS treated by myomectomy without morcellation and subsequent hysterectomy. Interestingly, evidence of muscle cells present in peritoneal fluid was found after myomectomies even before morcellation.[46] The need for adjuvant treatment in cases of inadvertent LMS morcellation is unknown, and one study found no benefit for adjuvant chemotherapy, chemoradiation, or radiation to improve survival or recurrence outcomes.[47]

Surgical Standard

uLMS is surgically staged according to the 2017 International Federation of Gynecology and Obstetrics (FIGO) staging for uLMS and endometrial stromal sarcomas **(Table 1)**. The surgery involves total hysterectomy,[39,44] with controversies surrounding need for lymphadenectomy and oophorectomy. If pathologic diagnosis occurs after hysterectomy, the NCCN recommends imaging with CT of the chest, abdomen, and pelvis, and to consider surgical reexploration.[44]

1. *Lymphadenectomy.* Lymphadenectomy is not usually necessary[38,44] given that the main LMS dissemination mechanism is hematogenous. The incidence of positive lymph nodes is low at 6.6% to 11% overall,[38,39,48] and less than 5% for early stages.[39] Omitting lymphadenectomy was not associated with decreased OS in the literature,[48] and a suggested surgical approach is to inspect and remove only grossly enlarged nodes.[39,40]
2. *Bilateral oophorectomy.* Oophorectomy is recommended for postmenopausal women, with improved OS demonstrated for patients older than 51 years in a National Cancer Database study.[48] NCCN and FIGO permit ovarian preservation in selected patients with early-stage LMS who wish to retain hormonal function.[38,44] This is controversial due to a speculative hormonal effect, because LMSs are often positive for ER and PR,[38,40] which contrasts with the cardiac and overall health beneficial effects of estrogen. In premenopausal women, oophorectomy for early LMS was not associated with an OS benefit.[39,48]
3. *Complete debulking and lung metastasectomy.* For patients with extrauterine resectable disease, complete surgical debulking is the recommended treatment by FIGO and NCCN.[38,44] Because LMS response to adjuvant treatment including

Table 1	
International Federation of Gynecology and Obstetrics staging for uterine sarcomas	
Stage	**Definition**
Leiomyosarcomas and endometrial stromal sarcomas	
I	Tumor limited to uterus
IA	<5 cm
IB	More than 5 cm
II	Tumor extends beyond the uterus within the pelvis
IIA	Adnexal involvement
IIB	Involvement of other pelvic tissues
III	Tumor invades abdominal tissues (not just protruding into the abdomen)
IIIA	One site
IIIB	More than 1 site
IIIC	Metastasis to pelvic and/or para aortic lymph nodes
IV	
IVA	Tumor invades bladder and/or rectum
IVB	Distant metastasis

systemic therapy and/or radiation is limited,[38,44] complete debulking to no gross residual disease, including resection of isolated pulmonary metastases, was shown in some studies to have a better outcome.[39,40] Similarly for recurrent uLMS, surgical resection when feasible was described to prolong survival with a median OS of 54 months (24–83 months) when complete resection was achieved.[49] Best candidates for secondary resection have localized recurrences and prolonged progression-free intervals of 12 to 18 months.[40] A recently explored avenue is the use of hyperthermic intraperitoneal chemotherapy for patients with primary or recurrent LMS sarcomatosis. A review including 68 patients showed a median OS of 29 to 37 months, but a perioperative death rate of 4%.[50]

SYSTEMIC THERAPY IN LEIOMYOSARCOMA
Adjuvant Chemotherapy

In LMS, approximately 50% of patients with localized disease will develop distant metastases and die of their disease, despite optimal local treatment.[51] The use of adjuvant chemotherapy, in an attempt to reduce the risk of disease recurrence in STS (which included patients with LMS) was evaluated in several trials with conflicting results. For example, a large randomized controlled trial (n = 351; EORTC STBSG 62931) compared adjuvant doxorubicin + ifosfamide versus observation in patients with STS. This study failed to demonstrate any impact in terms of both recurrence-free survival and OS.[52] In contrast, an Italian trial (n = 104) that randomized patients with STS to adjuvant epirubicin + ifosfamide versus observation demonstrated a 4-year OS benefit favoring chemotherapy use (69% vs 50%).[53] Unfortunately, these adjuvant STS trials suffer from the fact that treatment was deployed in a heterogeneous population of patients with STS, and some trials were also underpowered.

Meta-analysis of adjuvant chemotherapy studies in STS were not surprisingly encouraging for routine treatment. The initial meta-analysis by the Sarcoma Meta-Analysis Collaboration demonstrated no OS benefit with chemotherapy use.[54] However, an updated 2008 meta-analysis of 18 randomized trials (n = 1953) showed a significant benefit of OS favoring chemotherapy (OR for death 0.56; 95% CI, 0.36–0.85; P < .05).[55] This meta-analysis, however, did not include the EORTC STBSG 62931 mentioned previously. Subsequently, a pooled analysis of the 2 largest adjuvant chemotherapy EORTC studies (n = 819) failed to show OS benefit, apart from patients with R1 resection.[56]

Given the incongruous results, adjuvant chemotherapy use in STS (including LMS) varies across institutions and remains controversial. International guideline recommends discussing the option of adjuvant chemotherapy with patients affected by high-risk STS of extremity and trunk wall in the context of ambiguous evidence.[57]

Systemic Treatment Options in Metastatic Leiomyosarcoma

The rate of metastasis occurrence in patients with LMS treated for localized disease can vary by disease site of origin (31% in extremity, 58% in the abdomen, 53%–71% in the uterus).[12,38] In advanced or metastatic setting, the outcomes for patients with LMS are poor, with a varied median OS of 12 to 24 months.[58,59]

The main treatment option for patients with LMS with advanced/metastatic disease remains chemotherapy. No specific trials for LMS have been reported in first-line setting, but patients with LMS are represented in 20% to 40% of the STS trials population.[60–63] First-line chemotherapy for advanced, metastatic, or unresectable STS is typically based on doxorubicin monotherapy, with a response rate of 15% to 20%, with a further 30% to 40% of patients experiencing disease stabilization.[57,60–63] The median progression-free survival (PFS) of doxorubicin monotherapy is approximately 4.5 to 6 months.[60–63]

Several clinical studies comparing single-agent doxorubicin with doxorubicin combinations, such as doxorubicin + ifosfamide, doxorubicin + olaratumab, and gemcitabine + docetaxel, failed to show an OS advantage, although combination therapy may result in an improvement of response rates and PFS when compared with doxorubicin alone.[60] Combination treatments generally do come at a cost, as they are associated with elevated levels of toxicities and decreased treatment tolerability.[60–63] Despite this, it is worth noting that combination therapy is still routinely used in clinic. For example, gemcitabine and docetaxel combination, although not superior to doxorubicin, is commonly used in the first-line setting where doxorubicin cannot be used or in the second-line treatment setting.[3,64,65]

Several other regimens have also shown activity in LMS, beyond first-line treatment. These include agents such as trabectedin and eribulin. In a phase III trial, trabectedin demonstrated superiority over dacarbazine in PFS but failed to show advantage in OS.[66,67] In another phase III trial, OS superiority of eribulin, when compared with dacarbazine was reported in liposarcoma and LMS populations (median OS 13.5 vs 11.5 months; P = .0169), but this advantage is lost when analyzing the treatment effect in the LMS cohort alone.[68] Other treatment options for subsequent lines of therapy in LMS include dacarbazine, gemcitabine single agent, and liposomal doxorubicin[66–70] (**Table 2**).

When exploring nonchemotherapy, targeted treatment options for LMS, pazopanib (small-molecule inhibitor against vascular endothelial growth factor) demonstrated modest efficacy in STS, with PFS benefit alone.[71] In a subgroup analysis of patients with uLMS across 2 trials, a response rate of 11% PFS at 3 months and an OS of 17.5 months were observed).[72] Other nonchemotherapy options include antihormone therapies with ER/PR-positive LMS. These tumors may be characterized with indolent clinical course and demonstrated 12-week PFS rate of 50% with a median duration of treatment of 2.2 months, when treated with letrozole.[73,74]

Table 2
Chemotherapy types used for progressive lines of treatment in patients with advanced LMS

Study	Drug/ Combination Tested	Treatment Line	Phase	Number of Patients/ LMS Patients	RR (%)	PFS (month) >	OS (month)
Demetri et al,[66] 2012	Trabectedin vs Dacarbazine	>1	III	518/378	9.9 vs 6.9	4.2 vs 1.5	12.4 vs 12.9
Patel et al,[67] 2016	Trabectedin vs dacarbazine	>1	III	577/423	10 vs 7	4.3 vs 1.6	13.7 vs 13.1
Maki et al,[69] 2007	Gemcitabine vs gemcitabine + docetaxel	>1	IIR	122/38	8 vs 16	3 vs 6.2	11.5 vs 17.9
Schoffski et al,[68] 2016	Eribulin vs dacarbazine	>1	III	122/38	4 vs 5	2.6 vs 2.6	13.5 vs 11.5
Sutton et al,[70] 2005	Liposomal doxorubicin	>1	II	32/32*	16.1	NA	NA

Abbreviations: LMS, leiomyosarcoma; NA, not applicable; PFS, progression-free survival; OS, overall survival; RR, response rate.

Targeted agents are also recently or currently being evaluated in patients with LMS. Monotherapy with checkpoint inhibitors, such as pembrolizumab or nivolumab, showed low clinical activity in this tumor subtype with no responses and short-term clinical benefit were reported (PFS of 1.4–1.8 month).[75,76] Given the lack of activity in monotherapy trials, combination immunotherapy strategies are currently being explored. A recent retrospective study demonstrated a 45% overall response rate and a median PFS of 14.4 months among responders in patients with LMS treated with nivolumab and ipilimumab.[77] A prospective trial that included the preceding combination in STS has also been reported showing promising results of the combination.[78] In another study, combination therapy with durvalumab (PD L-1 inhibitor) with either olaparib (PARP inhibitor) or cediranib (anti-angiogenic inhibitor) resulted in disease stabilization in 30% of patients with LMS, some of whom were durable (DAPPER Trial-NCT03851614), again highlighting the value to exploring combination therapy with checkpoint inhibitors. Currently, there are several endeavors interrogating biomarkers that are associated with response or resistance to immunotherapy in sarcomas. These include genetic profiling to analyze tumor-immune micro-environment as well as inflammation signatures.[77–80] One other area of emerging interest, in terms of novel drug usage, is the discovery of homologous recombination defects in LMS, as previously discussed.[16] A recent phase 2 study demonstrated the combination of temozolamide and olaparib resulting in a response rate of 27% in heavily pre-treated patients with uLMS (NCT03880019). Together with the DAPPER study, there is now ample justification to explore PARP-inhibitor combinations in LMS.

In summary, the use of adjuvant chemotherapy in resected LMS remains uncertain and controversial. In the metastatic setting, first-line therapy is still dominated by doxorubicin-based therapies. In recent years, there has been an expansion of therapeutic options beyond first-line therapy to include agents such as trabectedin, eribulin, and pazopanib. Current trials are ongoing, with interrogation of immunotherapy combination strategies. In addition, PARP inhibition may be a useful and important therapeutic strategy for LMS.

FUTURE DIRECTIONS

As the biology of LMS becomes more comprehensively assessed by both histotype specific care and molecular profiling, the field has several promising directions to improve patient outcomes.[81] First, the diagnostic challenges of diagnosing uLMS has shown promise with the advent of circulating tumor DNA. Ongoing efforts by several groups to aid in establishing an accurate diagnosis are under way, and this approach could alleviate the challenges patients face when diagnosed postoperatively.[82–84] Second, our ability to determine higher versus low metastatic risk is also being addressed by cooperative group efforts.[83] We will learn more from the neoadjuvant STRASS 2 trial whether the use of neoadjuvant chemotherapy will benefit RP-LMS. Finally, because metastatic disease is the main clinical challenges patients face, new drug therapies are emerging in the DNA damage inhibitor space with promising phase 2 clinical trials.[85] Certainly, by understanding which patients with LMS require multidisciplinary therapy early in their course and by developing more effective systemic agents, improving patient outcomes should be realized in the future.

CLINICS CARE POINTS

- LMS can present as primary disease only, or with advanced disease.
- Diagnostic assessment should include a percutaneous biopsy.
- Staging workup should include a CT of chest/abdomen/pelvis, and/or MRI in pelvic or extremity tumors.
- Patients should be evaluated by an expert sarcoma multidisciplinary team to define the role of multimodal treatment.
- Surgery is the mainstay for curative intent treatment.
- Extent and complexity of these multivisceral resections may require multiple surgical teams, including surgical oncology, hepato-pancreato-biliary/transplant, and/or vascular surgery.
- Doxorubicin-based treatment is the mainstay for patients with metastatic LMS. The role of neoadjuvant regimens is currently under investigation.

DISCLOSURE

The authors have nothing to disclose.

REFERENCES

1. Gronchi A, Strauss DC, Miceli R, et al. Variability in patterns of recurrence after resection of primary retroperitoneal sarcoma (RPS): a report on 1007 patients from the multi-institutional collaborative RPS working group. Ann Surg 2016; 263(5):1002–9.
2. Serrano C, George S. Leiomyosarcoma. Hematol Oncol Clin North Am 2013; 27(5):957–74.
3. George S, Serrano C, Hensley ML, et al. Soft tissue and uterine leiomyosarcoma. J Clin Oncol 2018;36(2):144–50.
4. Hashimoto H, Tsuneyoshi M, Enjoji M. Malignant smooth muscle tumors of the retroperitoneum and mesentery: a clinicopathologic analysis of 44 cases. J Surg Oncol 1985;28(3):177–86.

5. Cancer IAfRo, editor. WHO classification of tumours of soft tissue and bone. 5 edition. Lyon (France)2020.

6. Gustafson P. Soft tissue sarcoma. Epidemiology and prognosis in 508 patients. Acta Orthop Scand Suppl 1994;259:1–31.

7. Amant F, Coosemans A, Debiec-Rychter M, et al. Clinical management of uterine sarcomas. Lancet Oncol 2009;10(12):1188–98.

8. Katz SC, DeMatteo RP. Gastrointestinal stromal tumors and leiomyosarcomas. J Surg Oncol 2008;97(4):350–9.

9. Svarvar C, Bohling T, Berlin O, et al. Clinical course of nonvisceral soft tissue leiomyosarcoma in 225 patients from the Scandinavian Sarcoma Group. Cancer 2007;109(2):282–91.

10. Berlin Ö, Stener B, Kindblom L-G, et al. Leiomyosarcomas of venous origin in the extremities. A correlated clinical, roentgenologic, and morphologic study with diagnostic and surgical implications. Cancer 1984;54(10):2147–59.

11. Clary BM, DeMatteo RP, Lewis JJ, et al. Gastrointestinal stromal tumors and leiomyosarcoma of the abdomen and retroperitoneum: a clinical comparison. Ann Surg Oncol 2001;8(4):290–9.

12. Gladdy RA, Qin LX, Moraco N, et al. Predictors of survival and recurrence in primary leiomyosarcoma. Ann Surg Oncol 2013;20(6):1851–7.

13. Fong Y, Coit DG, Woodruff JM, et al. Lymph node metastasis from soft tissue sarcoma in adults. Analysis of data from a prospective database of 1772 sarcoma patients. Ann Surg 1993;217(1):72–7.

14. Kleinerman RA, Schonfeld SJ, Sigel BS, et al. Bone and soft-tissue sarcoma risk in long-term survivors of hereditary retinoblastoma treated with radiation. J Clin Oncol 2019;37(35):3436–45.

15. Trojani M, Contesso G, Coindre JM, et al. Soft-tissue sarcomas of adults; study of pathological prognostic variables and definition of a histopathological grading system. Int J Cancer 1984;33(1):37–42.

16. Anderson ND, Babichev Y, Fuligni F, et al. Lineage-defined leiomyosarcoma subtypes emerge years before diagnosis and determine patient survival. Nat Commun 2021;12(1):4496.

17. Chudasama P, Mughal SS, Sanders MA, et al. Integrative genomic and transcriptomic analysis of leiomyosarcoma. Nat Commun 2018;9(1):144.

18. Cancer Genome Atlas Research Network. Comprehensive and integrated genomic characterization of adult soft tissue sarcomas. Cell 2017;171(4):950–965 e28.

19. Beck AH, Lee CH, Witten DM, et al. Discovery of molecular subtypes in leiomyosarcoma through integrative molecular profiling. Oncogene 2010;29(6):845–54.

20. Hemming ML, Fan C, Raut CP, et al. Oncogenic gene-expression programs in leiomyosarcoma and characterization of conventional, inflammatory, and uterogenic subtypes. Mol Cancer Res 2020;18(9):1302–14.

21. Crago AM, Brennan MF. Principles in management of soft tissue sarcoma. Adv Surg 2015;49:107–22.

22. O'Sullivan PJ, Harris AC, Munk PL. Radiological imaging features of non-uterine leiomyosarcoma. Br J Radiol 2008;81(961):73–81.

23. Benz MR, Dry SM, Eilber FC, et al. Correlation between glycolytic phenotype and tumor grade in soft-tissue sarcomas by 18F-FDG PET. J Nucl Med 2010;51(8):1174–81.

24. Van Houdt WJ, Schrijver AM, Cohen-Hallaleh RB, et al. Needle tract seeding following core biopsies in retroperitoneal sarcoma. Eur J Surg Oncol 2017;43(9):1740–5.

25. Berger-Richardson D, Burtenshaw SM, Ibrahim AM, et al. Early and late complications of percutaneous core needle biopsy of retroperitoneal tumors at two tertiary sarcoma centers. Ann Surg Oncol 2019;26(13):4692–8.

26. Swallow CJ, Strauss DC, Bonvalot S, et al. Management of primary retroperitoneal sarcoma (RPS) in the adult: an updated consensus approach from the Transatlantic Australasian RPS Working Group. Ann Surg Oncol 2021;28(12):7873–88.

27. Tseng WW, Barretta F, Conti L, et al. Defining the role of neoadjuvant systemic therapy in high-risk retroperitoneal sarcoma: a multi-institutional study from the Transatlantic Australasian Retroperitoneal Sarcoma Working Group. Cancer 2021;127(5):729–38.

28. D'Ambrosio L, Touati N, Blay JY, et al. Doxorubicin plus dacarbazine, doxorubicin plus ifosfamide, or doxorubicin alone as a first-line treatment for advanced leiomyosarcoma: a propensity score matching analysis from the European Organization for Research and Treatment of Cancer Soft Tissue and Bone Sarcoma Group. Cancer 2020;126(11):2637–47.

29. Bonvalot S, Gronchi A, Le Péchoux C, et al. Preoperative radiotherapy plus surgery versus surgery alone for patients with primary retroperitoneal sarcoma (EORTC-62092: STRASS): a multicentre, open-label, randomised, phase 3 trial. Lancet Oncol 2020;21(10):1366–77.

30. Fiore M, Colombo C, Locati P, et al. Surgical technique, morbidity, and outcome of primary retroperitoneal sarcoma involving inferior vena cava. Ann Surg Oncol 2012;19(2):511–8.

31. Bonvalot S, Miceli R, Berselli M, et al. Aggressive surgery in retroperitoneal soft tissue sarcoma carried out at high-volume centers is safe and is associated with improved local control. Ann Surg Oncol 2010;17(6):1507–14.

32. Gronchi A, Lo Vullo S, Fiore M, et al. Aggressive surgical policies in a retrospectively reviewed single-institution case series of retroperitoneal soft tissue sarcoma patients. J Clin Oncol 2009;27(1):24–30.

33. MacNeill AJ, Gronchi A, Miceli R, et al. Postoperative morbidity after radical resection of primary retroperitoneal sarcoma: a report from the Transatlantic RPS Working Group. Ann Surg 2018;267(5):959–64.

34. Ferraris M, Callegaro D, Barretta F, et al. Outcome of iliocaval resection and reconstruction for retroperitoneal sarcoma. J Vasc Surg Venous Lymphat Disord 2019;7(4):547–56.

35. Grilley-Olson JE, Webber NP, Demos DS, et al. Multidisciplinary management of oligometastatic soft tissue sarcoma. Am Soc Clin Oncol Educ Book 2018;38:939–48.

36. Wigge S, Heissner K, Steger V, et al. Impact of surgery in patients with metastatic soft tissue sarcoma: a monocentric retrospective analysis. J Surg Oncol 2018;118(1):167–76.

37. Tan MC, Brennan MF, Kuk D, et al. Histology-based classification predicts pattern of recurrence and improves risk stratification in primary retroperitoneal sarcoma. Ann Surg 2016;263(3):593–600.

38. Mbatani N, Olawaiye AB, Prat J. Uterine sarcomas. Int J Gynaecol Obstet 2018;143(Suppl 2):51–8.

39. Ricci S, Stone RL, Fader AN. Uterine leiomyosarcoma: epidemiology, contemporary treatment strategies and the impact of uterine morcellation. Gynecol Oncol 2017;145(1):208–16.

40. Martee L Hensley MML. Treatment and Prognosis of Uterine Leiomyosarcoma. UptoDate [Internet]. 2021.

41. Stewart EA. Uterine fibroids (leiomyomas): Differentiating fibroids from uterine sarcomas. UptoDate [Internet]. 2021.

42. Hinchcliff EM, Esselen KM, Watkins JC, et al. The role of endometrial biopsy in the preoperative detection of uterine leiomyosarcoma. J Minim Invasive Gynecol 2016;23(4):567–72.

43. Di Cello A, Borelli M, Marra ML, et al. A more accurate method to interpret lactate dehydrogenase (LDH) isoenzymes' results in patients with uterine masses. Eur J Obstet Gynecol Reprod Biol 2019;236:143–7.

44. National Comprehensive Cancer Network. Uterine Neoplasms. 2021. In: NCCN Clinical Practice Guidelines in Oncology [Internet].

45. Bogani G, Cliby WA, Aletti GD. Impact of morcellation on survival outcomes of patients with unexpected uterine leiomyosarcoma: a systematic review and meta-analysis. Gynecol Oncol 2015;137(1):167–72.

46. Toubia T, Moulder JK, Schiff LD, et al. Peritoneal washings after power morcellation in laparoscopic myomectomy: a pilot study. J Minim Invasive Gynecol 2016; 23(4):578–81.

47. Kim SI, Choi CH, Kim K, et al. Effectiveness of adjuvant treatment for morcellated, International Federation of Gynecology and Obstetrics stage I uterine leiomyosarcoma: a Korean multicenter study. J Obstet Gynaecol Res 2020;46(2):337–46.

48. Seagle BL, Sobecki-Rausch J, Strohl AE, et al. Prognosis and treatment of uterine leiomyosarcoma: a National Cancer Database study. Gynecol Oncol 2017;145(1):61–70.

49. Cybulska P, Sioulas V, Orfanelli T, et al. Secondary surgical resection for patients with recurrent uterine leiomyosarcoma. Gynecol Oncol 2019;154(2):333–7.

50. Matsuzaki S, Matsuzaki S, Chang EJ, et al. Surgical and oncologic outcomes of hyperthermic intraperitoneal chemotherapy for uterine leiomyosarcoma: a systematic review of literature. Gynecol Oncol 2021;161(1):70–7.

51. Gronchi A, Maki RG, Jones RL. Treatment of soft tissue sarcoma: a focus on earlier stages. Future Oncol 2017;13(1s):13–21.

52. Woll PJ, Reichardt P, Le Cesne A, et al. Adjuvant chemotherapy with doxorubicin, ifosfamide, and lenograstim for resected soft-tissue sarcoma (EORTC 62931): a multicentre randomised controlled trial. Lancet Oncol 2012;13(10):1045–54.

53. Frustaci S, Gherlinzoni F, De Paoli A, et al. Adjuvant chemotherapy for adult soft tissue sarcomas of the extremities and girdles: results of the Italian randomized cooperative trial. J Clin Oncol 2001;19(5):1238–47.

54. Adjuvant chemotherapy for localised resectable soft-tissue sarcoma of adults: meta-analysis of individual data. Lancet 1997;350(9092):1647–54.

55. Pervaiz N, Colterjohn N, Farrokhyar F, et al. A systematic meta-analysis of randomized controlled trials of adjuvant chemotherapy for localized resectable soft-tissue sarcoma. Cancer 2008;113(3):573–81.

56. Le Cesne A, Ouali M, Leahy MG, et al. Doxorubicin-based adjuvant chemotherapy in soft tissue sarcoma: pooled analysis of two STBSG-EORTC phase III clinical trials. Ann Oncol 2014;25(12):2425–32.

57. von Mehren M, Kane JM, Bui MM, et al. NCCN guidelines insights: soft tissue sarcoma, version 1.2021. J Natl Compr Canc Netw 2020;18(12):1604–12.

58. Van Glabbeke M, van Oosterom AT, Oosterhuis JW, et al. Prognostic factors for the outcome of chemotherapy in advanced soft tissue sarcoma: an analysis of 2,185 patients treated with anthracycline-containing first-line regimens–a European Organization for Research and Treatment of Cancer Soft Tissue and Bone Sarcoma Group Study. J Clin Oncol 1999;17(1):150–7.

59. Savina M, Le Cesne A, Blay JY, et al. Patterns of care and outcomes of patients with METAstatic soft tissue SARComa in a real-life setting: the METASARC observational study. BMC Med 2017;15(1):78.

60. Judson I, Verweij J, Gelderblom H, et al. Doxorubicin alone versus intensified doxorubicin plus ifosfamide for first-line treatment of advanced or metastatic soft-tissue sarcoma: a randomised controlled phase 3 trial. Lancet Oncol 2014; 15(4):415–23.

61. Tap WD, Wagner AJ, Schoffski P, et al. Effect of doxorubicin plus olaratumab vs doxorubicin plus placebo on survival in patients with advanced soft tissue sarcomas: the ANNOUNCE randomized clinical trial. JAMA 2020;323(13):1266–76.

62. Seddon B, Strauss SJ, Whelan J, et al. Gemcitabine and docetaxel versus doxorubicin as first-line treatment in previously untreated advanced unresectable or metastatic soft-tissue sarcomas (GeDDiS): a randomised controlled phase 3 trial. Lancet Oncol 2017;18(10):1397–410.

63. Tap WD, Papai Z, Van Tine BA, et al. Doxorubicin plus evofosfamide versus doxorubicin alone in locally advanced, unresectable or metastatic soft-tissue sarcoma (TH CR-406/SARC021): an international, multicentre, open-label, randomised phase 3 trial. Lancet Oncol 2017;18(8):1089–103.

64. Hensley ML, Blessing JA, Degeest K, et al. Fixed-dose rate gemcitabine plus docetaxel as second-line therapy for metastatic uterine leiomyosarcoma: a Gynecologic Oncology Group phase II study. Gynecol Oncol 2008;109(3):323–8.

65. Pautier P, Floquet A, Penel N, et al. Randomized multicenter and stratified phase II study of gemcitabine alone versus gemcitabine and docetaxel in patients with metastatic or relapsed leiomyosarcomas: a Federation Nationale des Centres de Lutte Contre le Cancer (FNCLCC) French Sarcoma Group Study (TAXOGEM study). Oncologist 2012;17(9):1213–20.

66. Demetri GD, von Mehren M, Jones RL, et al. Efficacy and safety of trabectedin or dacarbazine for metastatic liposarcoma or leiomyosarcoma after failure of conventional chemotherapy: results of a phase III randomized multicenter clinical trial. J Clin Oncol 2016;34(8):786–93.

67. Patel S, von Mehren M, Reed DR, et al. Overall survival and histology-specific subgroup analyses from a phase 3, randomized controlled study of trabectedin or dacarbazine in patients with advanced liposarcoma or leiomyosarcoma. Cancer 2019;125(15):2610–20.

68. Schöffski P, Chawla S, Maki RG, et al. Eribulin versus dacarbazine in previously treated patients with advanced liposarcoma or leiomyosarcoma: a randomised, open-label, multicentre, phase 3 trial. Lancet 2016;387(10028):1629–37.

69. Maki RG, Wathen JK, Patel SR, et al. Randomized phase II study of gemcitabine and docetaxel compared with gemcitabine alone in patients with metastatic soft tissue sarcomas: results of sarcoma alliance for research through collaboration study 002 [corrected]. J Clin Oncol 2007;25(19):2755–63.

70. Sutton G, Blessing J, Hanjani P, et al. Phase II evaluation of liposomal doxorubicin (Doxil) in recurrent or advanced leiomyosarcoma of the uterus: a Gynecologic Oncology Group study. Gynecol Oncol 2005;96(3):749–52.

71. van der Graaf WTA, Blay J-Y, Chawla SP, et al. Pazopanib for metastatic soft-tissue sarcoma (PALETTE): a randomised, double-blind, placebo-controlled phase 3 trial. The Lancet 2012;379(9829):1879–86.

72. Benson C, Ray-Coquard I, Sleijfer S, et al. Outcome of uterine sarcoma patients treated with pazopanib: a retrospective analysis based on two European Organisation for Research and Treatment of Cancer (EORTC) Soft Tissue and Bone

Sarcoma Group (STBSG) clinical trials 62043 and 62072. Gynecol Oncol 2016; 142(1):89–94.

73. George S, Feng Y, Manola J, et al. Phase 2 trial of aromatase inhibition with letrozole in patients with uterine leiomyosarcomas expressing estrogen and/or progesterone receptors. Cancer 2014;120(5):738–43.

74. O'Cearbhaill R, Zhou Q, Iasonos A, et al. Treatment of advanced uterine leiomyosarcoma with aromatase inhibitors. Gynecol Oncol 2010;116(3):424–9.

75. Ben-Ami E, Barysauskas CM, Solomon S, et al. Immunotherapy with single agent nivolumab for advanced leiomyosarcoma of the uterus: results of a phase 2 study. Cancer 2017;123(17):3285–90.

76. Tawbi HA, Burgess M, Bolejack V, et al. Pembrolizumab in advanced soft-tissue sarcoma and bone sarcoma (SARC028): a multicentre, two-cohort, single-arm, open-label, phase 2 trial. Lancet Oncol 2017;18(11):1493–501.

77. Monga V, Skubitz KM, Maliske S, et al. A retrospective analysis of the efficacy of immunotherapy in metastatic soft-tissue sarcomas. Cancers (Basel) 2020;12(7).

78. D'Angelo SP, Mahoney MR, Van Tine BA, et al. Nivolumab with or without ipilimumab treatment for metastatic sarcoma (Alliance A091401): two open-label, non-comparative, randomised, phase 2 trials. Lancet Oncol 2018;19(3):416–26.

79. Petitprez F, de Reynies A, Keung EZ, et al. B cells are associated with survival and immunotherapy response in sarcoma. Nature 2020;577(7791):556–60.

80. Danaher P, Warren S, Lu R, et al. Pan-cancer adaptive immune resistance as defined by the Tumor Inflammation Signature (TIS): results from The Cancer Genome Atlas (TCGA). J Immunother Cancer 2018;6(1):63.

81. Kasper B, Achee A, Schuster K, et al. Unmet medical needs and future perspectives for leiomyosarcoma patients-a position paper from the National LeioMyoSarcoma Foundation (NLMSF) and Sarcoma Patients EuroNet (SPAEN). Cancers (Basel) 2021;13(4).

82. Przybyl J, Spans L, Lum DA, et al. Detection of circulating tumor DNA in patients with uterine leiomyomas. JCO Precis Oncol 2019;3.

83. Hemming ML, Klega KS, Rhoades J, et al. Detection of circulating tumor DNA in patients with leiomyosarcoma with progressive disease. JCO Precis Oncol 2019; 2019.

84. Przybyl J, Chabon JJ, Spans L, et al. Combination approach for detecting different types of alterations in circulating tumor DNA in leiomyosarcoma. Clin Cancer Res 2018;24(11):2688–99.

85. Oza J, Doshi SD, Hao L, et al. Homologous recombination repair deficiency as a therapeutic target in sarcoma. Semin Oncol 2020;47(6):380–9.

Management of Synovial Sarcoma and Myxoid Liposarcoma

Nadia Hindi, MD[a,b,]*, Rick L. Haas, MD, PhD[c,d]

KEYWORDS

- Synovial sarcoma • Myxoid liposarcoma • Advanced soft tissue sarcoma
- Chemotherapy • Radiotherapy • Targeted therapy • Cellular therapy

KEY POINTS

- Synovial sarcoma (SS) and myxoid liposarcoma (MLS) are translocation-related sarcomas, frequently affecting young patients, with a high systemic risk and sensitivity to chemo and radiotherapy.
- Surgery is the mainstay of treatment of localized disease, frequently complemented with perioperative radiotherapy, and chemotherapy in high-risk patients.
- In the advanced setting, when local therapies such as metastasectomy or SBRT are not feasible, systemic therapy with anthracyclines (frequently in combination) is the standard first-line therapy.
- Recently, systemic therapy in advanced disease is more tailored, prioritizing those drugs more active, such as ifosfamide in SS and trabectedin in MLS.
- New strategies, based on a better knowledge of the molecular background, are being developed in these histologic types.

Often confessed, but not frequently practiced, soft tissue sarcomas (STS) should be treated on an individual basis. All entities described in the recent World Health Organization textbook[1] deserve an in-depth knowledge of their clinical behavior, clinical course, and sensitivity to both chemotherapy and radiotherapy (RT). In this article, the management of 2 distinct diseases is described, synovial sarcomas (SSs) and myxoid liposarcomas (MLS). Of note, even these 2 diagnoses can be further subdivided, SS into a monophasic and a biphasic variant and MLS into a

[a] Department of Oncology, Fundación Jimenez Diaz University Hospital and Hospital General de Villalba, Madrid, Spain; [b] Health Research Institute Fundación Jimenez Diaz, Universidad Autonoma de Madrid (IIS-FJD, UAM), Madrid, Spain; [c] Department of Radiotherapy at the Netherlands Cancer Institute, Amsterdam, the Netherlands; [d] Department of Radiotherapy at the Leiden University Medical Center, Leiden, the Netherlands
* Corresponding author. Department of Oncology, Fundación Jimenez Diaz University Hospital, Av Reyes Católicos, 2, Madrid 28040, Spain.
E-mail address: nhindi@atbsarc.org

Surg Oncol Clin N Am 31 (2022) 547–558
https://doi.org/10.1016/j.soc.2022.03.012
1055-3207/22/© 2022 Elsevier Inc. All rights reserved.

classic/low-grade and a cellular/high-grade variant. Even those subdivisions may correlate to clinical behavior and aggressiveness, especially for MLS with a greater than 5% cellular component.

These 2 entities share some common features. First, from the molecular point of view, both entities are translocation-related sarcomas. The fusion transcript product from specific genetic rearrangements (*SYT-SSX* in the case of SS[2] and *FUS-CHOP*[3] or less frequently, *EWS-CHOP*[4] in MLS) has a relevant role in the pathogenesis of these histologic types. Second, both entities also share their sensitivity to treatments. Both exhibit higher response rates to chemotherapy than STS in general,[5–7] and MLS also has an exquisite sensitivity to radiation.[8–12] Third, where the median age of all patients with STS is greater than 60 years and 40% of them are even older than 70 years, both patients with SS and MLS are significantly younger, on average well less than 50 years or even less than 40 years.[5,13,14] This age difference most likely coincides with a lower comorbidity profile and a higher performance status, opening the opportunity to more intense treatment regimens, where better outcomes can be expected.

RADIATION SENSITIVITY IN MYXOID LIPOSARCOMAS

Since the publication of the results of the Canadian SR-2 trial in 2002[15] and the subsequent gradual shift from postoperative to preoperative RT,[16] radiation oncologists have been able to observe the tumor responses on treatment from a volumetric point of view,[9,11] posttreatment from a pathologic point of view,[11–13,17] and, more importantly during follow-up, where high local control rates have been reported.[10,13,14] All these observations have led to the design of several clinical studies among which the SR-2 trial-derived gold standard of 50 Gy in 5 weeks was modified. Kosela-Paterczyk and coworkers[18] have treated 32 patients with MLS with a hypofractionated regimen of 5 × 4 to 5 Gy preoperative RT followed by immediate surgery, 3 to 7 days after the last fraction. The 5-year local relapse-free survival (LRFS) rate was 90%, and overall survival (OS) was 68%. In all analyzed surgical specimens RT response features (hyalinization, fibrosis, paucicellularity, hemorrhage, dilatation of vessels) were detected. The postoperative complication rate was 22% (7 of 31; 3 with wound infection requiring oral antibiotics, 2 with wound dehiscence, and 5 with prolonged wound healing). Lansu and colleagues[13] treated 79 patients with MLS with a conventionally fractionated, yet reduced total dose schedule of 18 × 2 Gy preoperative RT followed by surgery after a median of 44 days. In this "DOREMY" trial (NCT02106312), a 2-year local control rate of 100% and an extensive pathologic treatment response rate of 91% was observed. Interestingly, this reduced RT dose was associated with a relatively low rate of wound complication requiring intervention in only 17%, and the rate of grade 2 or higher late side effects was 14%. The overview of Moreau and colleagues[14] reporting on 418 patients with primary MLS confirmed the benefit in terms of local control by the addition of RT. Their 5-year local recurrence-free rates were 82% with surgery alone and 96% with the addition of RT. Local relapses were significantly prevented (sevenfold) by RT ($P < .001$) especially in patients with positive margins ($P < .05$).

Results from all these initiatives and clinical results have led to the design of an international registry (NCT04699292) where the outcome after several RT dose schedules (25, 36, and 50 Gy preoperative RT; 60–66 Gy postoperative RT; and no RT at all) is prospectively collected in conjunction with quality of life data.

The TRASTS phase I study (NCT02275286) investigated the feasibility of combining trabectedin with RT for MLS. The study showed a mild and manageable toxicity profile and a high in-field response rate, despite a relatively low RT dose of 10 × 3 Gy in the metastatic setting and 25 × 1.8 Gy in the localized MLS cohort.[19,20]

Finally, recently the results from a sarcoma radiobiological project were published.[21] In a panel of 14 cell lines, 3 were MLS derived. Although these cells showed a fairly homogeneous radiation response with SF2 values between 0.64 and 0.67, they were not the most radiation-sensitive ones, suggesting an interplay between the cells and their microenvironment to explain the exquisite clinically observed radiation sensitivity.

RADIATION SENSITIVITY IN SYNOVIAL SARCOMA

Patients with primary SS may also benefit from the addition of RT to their management. A National Cancer Database analysis by Gingrich and colleagues[22] identified 1216 patients with SS (aged ≥18 years) from 2004 to 2012 undergoing surgery. In this study, when performed, the timing of RT was mostly postoperative. On multivariate analysis, RT remained associated with improved OS (hazard ratio [HR], 0.676; $P = .004$; absolute gain of approximately 10% at 5 years). Naing and colleagues[23] identified 1189 patients with primary SS from the Surveillance, Epidemiology, and End Results (SEER) database with data on site and extent of surgery. Among patients receiving RT, an approximate 8% improvement in 5-year OS from 64.1% ± 4.8% without RT to 72.5% ± 3.8% with RT ($P = .003$) was observed. Similarly, an approximate 8% improvement in 5-year disease-specific survival (DSS) from 67.7% ± 4.8% without RT to 75.4% ± 3.8% with RT ($P = .015$) was shown. Song and coworkers[24] reported that adjuvant RT was a prognostic factor for better progression-free survival (PFS) and LRFS ($P = .006$ and .028, respectively) in a dataset of 103 patients with primary SS. Of particular interest for its very long median follow-up (13.2 years) is the study by Guadagnolo and colleagues[25] on 150 patients with SS treated at the University of Texas MD Anderson Cancer Center. Local control rates in this analysis did not differ between preoperative and postoperative RT. From a cellular point of view, SS-derived cells, as a group, showed the lowest SF2 values (mean 0.35) and were significantly more radiosensitive than MLS and leiomyosarcomas cells ($P = .0084$ and .024, respectively).[21]

COUNSELING INDIVIDUALLY MYXOID LIPOSARCOMAS AND SYNOVIAL SARCOMA

Nomograms have historically been developed to inform clinical decisions. In the last few years, several validated nomograms with useful downloadable apps have been developed and are being increasingly used in daily practice. From the Leiden University Medical Center, the PERSARC app was developed and is currently available in the app-store for various devices.[26] The app first asks to enter individual prognostic patient characteristics, like age, sex, size, tumor depth, histotype, and grade. In addition, treatment-related characteristics are entered, including the surgical margins, the addition of RT (before surgery, after surgery, or not at all), and the addition of chemotherapy (before surgery, after surgery, or not at all). The 5-year OS, local recurrence, and distant metastasis (DM) rates can be calculated for that specific patient. In this app, the timing of RT can be selected and its influence on local control estimated. Caregivers may use these data to balance oncological outcome estimates to expected toxicity. Similarly, colleagues from the Istituto Nazionale dei Tumori from Milan have developed another nomogram (Sarculator), able to estimate the 5- and 10-year DM risk and OS based on age, size, histotype, and grade at diagnosis.[27] As an improvement with regard to historical nomograms, both apps are able to calculate the dynamic OS risk during follow-up.[28]

MANAGEMENT OF LOCALIZED DISEASE

The cornerstone of therapy in the localized setting is to achieve a complete surgical resection with negative microscopic margins. In addition to the administration of perioperative RT (as already discussed), given their chemosensitivity, patients with SS and MLS are often evaluated for perioperative chemotherapy. The value of adjuvant chemotherapy has historically been a controversial issue due to conflicting results in clinical trials.[29] However, with the better selection of patients included in the most recent studies, it is clear that there is a subset of high-risk patients who do benefit from the addition of preoperative chemotherapy. Several clinical trials, developed by the Italian Sarcoma Group (ISG), in collaboration with the French and Spanish Group for Research on Sarcoma (GEIS) , showed the benefit of 3 cycles of full doses of epirubicin and ifosfamide (EI) in selected high-risk (defined as deep seated, high grade, and >5 cm) patients with STS with tumors arising in limbs and trunk wall.[30–32] In the most recent study, the ISG-10-01, the estimated gain in OS with 3 cycles of EI was around 10% at 5 years when compared with histotype-driven chemotherapy. The application of the nomogram was able to identify the subgroup of patients with the greatest benefit from preoperative chemotherapy. In detail, those patients with a risk of death due to sarcoma higher than 40% at 10 years who received 3 cycles of EI had a better OS (HR, 1.91; 95% confidence interval [CI], 1.00–3.66; $P = .05$) than those patients treated with histotype-driven chemotherapy.[33] In the case of SS, high-dose ifosfamide, an active regimen in the advanced setting,[34] was not superior to the EI standard, whereas in the experimental arm in MLS, trabectedin did not show inferiority in the third interim analysis of the study (HR for disease-free survival, 1.03; 95% CI, 0.24–4.39). Consequently, this cohort continued the recruitment and randomization of patients between 3 cycles of preoperative EI and 3 cycles of preoperative trabectedin. The results of this cohort are expected for 2022 and could potentially represent a change in standard of care. As already discussed, the combination of RT (45 Gy in 25 fractions) and trabectedin has been shown to be safe and active in the neoadjuvant setting of locally advanced MLS.[19] Another strategy known to be active in the preoperative setting, is the addition of hyperthermia to preoperative chemotherapy. This regimen shown an absolute 10-11% increase in the 5 and 10 year-OS in those patients receiving hyperthermia added to chemotherapy when compared with those only receiving chemotherapy in a large European Phase III study, with more that 340 patients (including more than 40 patients with SS). This could be an alternative in centers with the needed infrastructure.[35]

MANAGEMENT OF ADVANCED DISEASE

The development of distant metastasis significantly impacts the prognosis of patients with sarcoma. Although in the last decades, the survival of patients with metastatic sarcoma has increased due to the development of second-line options, and even if there were a small subset of metastatic patients with prolonged survival,[36] the median OS in this population is currently around 18 to 20 months.[37,38]

Surgical resection of metastatic disease can be indicated, especially in those patients with oligometastatic resectable lung disease and with a prolonged disease-free interval (>12 months).[39] Excluding extrapulmonary disease is indicated, and is especially necessary in MLS, which has a tendency to develop metastasis in other sites, such as soft tissue, bone, or abdominal cavity.[40] Stereotactic body radiation therapy can be an alternative in selected patients.[41]

In patients with unresectable metastasis, systemic therapy is the preferred treatment choice. In general, the aim of systemic therapy in the advanced setting is disease control while maintaining quality of life, and thus, the balance between benefit and side effects is critical. As described previously, SS and MLS are chemosensitive entities. As in other STS, first-line therapy is based on anthracyclines. Although anthracycline combinations have not shown superiority to doxorubicin alone in terms of OS,[42] in this chemosensitive population, anthracyclines (doxorubicin or epirubicin) plus ifosfamide can represent a reasonable alternative, because the combination is more active both in terms of overall response rate (ORR) and PFS; this is of special interest in patients in whom a tumoral response is needed, for example, in symptomatic patients or in those with potentially resectable disease. In detail, the combination of doxorubicin and ifosfamide in advanced MLS is very active, with ORR of 54.5% and median time to progression of 23 months in a retrospective series from MD Anderson Cancer Center.[43] In the same vein, first-line combinations of doxorubicin plus ifosfamide showed ORR of 58.6% in a retrospective analysis with more than 100 patients with SS from the Royal Marsden Hospital.[44] Indeed, patients with SS were those who benefit the most from ifosfamide-containing first-line regiments in a large analysis from the European Organization for Research and Treatment of Cancer (EORTC), which analyzed data from 1337 patients with sarcoma.[45] For specific SS populations, such as children, adolescent, and young adults, the combination could be considered the standard in first line.[46] Of course, as the combination is more toxic, a careful patient selection is needed.

Beyond first line, there are several currently approved or standardly used second-line options in patients with advanced STS. At present, molecular predictive factors to second-line options are still lacking, but histologic subtype is usually helpful in predicting sensitivity to certain drugs.

In SS, ifosfamide is, in addition to anthracyclines, the most active drug, and generally constitutes the choice for the second line. Multiple studies have shown a high ORR of SS to ifosfamide, ranging from 28.6% to 100%.[34,47–49] Higher doses (greater than 12 g/m^2) in general are able to induce higher ORR and can be useful as rescue regimens, even after previous treatment with standard doses of ifosfamide.[50–52] The continuous infusion of 14 g/m^2, during 14 days every 28 days is a well-tolerated and active regimen. Although in combination with anthracyclines, ifosfamide is able to induce a higher ORR in the first line in patients with MLS, the activity of high-dose ifosfamide in MLS is not so convincing.[53]

Trabectedin, a drug approved in the treatment of patients with advanced sarcoma after doxorubicin and ifosfamide, has multiple mechanisms of action. Among them, trabectedin is able to block the binding to DNA of the oncogenic fusion protein product of specific rearrangements in translocation-related sarcomas. This mechanism of action is specially active in MLS,[54] in which trabectedin prevents FUS-CHOP union to DNA, reverting the effect on gene transcription of the chimera. As a result, adipocytic differentiation is restored, a very characteristic phenomenon observed in trabectedin- (and radiation-) pretreated MLS specimens. The activity of trabectedin in MLS is well known, as already shown in 2007 in a multicentric retrospective series, with ORR of 51% and median PFS of 14 months.[55] Activity of trabectedin in SS has also been reported, with ORR of 15% and median PFS of 3 months in a multicentric retrospective series.[56] Interestingly, in those patients achieving a response, the median duration of response (DOR) was 7 months, in line with the DOR reported in the pivotal phase 3 trial of trabectedin in L-sarcomas.

Tyrosine kinase inhibitors, with antiangiogenic activity, have shown activity in patients with SS. Pazopanib, approved in the treatment of patients with pretreated advanced STS based on the results of the PALETTE study,[57] showed an improvement in PFS (4.6 months vs 1.6 months, $P < .0001$) when compared with placebo in patients with STS, including patients with SS. Indeed, in the previous phase 2 trial patients with SS have shown the best 3-month PFS rate (49%) and have achieved 5 of the 9 reported responses.[58] Regorafenib was also active in SS, as shown by the REGOSARC randomized phase 2 trial, with a median PFS in the SS cohort of 5.6 months.[59] Similarly, signs of activity in SS have been shown for anlotinib, with 75% of patients free of progression at 12 weeks, and a median PFS of 7.7 months in a phase 2 study including a cohort with 47 patients.[60] Retrospective series also suggest the activity in SS of apatinib.[61]

Eribulin is approved for the therapy for advanced liposarcomas, including MLS, based on the superior results in OS with eribulin when compared with dacarbazine in a phase 3 trial.[62] The specific activity of eribulin in MLS is not well established, and in the subgroup analysis for patients with liposarcoma included in the trial, differences in PFS and OS between eribulin and dacarbazine, although numerically superior, were not statistically significant in patients with MLS.[63]

Gemcitabine-based regimens are other available options for the treatment of patients with advanced sarcoma. However, neither the combination of gemcitabine-docetaxel[64,65] nor the better tolerated gemcitabine-dacarbazine[66] have shown especially interesting results in SS or MLS, so other more active drugs should be prioritized.

UPCOMING OPTIONS

In the past few years, several therapeutic strategies are being developed in advanced SS and MLS, based in specific molecular pathways or molecular characteristics.

Contrary to oncogenic fusions in MLS, *SS18-SSX* fusions do not contain DNA-binding domains, and its effects on gene transcription occur indirectly, acting as epigenetic modifiers. SS18-SSX protein is able to interact and modify the activity of chromatin remodeling complexes (SWItch/Sucrose Non-Fermentable [SWI/SNF] and the Polycomb Repressive Complexes [PRC])[67]; this served as a rational for the potential activity of EZH2 inhibitors, such as tazemetostat, which indeed showed activity in preclinical models of SS.[68] Unfortunately, in the cohort of 33 patients with SS treated with tazemetostat in a phase 2 trial, although 15% of patients had disease control lasting more than 16 weeks, the cohort did not achieve the prespecified criteria for success.[69] BDR9 inhibitors (another component of SWI/SNF complex) are also currently being tested in SS (NCT04965753).[70]

Lastly, cellular immunotherapy has emerged in the last years as a promising therapeutic option in SS and MLS. Genetically modified T lymphocytes, with the introduction of T cell receptors (TCRs) able to target specific tumor antigens, is an interesting therapeutic strategy in development. New York Esophageal Tumor Antigen-1 (NY-ESO-1) and Melanoma Antigen A4 (MAGE-A4) are currently the cancer-testis antigens with the highest interest in sarcoma. NY-ESO-1 has been described to be expressed in 49% to 100% of SS[71,72] and 88% to 100% of MLS,[73,74] whereas MAGE-A4 is expressed in 53% to 82% of SS.[75,76] One of the main limitations of this technology is the restriction of candidate patients to those with HLA:02 haplotype. Several clinical trials are currently ongoing, with promising early results, in the form of frequent partial responses and some prolonged responses in patients with pretreated SS and MLS.[77–79] The best conditioning regimens, strategies to prolong the presence of TCR cells, and moreover the need of new technologies to translate this strategy to patients with other HLA haplotypes are current challenges of cellular immunotherapy in sarcoma. The prolonged time for T-cell manufacturing and the expected high marketing price are other limits of these therapies.

To conclude, the management of patients with SS and MLS is being refined in the last decades based on the better knowledge of the molecular basis of both histologic subtypes, and on the cumulative evidence on the differential sensitivity to the several available therapeutic options. The emergence of new therapeutic options, as well as this personalized approach, will is hoped to translate, as occurs in other STS, into prolonged OS in this population.

CLINICS CARE POINTS

- SS and liposarcomas (MLS) are translocation-related sarcoma, and the identification of the rearrangement confirms their diagnosis.

- Surgery with negative margins is the mainstay of therapy in localized disease. The addition of RT has shown to improve local control, and the addition of preoperative chemotherapy has shown an increase in OS in high-risk patients.

- Combination therapy with full doses of epirubicin/doxorubicin and ifosfamide is the standard perioperative regimen, although trabectedin could represent an alternative in MLS if the preliminary results from ISG 10-01 are confirmed.

- In the metastatic setting, combination chemotherapy with doxorubicin plus ifosfamide has not formally demonstrated better results in terms of OS, but in these chemosensitive entities this is frequently considered due to a better ORR and longer PFS.

- Beyond anthracyclines, ifosfamide and trabectedin achieve the best results in advanced disease in SS and MLS, respectively. New active options are eagerly needed.

- Cellular therapy has shown preliminary promising results. However, the restriction in haplotypes as well as the time to produce the modified T lymphocytes are challenges to this new therapeutic option.

DISCLOSURE

N. Hindi has received honoraria from PharmaMar (expert testimony and invited speaker) and performs work in clinical trials or contracted research for which her institution received financial support from PharmaMar, Eli Lilly and Company, Adaptimmune Therapeutics, AROG, Bayer, Eisai, Lixte, Karyopharm, Deciphera, GSK, Novartis, Blueprint, Nektar, Forma, Amgen, and Daiichi Sankyo. R.L. Haas has no conflicts of interest to declare.

REFERENCES

1. Soft tissue and bone tumors, WHO classification of tumours, 5th edition. vol. 3: Lyon, France: IARC; 2020.
2. Clark J, Rocques PJ, Crew AJ, et al. Identification of novel genes, SYT and SSX, involved in the t(X;18)(p11.2;q11.2) translocation found in human synovial sarcoma. Nat Genet 1994;7(4):502–8.
3. Aman P, Ron D, Mandahl N, et al. Rearrangement of the transcription factor gene CHOP in myxoid liposarcomas with t(12;16)(q13;p11). Genes Chromosomes Cancer 1992;5(4):278–85.
4. Panagopoulos I, Hoglund M, Mertens F, et al. Fusion of the EWS and CHOP genes in myxoid liposarcoma. Oncogene 1996;12(3):489–94.
5. Vlenterie M, Ho VK, Kaal SE, et al. Age as an independent prognostic factor for survival of localised synovial sarcoma patients. Br J Cancer 2015;113(11): 1602–6.

6. Stacchiotti S, Van Tine BA. Synovial Sarcoma: Current Concepts and Future Perspectives. J Clin Oncol 2018;36(2):180–7.

7. Desar IME, Fleuren EDG, van der Graaf WTA. Systemic Treatment for Adults with Synovial Sarcoma. Curr Treat Options Oncol 2018;19(2):13.

8. Lansu J, Bovee J, Braam P, et al. Dose Reduction of Preoperative Radiotherapy in Myxoid Liposarcoma: A Nonrandomized Controlled Trial. JAMA Oncol 2021;7(1):e205865.

9. Betgen A, Haas RL, Sonke JJ. Volume changes in soft tissue sarcomas during preoperative radiotherapy of extremities evaluated using cone-beam CT. J Radiat Oncol 2013;2(1):55–62.

10. Chung PW, Deheshi BM, Ferguson PC, et al. Radiosensitivity translates into excellent local control in extremity myxoid liposarcoma: a comparison with other soft tissue sarcomas. Cancer 2009;115(14):3254–61.

11. Engstrom K, Bergh P, Cederlund CG, et al. Irradiation of myxoid/round cell liposarcoma induces volume reduction and lipoma-like morphology. Acta Oncol 2007;46(6):838–45.

12. Pitson G, Robinson P, Wilke D, et al. Radiation response: an additional unique signature of myxoid liposarcoma. Int J Radiat Oncol Biol Phys 2004;60(2):522–6.

13. Lansu J, Van Houdt WJ, Schaapveld M, et al. Time Trends and Prognostic Factors for Overall Survival in Myxoid Liposarcomas: A Population-Based Study. Sarcoma 2020;2020:2437850.

14. Moreau LC, Turcotte R, Ferguson P, et al. Myxoid\round cell liposarcoma (MRCLS) revisited: an analysis of 418 primarily managed cases. Ann Surg Oncol 2012;19(4):1081–8.

15. O'Sullivan B, Davis AM, Turcotte R, et al. Preoperative versus postoperative radiotherapy in soft-tissue sarcoma of the limbs: a randomised trial. Lancet 2002;359(9325):2235–41.

16. Van Meekeren M, Fiocco M, Ho VKY, et al. Patterns of Perioperative Treatment and Survival of Localized, Resected, Intermediate- or High-Grade Soft Tissue Sarcoma: A 2000-2017 Netherlands Cancer Registry Database Analysis. Sarcoma 2021;2021:9976122.

17. de Vreeze RS, de Jong D, Haas RL, et al. Effectiveness of radiotherapy in myxoid sarcomas is associated with a dense vascular pattern. Int J Radiat Oncol Biol Phys 2008;72(5):1480–7.

18. Kosela-Paterczyk H, Szumera-Cieckiewicz A, Szacht M, et al. Efficacy of neoadjuvant hypofractionated radiotherapy in patients with locally advanced myxoid liposarcoma. Eur J Surg Oncol 2016;42(6):891–8.

19. Gronchi A, Hindi N, Cruz J, et al. Trabectedin and RAdiotherapy in Soft Tissue Sarcoma (TRASTS): Results of a Phase I Study in Myxoid Liposarcoma from Spanish (GEIS), Italian (ISG), French (FSG) Sarcoma Groups. EClinicalMedicine 2019;9:35–43.

20. Martin-Broto J, Hindi N, Lopez-Pousa A, et al. Assessment of Safety and Efficacy of Combined Trabectedin and Low-Dose Radiotherapy for Patients With Metastatic Soft-Tissue Sarcomas: A Nonrandomized Phase 1/2 Clinical Trial. JAMA Oncol 2020;6(4):535–41.

21. Haas RL, Floot BGJ, Scholten AN, et al. Cellular Radiosensitivity of Soft Tissue Sarcoma. Radiat Res 2021;196(1):23–30.

22. Gingrich AA, Marrufo AS, Liu Y, et al. Radiotherapy is Associated With Improved Survival in Patients With Synovial Sarcoma Undergoing Surgery: A National Cancer Database Analysis. J Surg Res 2020;255:378–87.

23. Naing KW, Monjazeb AM, Li CS, et al. Perioperative radiotherapy is associated with improved survival among patients with synovial sarcoma: A SEER analysis. J Surg Oncol 2015;111(2):158–64.
24. Song S, Park J, Kim HJ, et al. Effects of Adjuvant Radiotherapy in Patients With Synovial Sarcoma. Am J Clin Oncol 2017;40(3):306–11.
25. Guadagnolo BA, Zagars GK, Ballo MT, et al. Long-term outcomes for synovial sarcoma treated with conservation surgery and radiotherapy. Int J Radiat Oncol Biol Phys 2007;69(4):1173–80.
26. van Praag VM, Rueten-Budde AJ, Jeys LM, et al. A prediction model for treatment decisions in high-grade extremity soft-tissue sarcomas: Personalised sarcoma care (PERSARC). Eur J Cancer 2017;83:313–23.
27. Callegaro D, Miceli R, Bonvalot S, et al. Development and external validation of two nomograms to predict overall survival and occurrence of distant metastases in adults after surgical resection of localised soft-tissue sarcomas of the extremities: a retrospective analysis. Lancet Oncol 2016;17(5):671–80.
28. Callegaro D, Miceli R, Bonvalot S, et al. Development and external validation of a dynamic prognostic nomogram for primary extremity soft tissue sarcoma survivors. EClinicalMedicine 2019;17:100215.
29. Woll PJ, Reichardt P, Le Cesne A, et al. Adjuvant chemotherapy with doxorubicin, ifosfamide, and lenograstim for resected soft-tissue sarcoma (EORTC 62931): a multicentre randomised controlled trial. Lancet Oncol 2012;13(10):1045–54.
30. Frustaci S, Gherlinzoni F, De Paoli A, et al. Adjuvant chemotherapy for adult soft tissue sarcomas of the extremities and girdles: results of the Italian randomized cooperative trial. J Clin Oncol 2001;19(5):1238–47.
31. Gronchi A, Ferrari S, Quagliuolo V, et al. Histotype-tailored neoadjuvant chemotherapy versus standard chemotherapy in patients with high-risk soft-tissue sarcomas (ISG-STS 1001): an international, open-label, randomised, controlled, phase 3, multicentre trial. Lancet Oncol 2017;18(6):812–22.
32. Gronchi A, Frustaci S, Mercuri M, et al. Short, full-dose adjuvant chemotherapy in high-risk adult soft tissue sarcomas: a randomized clinical trial from the Italian Sarcoma Group and the Spanish Sarcoma Group. J Clin Oncol 2012;30(8):850–6.
33. Gronchi A, Palmerini E, Quagliuolo V, et al. Neoadjuvant Chemotherapy in High-Risk Soft Tissue Sarcomas: Final Results of a Randomized Trial From Italian (ISG), Spanish (GEIS), French (FSG), and Polish (PSG) Sarcoma Groups. J Clin Oncol 2020;38(19):2178–86.
34. Nielsen OS, Judson I, van Hoesel Q, et al. Effect of high-dose ifosfamide in advanced soft tissue sarcomas. A multicentre phase II study of the EORTC Soft Tissue and Bone Sarcoma Group. Eur J Cancer 2000;36(1):61–7.
35. Issels RD, Lindner LH, Verweij J, et al. Effect of Neoadjuvant Chemotherapy Plus Regional Hyperthermia on Long-term Outcomes Among Patients With Localized High-Risk Soft Tissue Sarcoma: The EORTC 62961-ESHO 95 Randomized Clinical Trial. JAMA Oncol 2018;4(4):483–92.
36. Blay JY, van Glabbeke M, Verweij J, et al. Advanced soft-tissue sarcoma: a disease that is potentially curable for a subset of patients treated with chemotherapy. Eur J Cancer 2003;39(1):64–9.
37. Italiano A, Mathoulin-Pelissier S, Cesne AL, et al. Trends in survival for patients with metastatic soft-tissue sarcoma. Cancer 2011;117(5):1049–54.
38. Tap WD, Wagner AJ, Schoffski P, et al. Effect of Doxorubicin Plus Olaratumab vs Doxorubicin Plus Placebo on Survival in Patients With Advanced Soft Tissue Sarcomas: The ANNOUNCE Randomized Clinical Trial. JAMA 2020;323(13):1266–76.

39. Gronchi A, Miah AB, Dei Tos AP, et al. Soft tissue and visceral sarcomas: ESMO-EURACAN-GENTURIS Clinical Practice Guidelines for diagnosis, treatment and follow-up. Ann Oncol 2021;32(11):1348–65.

40. Visgauss JD, Wilson DA, Perrin DL, et al. Staging and Surveillance of Myxoid Liposarcoma: Follow-up Assessment and the Metastatic Pattern of 169 Patients Suggests Inadequacy of Current Practice Standards. Ann Surg Oncol 2021;28(12): 7903–11.

41. Navarria P, Ascolese AM, Cozzi L, et al. Stereotactic body radiation therapy for lung metastases from soft tissue sarcoma. Eur J Cancer 2015;51(5):668–74.

42. Judson I, Verweij J, Gelderblom H, et al. Doxorubicin alone versus intensified doxorubicin plus ifosfamide for first-line treatment of advanced or metastatic soft-tissue sarcoma: a randomised controlled phase 3 trial. Lancet Oncol 2014; 15(4):415–23.

43. Katz D, Boonsirikamchai P, Choi H, et al. Efficacy of first-line doxorubicin and ifosfamide in myxoid liposarcoma. Clin Sarcoma Res 2012;2(1):2.

44. Spurrell EL, Fisher C, Thomas JM, et al. Prognostic factors in advanced synovial sarcoma: an analysis of 104 patients treated at the Royal Marsden Hospital. Ann Oncol 2005;16(3):437–44.

45. Sleijfer S, Ouali M, van Glabbeke M, et al. Prognostic and predictive factors for outcome to first-line ifosfamide-containing chemotherapy for adult patients with advanced soft tissue sarcomas: an exploratory, retrospective analysis on large series from the European Organization for Research and Treatment of Cancer-Soft Tissue and Bone Sarcoma Group (EORTC-STBSG). Eur J Cancer 2010; 46(1):72–83.

46. Venkatramani R, Xue W, Randall RL, et al. Synovial Sarcoma in Children, Adolescents, and Young Adults: A Report From the Children's Oncology Group ARST0332 Study. J Clin Oncol 2021;39(35):3927–37.

47. Rosen G, Forscher C, Lowenbraun S, et al. Synovial sarcoma. Uniform response of metastases to high dose ifosfamide. Cancer 1994;73(10):2506–11.

48. Martin-Liberal J, Alam S, Constantinidou A, et al. Clinical activity and tolerability of a 14-day infusional Ifosfamide schedule in soft-tissue sarcoma. Sarcoma 2013; 2013:868973.

49. Buesa JM, Lopez-Pousa A, Martin J, et al. Phase II trial of first-line high-dose ifosfamide in advanced soft tissue sarcomas of the adult: a study of the Spanish Group for Research on Sarcomas (GEIS). Ann Oncol 1998;9(8):871–6.

50. Noujaim J, Constantinidou A, Messiou C, et al. Successful Ifosfamide Rechallenge in Soft-Tissue Sarcoma. Am J Clin Oncol 2018;41(2):147–51.

51. Lee SH, Chang MH, Baek KK, et al. High-dose ifosfamide as second- or third-line chemotherapy in refractory bone and soft tissue sarcoma patients. Oncology 2011;80(3–4):257–61.

52. Le Cesne A, Antoine E, Spielmann M, et al. High-dose ifosfamide: circumvention of resistance to standard-dose ifosfamide in advanced soft tissue sarcomas. J Clin Oncol 1995;13(7):1600–8.

53. Colia V, Fumagalli E, Provenzano S, et al. High-Dose Ifosfamide Chemotherapy in a Series of Patients Affected by Myxoid Liposarcoma. Sarcoma 2017;2017: 3739159.

54. Di Giandomenico S, Frapolli R, Bello E, et al. Mode of action of trabectedin in myxoid liposarcomas. Oncogene 2014;33(44):5201–10.

55. Grosso F, Jones RL, Demetri GD, et al. Efficacy of trabectedin (ecteinascidin-743) in advanced pretreated myxoid liposarcomas: a retrospective study. Lancet Oncol 2007;8(7):595–602.

56. Sanfilippo R, Dileo P, Blay JY, et al. Trabectedin in advanced synovial sarcomas: a multicenter retrospective study from four European institutions and the Italian Rare Cancer Network. Anticancer Drugs 2015;26(6):678–81.

57. van der Graaf WT, Blay JY, Chawla SP, et al. Pazopanib for metastatic soft-tissue sarcoma (PALETTE): a randomised, double-blind, placebo-controlled phase 3 trial. Lancet 2012;379(9829):1879–86.

58. Sleijfer S, Ray-Coquard I, Papai Z, et al. Pazopanib, a multikinase angiogenesis inhibitor, in patients with relapsed or refractory advanced soft tissue sarcoma: a phase II study from the European organisation for research and treatment of cancer-soft tissue and bone sarcoma group (EORTC study 62043). J Clin Oncol 2009;27(19):3126–32.

59. Mir O, Brodowicz T, Italiano A, et al. Safety and efficacy of regorafenib in patients with advanced soft tissue sarcoma (REGOSARC): a randomised, double-blind, placebo-controlled, phase 2 trial. Lancet Oncol 2016;17(12):1732–42.

60. Chi Y, Fang Z, Hong X, et al. Safety and Efficacy of Anlotinib, a Multikinase Angiogenesis Inhibitor, in Patients with Refractory Metastatic Soft-Tissue Sarcoma. Clin Cancer Res 2018;24(21):5233–8.

61. Wang Y, Lu M, Zhou Y, et al. The Efficacy and Safety of Apatinib in Advanced Synovial Sarcoma: A Case Series of Twenty-One Patients in One Single Institution. Cancer Manag Res 2020;12:5255–64.

62. Schoffski P, Chawla S, Maki RG, et al. Eribulin versus dacarbazine in previously treated patients with advanced liposarcoma or leiomyosarcoma: a randomised, open-label, multicentre, phase 3 trial. Lancet 2016;387(10028):1629–37.

63. Demetri GD, Schoffski P, Grignani G, et al. Activity of Eribulin in Patients With Advanced Liposarcoma Demonstrated in a Subgroup Analysis From a Randomized Phase III Study of Eribulin Versus Dacarbazine. J Clin Oncol 2017;35(30): 3433–9.

64. Seddon B, Strauss SJ, Whelan J, et al. Gemcitabine and docetaxel versus doxorubicin as first-line treatment in previously untreated advanced unresectable or metastatic soft-tissue sarcomas (GeDDiS): a randomised controlled phase 3 trial. Lancet Oncol 2017;18(10):1397–410.

65. Maki RG, Wathen JK, Patel SR, et al. Randomized phase II study of gemcitabine and docetaxel compared with gemcitabine alone in patients with metastatic soft tissue sarcomas: results of sarcoma alliance for research through collaboration study 002 [corrected]. J Clin Oncol 2007;25(19):2755–63.

66. Garcia-Del-Muro X, Lopez-Pousa A, Maurel J, et al. Randomized phase II study comparing gemcitabine plus dacarbazine versus dacarbazine alone in patients with previously treated soft tissue sarcoma: a Spanish Group for Research on Sarcomas study. J Clin Oncol 2011;29(18):2528–33.

67. Hale R, Sandakly S, Shipley J, et al. Epigenetic Targets in Synovial Sarcoma: A Mini-Review. Front Oncol 2019;9:1078.

68. Kawano S, Grassian AR, Tsuda M, et al. Preclinical Evidence of Anti-Tumor Activity Induced by EZH2 Inhibition in Human Models of Synovial Sarcoma. PLoS One 2016;11(7):e0158888.

69. Schoffski PAM, Stacchiotti S, Davis LE, et al. Phase 2 multicenter study of the EZH2 inhibitor tazemetostat in adults with synovial sarcoma. J Clin Oncol 2017; 35(15_suppl):1057–11057.

70. NCT04965753. 2022. Available at: https://clinicaltrials.gov/ct2/show/NCT04965753. Accessed February 17, 2022.

71. Endo M, de Graaff MA, Ingram DR, et al. NY-ESO-1 (CTAG1B) expression in mesenchymal tumors. Mod Pathol 2015;28(4):587–95.

72. Jungbluth AA, Antonescu CR, Busam KJ, et al. Monophasic and biphasic synovial sarcomas abundantly express cancer/testis antigen NY-ESO-1 but not MAGE-A1 or CT7. Int J Cancer 2001;94(2):252–6.
73. Hemminger JA, Ewart Toland A, Scharschmidt TJ, et al. The cancer-testis antigen NY-ESO-1 is highly expressed in myxoid and round cell subset of liposarcomas. Mod Pathol 2013;26(2):282–8.
74. Pollack SM, Jungbluth AA, Hoch BL, et al. NY-ESO-1 is a ubiquitous immunotherapeutic target antigen for patients with myxoid/round cell liposarcoma. Cancer 2012;118(18):4564–70.
75. Kakimoto T, Matsumine A, Kageyama S, et al. Immunohistochemical expression and clinicopathological assessment of the cancer testis antigens NY-ESO-1 and MAGE-A4 in high-grade soft-tissue sarcoma. Oncol Lett 2019;17(4):3937–43.
76. Iura K, Maekawa A, Kohashi K, et al. Cancer-testis antigen expression in synovial sarcoma: NY-ESO-1, PRAME, MAGEA4, and MAGEA1. Hum Pathol 2017;61: 130–9.
77. D'Angelo SP, Melchiori L, Merchant MS, et al. Antitumor Activity Associated with Prolonged Persistence of Adoptively Transferred NY-ESO-1 (c259)T Cells in Synovial Sarcoma. Cancer Discov 2018;8(8):944–57.
78. Mitchell G, Pollack SM, Wagner MJ. Targeting cancer testis antigens in synovial sarcoma. J Immunother Cancer 2021;9(6):e002072.
79. Martin-Broto J, Moura DS, Van Tine BA. Facts and Hopes in Immunotherapy of Soft-Tissue Sarcomas. Clin Cancer Res 2020;26(22):5801–8.

The Cancer Genome Atlas
Impact and Future Directions in Sarcoma

Jessica Burns, MS[a,1], Jeffrey M. Brown, BS[b,1],
Kevin B. Jones, MD[b,2,*], Paul H. Huang, PhD[a,2]

KEYWORDS

• TCGA • Sarcoma • Multiomics • Profiling

KEY POINTS

- The Cancer Genome Atlas initiative in soft tissue sarcoma (STS) spurred improvements in biological understanding of disease and continues to act as a valuable resource of molecular profiling data in STS.
- The design of molecular profiling studies in sarcoma varies greatly, and itself plays an important role in the interpretation and conclusions made in a study.
- Molecular profiling in sarcoma can identify candidate drug targets and reveal biomarkers, therefore facilitating translational research.

INTRODUCTION

The Cancer Genome Atlas (TCGA) project is a large-scale effort to comprehensively profile tumor samples from multiple cancer types.[1] Conceptualized in 2005 by The National Cancer Advisory Board's working group on biomedical technology in the United States, the overarching intent in establishing TCGA was to "improve our ability to diagnose, treat, and prevent cancer."[2] Specifically, the TCGA aims to catalog cancer-specific profiles through genome sequencing methods that encompass multiple molecular modalities such as the genome, transcriptome, and methylome.

TCGA is jointly coordinated by the National Cancer Institute and the National Human Genome Research Institute, and is facilitated by numerous research centers.[3] The project therefore leverages the collaborative nature of scientific research, and in doing so, collates sophisticated and comprehensive genome data at a scale inaccessible to individual research groups.

Since 2005, TCGA has initiated studies spanning 33 cancer types.[4] The inclusion of specific cancer types was selective and based on their "poor prognosis," the potential

[a] Division of Molecular Pathology, Institute of Cancer Research, 15 Cotswold Rd, London SM2 5NG, United Kingdom; [b] Department of Orthopaedics and Oncological Sciences, Huntsman Cancer Institute, University of Utah School of Medicine, 2000 Circle of Hope Drive, Salt Lake City, UT, 84108, USA
[1] Joint first authors.
[2] Joint corresponding authors.
* Corresponding author.
E-mail address: Kevin.Jones@hci.utah.edu

Surg Oncol Clin N Am 31 (2022) 559–568
https://doi.org/10.1016/j.soc.2022.03.013
1055-3207/22/© 2022 Elsevier Inc. All rights reserved.

"overall public health impact," and the "availability of human tumor and matched normal samples" for analysis.[5] Sarcoma is a disease of unmet need, with a poor prognosis and limited therapeutic options in the advanced setting.[6] Furthermore, first-line intervention for primary disease is surgical resection, and thus there is often abundant tumor material available.[7] As such, sarcoma satisfied all criteria for selection, and was included in TCGA profiling efforts.

In this article, a short overview of the TCGA study in soft tissue sarcoma (STS) (TCGA-SARC) is provided, and its major findings and importance within the domain are reviewed.[8] In addition, the future of molecular profiling in sarcoma in reference to work performed by TCGA-SARC and other multiomic studies is explored. The different approaches to molecular profiling, encompassing both methodology and study design, are assessed and the utility of molecular profiling is discussed, to provide a perspective on the future directions of molecular profiling studies in sarcoma.

Summary and Initial Impact of TCGA-SARC

Establishment of TCGA-SARC marked the largest and most comprehensive attempt to perform sarcoma genomics.[8] In total, there were 206 tumors representing 6 histologic types (leiomyosarcoma [LMS], dedifferentiated liposarcoma [DDLPS], undifferentiated pleomorphic sarcoma [UPS], myxofibrosarcoma [MFS], malignant peripheral nerve sheath tumor [MPNST], synovial sarcoma [SS]). Samples were profiled over a range of different platforms encompassing single nucleotide polymorphism-based copy number analysis, whole-exome sequencing (WES), whole-genome sequencing, RNA sequencing (RNA-seq), microRNA (miRNA) sequencing, methylation analysis, and reverse-phase protein array.

Based on these multiplatform analyses, TCGA-SARC reported 3 major observations. First, LMS, DDLPS, UPS, MFS, and MPNST were characterized by a low somatic mutational burden and frequent copy number alterations. There were very few recurrent mutations across samples, and this coupled with the low mutational burden demonstrated that the genomic profile of these sarcoma types starkly contrasted that of the many epithelial tumors profiled by TCGA.

Second, through integrated intrasubtype analysis, stratification of patients based solely on molecular profiles was shown to associate with outcome. Specifically, unsupervised clustering of 50 patients with DDLPS based on somatic copy number alterations (SCNA) identified 3 clusters with differing outcomes. Patients with SCNA profiles in which Jun proto-oncogene (*JUN*) amplification or telomerase reverse transcriptase (*TERT*) amplification and chromosome instability was present had significantly worse disease-specific survival (DSS) than other patients. Patients with DDLPS could also be stratified for DSS based on methylation status, with hypermethylated status correlating with a significantly shorter DSS than hypomethylated status. Integration of SCNA and methylation clusters facilitated further patient stratification with different DSS, and interestingly identified an integrative cluster with an estimated low immature dendritic cell (DC) score (inferred from the methylation data) to have the poorest DSS. Overall, integrative analysis highlighted the presence of extensive intrasubtype genomic heterogeneity and alluded to the importance of immune activity in sarcoma.

Finally, inference of immune microenvironment profiles from DNA methylation and RNA-seq data revealed an association between immune composition and outcome. In LMS, high scores for natural killer (NK) cells, CD8, and mast cells were associated with a favorable DSS; in UPS and MFS, NK cells, DC, and immature DC were also associated with a favorable DSS; and in DDLPS, an elevated T helper cell type 2 signature was associated with a poorer DSS. Despite the prior identification of an integrative DDLPS cluster with low immature DC score and poor DSS, no association was found between immature DC score and DSS in patients with DDLPS. In general, DDLPS, UPS, and MFS showed high expression of immune markers relative to other subtypes, which may explain why some patients with these diagnoses have responded favorably to immune checkpoint inhibition.[9–11]

TCGA achieved remarkable genomic coverage in several sarcoma types.[8] However, there was an absence of any in-depth proteomic or metabolomic assessment, which may have offered additional, complementary, or contrasting information. Although assessing molecular profiles beyond the genomic level is beyond the scope of TCGA, it is critical not to underestimate the importance of capturing multiomic tumor profiles that are as complete as possible. In addition, although the study captured an impressive 6 different subtypes, it is notable that these were the more common entities, and that none were bone sarcomas. As a disease comprising more than 100 different histologies, inclusion of all subtypes is not feasible; however, including some ultrarare sarcoma subtypes and bone sarcomas may have offered a more complete and diverse profile of sarcoma genomics.[12]

Overall, the TCGA-SARC study revealed insights into the biological basis of sarcoma, highlighted how biology is associated with outcome in sarcoma, and suggested that stratification of patients based on immune profiles may serve to guide treatment approaches in the future.[8] Yet, the impact of TCGA in the sarcoma research field has reached far beyond the initially reported findings. Owing to TCGA's commitment to making all data publicly available, many subsequent studies have since used TCGA data, some of which are discussed in later sections of this article.

Approaches to Molecular Profiling in Sarcoma

There are 3 major considerations in the design of a molecular profiling study in sarcoma: first, whether the study will focus on a particular subtype or include multiple subtypes; second, whether a single method (eg, WES) or multiple methods for profiling will be used; and third, whether the study will be retrospective or prospective in nature. TCGA-SARC was a multisubtype, multimodal, retrospective study; however, across the sarcoma research field many different study designs exist, each with their own benefits and caveats discussed herein.

Histology is central to the field of sarcoma, with histopathologic review being the gold standard for diagnosis.[7,12] It is therefore unsurprising that many sarcoma studies focus on a single histologic type. Single type analyses allow resources to be focused for in-depth type profiling and are vital in exploring heterogeneity within subtypes. This fact can be evidenced by LMS genomic studies, which have identified 3 transcriptomic subtypes. The first study to reveal 3 LMS subgroups was reported in 2010, and used DNA microarrays to assess 51 LMS samples.[13] Of the 3 subgroups identified, 1 was enriched in muscle-related ontologies and 1 was composed mostly of gynecologic tumors. These subgroups were most recently recapitulated in 2021 by Anderson and colleagues.[14] The investigators assessed 70 LMS genomes and 130 LMS transcriptomes (including TCGA data) to uncover the 3 molecular subgroups of LMS referred to as dedifferentiated LMS, gynecologic LMS, and abdominal LMS. In addition to recapitulating the originally reported subgroups, this study showed that the dedifferentiated and primarily gynecologic subgroups have high immune infiltrates, and were associated with a poorer overall survival. The study also used phylogenetic analysis to reveal that LMS subgroups are defined early in tumor evolution and that metastatic seeds of LMS are likely established many years before diagnosis. Such in-depth analyses may not have been possible if resources were directed to the inclusion of multiple types. However, STSs are frequently managed in a "one size fits all" manner in the clinic. For the vast majority of STS diagnoses, surgical resection is the treatment of choice for primary disease, and conventional chemotherapy is administered for advanced disease. To move clinical management toward a more personalized approach for STS treatment, it may be necessary for multiple types to be molecularly assessed to make findings that may bear more relevance to current clinical management, facilitating future translation to the clinic. Numerous trials in sarcoma have shown varied responses to treatment approaches both across and within types. For example, the PALETTE phase 3 trial that assessed pazopanib in non-adipocytic sarcomas showed 67% of patients to achieve stable disease with pazopanib, versus 38% on placebo.[15] However, histology was not significantly associated with progression-free survival, suggesting a type-independent response to treatment. We hypothesize that commonalities observed in clinical response across types may be explained by shared tumor biology potentially independent of type. Investigating such shared tumor biology requires molecular studies across multiple types to be conducted.

As well as being a multitype study, TCGA-SARC covered multiple molecular profiling modalities.[8] Integration of multiple data types represents a huge challenge for analysts. Data integration in the context of cancer omics aims to provide information on a tumor that is free of redundancy, unified, and readily interpretable. However, the reality of biological data complicates this in several ways. First, concordance between different omic datasets at the molecular level is often poor, restricting unified conclusion from being made.[16,17] Second, combining data from different platforms requires data harmonization; this involves extensive scaling, normalization, and transformation of the data, and is compounded when multiple different data forms are present (eg, relative/absolute quantitation, continuous/categorical variables). Third, experimental design, the presence of batch effects, and nonstandardized experimental methodologies in molecular profiling can complicate integrative analyses that use publicly available data. In short, omic data integration is not trivial, and there is a lack of formally established procedures to handle such data. In addition to the informatics challenges, as the number of platforms increases, so does the amount of tissue required. Biopsies are therefore often unsuitable for multimodal analysis, and large surgical excision specimens are required. TCGA-SARC covered several profiling levels to generate a comprehensive genomic profile, permitting integrative analysis. Yet no comprehensive proteomic, phosphoproteomic, or metabolomic profiling was performed. Although the study of genomics in cancer has driven many improvements in disease understanding, proteomics, phosphoproteomics, and metabolomics offer a more in-depth perspective on the signaling activity and biological processes active within a tumor.[18–20] Proteomics, phosphoproteomics, and metabolomics can therefore better recapitulate the biological phenotype of a tumor compared with genomics. In addition, most drugs are targeted toward proteins, therefore proteomics is uniquely geared toward the study of candidate drug targets.[21] Each different molecular profile offers unique information; therefore integrating multiple profiles is key in establishing a comprehensive understanding of tumor biology (**Fig. 1**). In line with this, the Clinical Proteomic Tumor Analysis Consortium (CPTAC) project has been initiated.[22] CPTAC is a multi-institutional effort focused on the integrative analysis of genomic and proteomic data (proteogenomics) in specific cancer types. The CPTAC project in STS has been announced; however, the results are yet to be published.

Molecular profiling is often used in retrospective studies, in which cohorts of patients are established based on archival tissue. TCGA-SARC was retrospective, and was therefore able to accumulate a large number of tumors for analysis.[8] Achieving large cohorts for a rare cancer is a challenging feat. As a result, retrospective studies that are able to exploit archival resources to maximize tumor collection are critical to

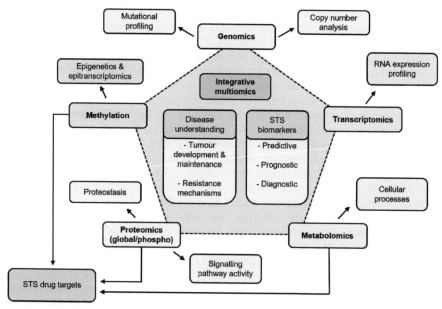

Fig. 1. The utility of mutliomic profiling in STS research. Genomics (*blue*), transcriptomics (*orange*), proteomics (*yellow*), metabolomics (*green*), and methylation analysis (*purple*) each offer unique insights into tumor biology, and together can develop a comprehensive understanding of STS and provide opportunities to drive improvements in clinic.

sarcoma research. However, retrospective studies do have caveats. These studies are often hampered by poor quality and incomplete clinical data. In contrast, in prospective studies, the data collection and subsequent analyses are coordinated and centered on predefined study objectives. Using molecular profiling approaches within prospective studies therefore establishes comprehensive and high-quality datasets, which can then be interrogated for biomarkers. For example, miRNA analysis of tumor samples from patients in the EORTC 62052 phase 2 trial assessing eribulin in STS revealed that miR-106a, miR-17, and miR-34a levels differ between responders and nonresponders,[23] thereby highlighting a potential method of patient stratification for eribulin treatment. However, there are also challenges associated with prospective studies. These studies are often limited in cohort size due to study enrollment and inclusion criteria. Moreover, in prospective studies there is a lag time between when the study commences, when the primary end point is reached, and when subsequent events such a recurrence occurs. As a result, translational research and molecular studies can only be undertaken only when these end points are met.

Utility of Molecular Profiling in Sarcoma

As methods of molecular profiling have advanced and expanded into clinical care, sarcomas, and cancers in general, are increasingly understood and categorized as a disease of specific genomic aberrations, rather than their clinical or histopathologic appearance.[24] Understanding sarcoma biology at the genomic and proteomic level profoundly influences future developments in sarcoma detection and clinical management.

The molecular profiling of sarcoma is therefore of diagnostic, therapeutic, and prognostic value and has become an increasingly important aspect of sarcoma research. As summarized previously, TCGA for sarcoma was a longitudinal, multi-institutional effort to molecularly characterize 6 subtypes of STS.[8] One sarcoma type—SS—is a simple karyotype, translocation-dependent malignancy, whereas the other 5 types were complex genome sarcomas including DDLPS, LMS, UPS, MFS, and MPNST. No bone sarcomas were reviewed as part of this initiative.

One of the aims of genomic assessment from studies like TCGA for sarcoma is the identification of novel molecular mechanisms driving oncogenesis, and subsequently, actionable drug targets. A prominent example of this type of precision medicine was the identification of neurotrophic tyrosine receptor kinase (NTRK) gene fusions as oncogenic drivers in multiple cancers, as well as certain sarcomas. Infantile fibrosarcomas are a notable example, with approximately 90% involving NTRK fusions.[25] Identification of this mechanism of disease led to the creation of TRK inhibitors larotrectinib and entrectinib, which have demonstrated robust efficacy and minimal side effect profiles in NTRK fusion sarcomas and other cancers.[26] With this context, a limitation of profiling data derived from TCGA was the lack of novel oncogenic mechanisms identified in the 5 complex genome sarcomas evaluated, and a corresponding lack of new pharmacologic targets.

While identification of new therapeutic targets remains an issue of ongoing research in sarcoma, molecular profiling has also been proved to be tremendously useful in guiding sarcoma prognosis. As mentioned previously, part of TCGA involved clustering DDLPS tumors by amplified small copy number alterations and DNA methylation patterns, which revealed significantly worse DSS in hypermethylated tumors compared with those with hypomethylation, and increased survival in 6q25.1 amplification compared with JUN or TERT amplifications.[8] Similarly, Bertucci and colleagues[27] evaluated the role of the Genomic Grade Index (GGI) in STS by correlating mRNA expression and clinical outcomes for 678 resected STS, 433 of which were complex genome sarcomas (UPS, LMS). The high GGI signature was associated with poorer prognosis than low GGI STS, and the 5-year survival was 53% for "GGI-high" samples compared with 78% for "GGI-low" tumors. The prognostic findings of this genomic grade assessment were significant on multivariate evaluation, whereas interestingly, histopathologic grade was not.

Additionally, Le Guellec and colleagues[28] reported validation of the Complexity Index in Sarcomas (CINSARC), a prognostic gene expression signature in sarcomas. The investigators described the capacity to predict metastatic outcome using CINSARC, which outperformed the use of histologic grade as a prognostic factor. CINSARC designates 2 grades: a sarcoma with low CINSARC score (good prognosis) would be labeled C1 and a sarcoma with higher CINSARC score (poor prognosis) would be labeled C2. The metastasis-free survival for the C1 and C2 groups in the initial cohort was 75% and 35%, respectively. Importantly, this grading method proved useful in discriminating tumors described as "grade 2" by conventional histopathology, an intermediate grade group often associated with prognostic ambiguity. GGI, CINSARC, and other molecular signatures require further validation but will likely serve a larger role in providing prognostic information for clinicians and their patients in the future.[29]

Beyond providing a more accurate and nuanced prognostic picture of STS, genomic assessment also has predictive value, informing the response to a given therapy. The presence of immune cells is known to inversely correlate with tumor progression and recurrence.[30] Using the TCGA and other molecular datasets, Petitprez and colleagues[31] reported B cells to be the strongest prognostic factor in their immune cell deconvolution analysis of 608 STS gene expression profiles. Using samples from the SARC0208 trial, the investigators demonstrated that B cell presence likewise predicted response to PD1 blockade.[31] In summary, the response to a specific medical therapy may vary widely depending on measurable gene-level aberrations and subsequent expression for a given sarcoma, as well as features of the immune microenvironment. In addition, the gene expression signatures described previously also may have predictive value. The role of perioperative chemotherapy in STS remains controversial, with current consensus recommending neoadjuvant chemotherapy in "high-risk" STS.[32] Expression signatures such as CINSARC or GGI may be useful in identifying these "high-risk" patients with higher likelihood of responding to the chemotherapy, and CINSARC is being currently evaluated in this capacity.[29]

With knowledge of the predictive and prognostic impact of sarcoma profiling, genomic and proteomic assessment of STS may play an increasingly important role in future clinical trial design, and findings of previous molecular profiling studies have been used to inform ongoing trials. For example, CINSARC has been used in 2 phase 3 trials to stratify patients and assess the role of chemotherapy in C2 (poor prognosis) resectable STS (NCT03805022, NCT04307277). In both trials, C1- (good prognosis) and C2-graded patients with varying therapeutic intervention are included for comparison, highlighting the importance of genomic assessment in these studies. A related prospective observational study aims to validate CINSARC and determine its predictive value by classifying patients with CINSARC before neoadjuvant chemotherapy and surgical resection (NCT02789384).

However whether these genomic signatures (GGI/CINSARC) provide prognostic and predictive information better than clinical nomograms such as Sarculator[33–36] is left to be understood. Future studies should possibly combine modalities to refine the calculation of the risk and predict the response to therapy.

Aside from gene expression signatures, proteomic assessment of STS also has influenced clinical trial design. Noting that argininosuccinate synthetase 1 (ASS1), the rate-limiting enzyme of arginine biosynthesis, is silenced in about 90% of sarcomas and associated with worse survival, Van Tine and collaborators[37] have conducted a phase 2 clinical trial for STS with use of pegylated arginine deiminase (ADI-PEG20) in combination with gemcitabine and docetaxel. ASS1-deficient tumors are sensitive to arginine deprivation via ADI-PEG20, which converts arginine to citrulline and increases efficacy of gemcitabine in concert with docetaxel.[38] This trial serves as an example of how an increased understanding of sarcoma molecular biology may lead to novel therapeutic approaches.

SUMMARY

TCGA initiative and related studies serve an invaluable role in laying a foundational understanding of the genomic landscape of sarcoma, upon which future advances in clinical management will be built. TCGA demonstrates that copy number alterations of key regulatory genes (TP53, RB1) are heavily involved in the 5 complex-genome sarcomas surveyed (DDLPS, LMS, UPS, MFS, and MPNST); this contrasts with SS, the single simple karyotype, translocation-driven sarcoma evaluated by TCGA. Novel molecular mechanisms and targets were not identified through TCGA assessment, but genomic markers of prognosis, such as methylation patterns, and the influence of the immune microenvironment were described. Classification of STS by gene expression signature has an increasingly important role in the clinical domain by imparting a more accurate prognostic picture and by influencing clinical trial design. Sarcoma remains a devastating clinical condition, and although considerable advances have been made in understanding the molecular basis of sarcoma pathophysiology, additional diagnostic and therapeutic challenges remain. Further understanding of the genetic and immunologic features of sarcomagenesis is vital for directing future research endeavors, which are hoped to lead to clinically applicable insights that may lessen the impact of sarcoma on patients diagnosed with this rare group of malignancies.

REFERENCES

1. The Cancer Genome Atlas Program - National Cancer Institute [Internet]. Available at: https://www.cancer.gov/about-nci/organization/ccg/research/structural-genomics/tcga. Accessed August 26, 2021.
2. The Cancer Genome Atlas - Timeline and Milestones - National Cancer Institute [Internet]. Available at: https://www.cancer.gov/about-nci/organization/ccg/research/structural-genomics/tcga/history/timeline. Accessed August 26, 2021.
3. The Cancer Genome Atlas - Molecular Characterization Platforms - National Cancer Institute [Internet]. Available at: https://www.cancer.gov/about-nci/organization/ccg/research/structural-genomics/tcga/using-tcga/technology. Accessed September 20, 2021.
4. The Cancer Genome Atlas - Publications - National Cancer Institute [Internet]. Available at: https://www.cancer.gov/about-nci/organization/ccg/research/structural-genomics/tcga/publications. Accessed August 26, 2021.
5. The Cancer Genome Atlas - Cancers Selected for Study - National Cancer Institute [Internet]. Available at: https://www.cancer.gov/about-nci/organization/ccg/research/structural-genomics/tcga/studied-cancers. Accessed August 26, 2021.
6. Schöffski P, Cornillie J, Wozniak A, et al. Soft tissue sarcoma: an update on systemic treatment options for patients with advanced disease. Oncol Res Treat 2014;37(6):355–62.
7. Dangoor A, Seddon B, Gerrand C, et al. UK guidelines for the management of soft tissue sarcomas. Clin Sarcoma Res 2016;6(1):1–26.
8. Abeshouse A, Adebamowo C, Adebamowo SN, et al. Comprehensive and integrated genomic characterization of adult soft tissue sarcomas. Cell 2017; 171(4):950–65.e28.
9. D'Angelo SP, Mahoney MR, Van Tine BA, et al. Nivolumab with or without ipilimumab treatment for metastatic sarcoma (Alliance A091401): two open-label, non-comparative, randomised, phase 2 trials. Lancet Oncol 2018;19(3):416–26.
10. Tawbi HA, Burgess M, Bolejack V, et al. Pembrolizumab in advanced soft-tissue sarcoma and bone sarcoma (SARC028): a multicentre, two-cohort, single-arm, open-label, phase 2 trial. Lancet Oncol 2017;18(11):1493–501.
11. Wagner M, He Q, Zhang Y, et al. 796 A phase I/II trial combining avelumab and trabectedin for advanced liposarcoma and leiomyosarcoma. J Immunother Cancer 2020;8(Suppl 3):A844.
12. Jo VY, Fletcher CDM. WHO classification of soft tissue tumours: an update based on the 2013 (4th) edition. Pathology 2014;46(2):95–104.
13. Beck AH, Lee C-H, Witten DM, et al. Discovery of molecular subtypes in leiomyosarcoma through integrative molecular profiling. Oncogene 2010;29(6):845–54.
14. Anderson ND, Babichev Y, Fuligni F, et al. Lineage-defined leiomyosarcoma subtypes emerge years before diagnosis and determine patient survival. Nat Commun 2021;12(1):1–14.
15. Van Der Graaf WTA, Blay JY, Chawla SP, et al. Pazopanib for metastatic soft-tissue sarcoma (PALETTE): a randomised, double-blind, placebo-controlled phase 3 trial. Lancet 2012;379(9829):1879–86.
16. Krassowski M, Das V, Sahu SK, et al. State of the Field in Multi-Omics Research: From Computational Needs to Data Mining and Sharing. Front Genet 2020;0: 1598.

17. Gomez-Cabrero D, Abugessaisa I, Maier D, et al. Data integration in the era of omics: current and future challenges. BMC Syst Biol 2014;8(2):1–10.

18. Schmidt DR, Patel R, Kirsch DG, et al. Metabolomics in cancer research and emerging applications in clinical oncology. CA Cancer J Clin 2021;71(4):333–58.

19. Noujaim J, Payne LS, Judson I, et al. Phosphoproteomics in translational research: a sarcoma perspective. Ann Oncol 2016;27(5):787–94.

20. Burns J, Wilding CP, Jones RL, et al. Proteomic research in sarcomas – current status and future opportunities. Semin Cancer Biol 2020;61:56–70. Academic Press.

21. Santos R, Ursu O, Gaulton A, et al. A comprehensive map of molecular drug targets. Nat Rev Drug Discov 2017;16(1):19.

22. Clinical Proteomic Tumor Analysis Consortium (CPTAC) | NCI Genomic Data Commons [Internet]. Available at: https://gdc.cancer.gov/about-gdc/contributed-genomic-data-cancer-research/clinical-proteomic-tumor-analysis-consortium-cptac. Accessed October 12, 2021.

23. Wiemer EAC, Wozniak A, Burger H, et al. Identification of microRNA biomarkers for response of advanced soft tissue sarcomas to eribulin: Translational results of the EORTC 62052 trial. Eur J Cancer 2017;75:33–40.

24. Verweij J, Baker L. Future treatment of soft tissue sarcomas will be driven by histological subtype and molecular aberrations. Eur J Cancer 2010;46(5):863–8.

25. Bourgeois J, Knezevich S, Mathers J, et al. Molecular detection of the ETV6-NTRK3 gene fusion differentiates congenital fibrosarcoma from other childhood spindle cell tumors. Am J Surg Pathol 2000;24(7):937–46.

26. Demetri G, Antonescu C, Bjerkehagen B, et al. Diagnosis and management of tropomyosin receptor kinase (TRK) fusion sarcomas: expert recommendations from the World Sarcoma Network. Ann Oncol 2020;31(11):1506–17.

27. Bertucci F, De Nonneville A, Finetti P, et al. The Genomic Grade Index predicts postoperative clinical outcome in patients with soft-tissue sarcoma. Ann Oncol 2018;29(2):459–65.

28. Le Guellec S, Lesluyes T, Sarot E, et al. Validation of the Complexity INdex in SARComas prognostic signature on formalin-fixed, paraffin-embedded, soft-tissue sarcomas. Ann Oncol 2018;29(8):1828–35.

29. Merry E, Thway K, Jones RL, et al. Predictive and prognostic transcriptomic biomarkers in soft tissue sarcomas. NPJ Precis Oncol 2021;5(1).

30. Bindea G, Mlecnik B, Tosolini M, et al. Spatiotemporal dynamics of intratumoral immune cells reveal the immune landscape in human cancer. Immunity 2013; 39(4):782–95.

31. Petitprez F, de Reyniès A, Keung EZ, et al. B cells are associated with survival and immunotherapy response in sarcoma. Nat 2020;577(7791):556–60.

32. Casali P, Abecassis N, Aro H, et al. Soft tissue and visceral sarcomas: ESMO-EURACAN Clinical Practice Guidelines for diagnosis, treatment and follow-up. Ann Oncol Off J Eur Soc Med Oncol 2018;29(Suppl 4):iv51–67.

33. Callegaro D, Miceli R, Bonvalot S, et al. Development and external validation of two nomograms to predict overall survival and distant metastases after surgical resection of localised soft tissue sarcomas of the extremities: a retrospective analysis. Lancet Oncol 2016;17:671–80.

34. Callegaro D, Miceli R, Bonvalot S, et al. Development and external validation of a dynamic prognostic nomogram for primary extremity soft tissue sarcoma survivors. EClinicalMedicine 2019;17:100215.

35. Pasquali S, Pizzamiglio S, Touati N, et al. The impact of chemotherapy on survival of patients with extremity and trunk wall soft tissue sarcoma: revisiting the results of the EORTC-STBSG 62931 randomized trial. Eur J Cancer 2019;109:51–60.

36. Pasquali S, Palmerini E, Quagliuolo V, et al. Neoadjuvant chemotherapy in high risk soft tissue sarcomas: a sarculator-based risk stratification analysis of the randomized trial ISG-STS 1001. Cancer 2022;128(1):85–93.

37. NCT03449901. https://www.clinicaltrials.gov/ct2/show/NCT03449901?term=brian+van+tine&draw=3&rank=22.

38. Prudner BC, Rathore R, Robinson AM, et al. Arginine Starvation and Docetaxel Induce c-Myc–Driven hENT1 Surface Expression to Overcome Gemcitabine Resistance in ASS1-Negative Tumors. Clin Cancer Res 2019;25(16):5122–34.

Printed and bound by CPI Group (UK) Ltd, Croydon, CR0 4YY

03/10/2024

01040480-0008